ENDORPHINS

MODERN PHARMACOLOGY-TOXICOLOGY

A Series of Monographs and Textbooks

1 A Guide to Molecular Pharmacology-Toxicology, Parts I and II *Edited by R. M. Featherstone*

2 Psychopharmacological Treatment: Theory and Practice *Edited by Herman C. B. Denber*

3 Pre- and Postsynaptic Receptors *Edited by Earl Usdin and William E. Bunney, Jr.*

4 Synaptic Receptors: Isolation and Molecular Biology *Eduardo De Robertis*

5 Methods in Narcotics Research *Edited by Seymour Ehrenpreis and Amos Neidle*

6 Horizons in Clinical Pharmacology *Edited by Roger F. Palmer*

7 Synthetic Antidiarrheal Drugs: Synthesis–Preclinical and Clinical Pharmacology *Edited by Willem Van Bever and Harbans Lal*

8 Receptors and Mechanism of Action of Steroid Hormones, Parts I and II *Edited by Jorge R. Pasqualini*

9 Hormone-Receptor Interaction: Molecular Aspects *Edited by Gerald S. Levey*

10 Structure and Function of Monoamine Enzymes *Edited by Earl Usdin, Norman Weiner, and Moussa B. H. Youdin*

11 Receptors in Pharmacology *Edited by John R. Smythies and Ronald J. Bradley*

12 Noncatecholic Phenylethylamines (in two parts) *Edited by Aron D. Mosnaim and Marion E. Wolf*

13 Biochemistry of Mental Disorders: New Vistas *Edited by Earl Usdin and Arnold J. Mandell*

14 Developments in Opiate Research *Edited by Albert Herz*

15 Cadmium Toxicity *Edited by John H. Mennear*

16 Body Temperature: Regulation, Drug Effects, and Therapeutic Implications *Edited by Peter Lomax and Edward Schönbaum*

17 Interferon and Interferon Inducers: Clinical Applications *Edited by Dale A. Stringfellow*

18 The Spinal Cord and Its Reaction to Traumatic Injury: Anatomy–Physiology–Pharmacology–Therapeutics *Edited by William F. Windle*

19 Hypertension Research: Methods and Models *Edited by Frederick M. Radzialowski*

20 Endorphins: Chemistry, Physiology, Pharmacology, and Clinical Relevance *Edited by Jeffrey B. Malick and Robert M. S. Bell*

ENDORPHINS

Chemistry, Physiology, Pharmacology, and Clinical Relevance

EDITED BY

Jeffrey B. Malick, Ph.D.
Stuart Pharmaceuticals
Division of ICI Americas Inc.
Wilmington, Delaware

Robert M. S. Bell, M.D.
Rama Medical Clinic
Charlotte, North Carolina

MARCEL DEKKER, INC. New York and Basel

Library of Congress Cataloging in Publication Data
Main entry under title:

Endorphins: chemistry, physiology, pharmacology, and clinical relevance.

(Modern pharmacology-toxicology)
Includes indexes.
1. Endorphins. I. Malick, Jeffrey B. II. Bell, Robert M. S.
[DNLM: 1. Endorphins. W1 MO167T v. 20 / QU68 E55]
QP951.E5E5 612'.814 81-22214
ISBN 0-8247-1687-6 AACR2

Marcel Dekker, Inc.
270 Madison Avenue, New York, New York 10016

Current Printing (last digit):
10 9 8 7 6 5 4 3 2 1

Printed in the United States of America

To Our Wives and Parents

Preface

. . . dreams out of the ivory gate,
and visions before midnight.

Sir Thomas Browne, *On Dreams*

The ancient Sumerians referred to the poppy as the "joy plant." It seems probable that they were aware of the mood-elevating properties of the sticky juices, later called opium, that oozed from the flower seed capsule. Greek and then Roman physicians from 300 B.C. onward were knowledgeable of its actions, prescribing it to their patients for various conditions. Since then opium has been used in most countries down through the ages, not only for its medicinal properties (e.g., pain relief) but also as a social drug that provided a sense of well-being, a dreamlike state, and a calming effect. It was the latter effects that often led to addiction and antisocial drug-seeking behavior. Of all the drugs that have been used, probably none has produced so much benefit and yet, paradoxically, so much despair as opium.

The modern impetus to opioid research can probably be dated to 1803, when Setürner isolated the morphine alkaloid from opium. He named the compound after Morpheus, the Greek god of dreams. Since that time, the drug has provided the basis of research for countless scientists. Their quest to conquer pain, to understand the pharmacological profiles of opioids, and to unravel their physiological actions has been relentless. This pursuit was fired not only by the zeal of their calling but also by public pressure to rid society of the problems arising from the abuse of such compounds.

This book takes up the story in the 1970s, when it was demonstrated that morphine receptors were present in the brain of vertebrate animals, and carries it forward into the early 1980s. The discovery of opiate receptors prompted a provocative question: If there were receptors, shouldn't there be endogenous substances which would bind with them? The answer was soon forthcoming with the discovery of the endorphins, which included β-endorphin and methionine- and leucine-enkephalin. With these discoveries, a whole new era of narcotic research began. In these pages we document much of the work undertaken during the exciting early years following the identification of the morphine receptor. Hundreds of scientific papers have been produced in what has been an avalanche of information. With each new paper there has been a general furthering of our understanding of what lies beneath each of nature's veils.

Where this exponential quest for knowledge is taking us is not easy to see. The early hopes of discovering a nonaddictive morphine substitute with fewer side effects have not been fulfilled. It seems that the naturally occurring opioid peptides and their synthetic congeners that have been made to date have properties similar to those of the ancient botanical alkaloid. Many pharmaceutical companies and research institutions are testing synthetic polypeptides in an attempt to find analgesics that are improvements on currently available drugs. We hope that the effort is rewarded. However, although the endorphins have been shown to be analgesics in humans, they do not appear to offer significant advantages over existing poppy derivatives since they exhibit tolerance, physical-dependence liability, and cross-tolerance to morphine, produce respiratory depression, and are self-administered by animals. Thus, unless some advantage other than potency can be discovered, it appears highly unlikely that the endorphins will be used widely as antinociceptive agents.

The function of endorphins in the body and their significance in disease states are slowly unfolding. Their role in psychiatric disorders has been one of the areas more aggressively pursued and many claims are currently being made. Endorphins are distributed widely throughout the body and one can speculate that they may eventually be shown to be involved in many other functions, such as blood pressure control, sleep regulation, and gastrointestinal function, just to mention a few. In addition, they may help solve many of the other enigmas of both medicine and physiology. However, like Morpheus, it is easy to dream.

We would like to thank all the authors who have made this volume possible, our secretaries for making it happen, and our wives for their great patience and for insisting that we persevere.

Robert M. S. Bell
Jeffrey B. Malick

Contributors

*Eugene R. Baizman, Ph. D.** Addiction Research Foundation, Pala Alto, California

Floyd E. Bloom, M. D. A. V. Davis Center for Behavioral Neurobiology, The Salk Institute, San Diego, California

Brian M. Cox, Ph. D.† Addiction Research Foundation, Palo Alto, California

William L. Dewey, Ph. D. Department of Pharmacology, Medical College of Virginia, Virginia Commonwealth University, Richmond, Virginia

Jeffrey M Goldstein, Ph. D. Biomedical Research Department, Stuart Pharmaceuticals, Division of ICI Americas Inc., Wilmington, Delaware

John A. H. Lord, Ph. D. Pharmaceutical Division, Reckitt and Colman Ltd., Hull, England

Jeffrey B. Malick, Ph. D. Biomedical Research Department, Stuart Pharmaceuticals, Division of ICI Americas Inc., Wilmington, Delaware

Michael J. Rance, Ph.D. Pharmaceutical Division, Reckitt and Colman Ltd., Hull, England

Present Affiliation:
*Sterling-Winthrop Research Institute, Rensselaer, New York
†Department of Pharmacology, Uniformed Services University of the Health Sciences, Bethesda, Maryland

Jean P. Rossier, M. D., D. S. * A. V. Davis Center for Behavioral Neurobiology, The Salk Institute, San Diego, California

Eric J. Simon, Ph. D. Departments of Psychiatry and Pharmacology, New York University Medical Center, New York, New York

Colin F. C. Smith, Ph. D. Pharmaceutical Division, Reckitt and Colman Ltd., Hull, England

Derek G. Smyth, Ph. D. Laboratory of Peptide Chemistry, National Institute for Medical Research, Mill Hill, London, England

Lars Terenius, M. D. Department of Pharmacology, University of Uppsala, Uppsala, Sweden

Present Affiliation:
*Department of Neurophysiologic Research, C. N. R. S. Laboratories, Gif-sur-Yvette, France

Contents

chapter 1

History

Eric J. Simon

New York University Medical Center
New York, New York

I. INTRODUCTION

The editors have asked me to be the historian for this volume. I consider this invitation to be both an honor and a challenge. After some (but probably not enough) reflection I agreed to take on this task, aware of the not inconsiderable hazards involved in it, not to mention the obvious problem that other chapters contain certain aspects of the history of this field. Since the editors felt the need for a separate chapter covering the historical development of this rapidly moving and exciting field, I shall attempt to perform this task with all the objectivity and accuracy at my disposal.

II. DEVELOPMENTS THAT LED TO THE POSTULATION AND DISCOVERY OF OPIATE RECEPTORS

The modern era of opiate research is usually considered to have begun in 1973 with the demonstration of stereospecfic opiate receptors in the central nervous system of animals and humans. This discovery, like all discoveries, was not made in a vacuum. This section deals with developments that led to the recognition that such receptor sites must exist and to their ultimate discovery.

Opium is probably the oldest known medication and morphine has been known since the nineteenth century to be the major alkaloid responsible for most of its pharmacological and medicinal effects. The roots of the recent revolutionary developments in the opiate field are contained in the large body of research that was carried out over the last 50 years on the mode of action of morphine and related drugs and the large-scale efforts in many laboratories to synthesize a nonaddictive analgesic. Although this has not yet been achieved, thousands of compounds, more or less structurally related to morphine and many of them very useful, have been synthesized. A considerable amount of information on the structural requirements for analgesic action came out of this work. It was recognized that analgesic action resides in only one of the enantiomers of a racemic mixture, usually the levorotatory isomer. Furthermore, it became quickly apparent that parts of the morphine molecule could be altered drastically or dispensed with entirely without major changes in pharmacological potency. On the other hand, even small changes in certain parts of the molecule resulted in profound effects on its pharmacology. The best studied and most interesting such change is the substitution of the methyl group on the tertiary nitrogen by an allyl or cyclopropylmethyl group, which causes the resulting molecule to become a potent specific antagonist against many of the pharmacological effects of morphine and related opiates. Some of these antagonists retain some of their "agonist" properties (e.g., nalorphine, cyclazocine), whereas others are "pure" antagonists (e.g., naloxone and naltrexone).

The recognition of the remarkable stereospecificity and structural constraints placed on analgesic and other actions of opiates led to the receptor hypothesis. This hypothesis, held by investigators in this area for several decades, postulates that opiates must bind to specific sites in or on brain cells and that this binding triggers the physical and/or chemical steps that result in the responses observed. These sites or receptors, as they were termed in analogy to the hormone receptors, would permit only drugs with suitable structures and stereochemistry to bind—by far the easiest way to explain the observed specificities of opiate action.

Another important development in the opiate field was the development of in vitro bioassays for analgesic potency. The electrically evoked contractions of the isolated guinea pig ileum were shown by Paton (1) and Schaumann (2) to be inhibited by opiates at low concentrations. This system was studied in great detail in the laboratory of Hans Kosterlitz (3, 4). Remarkable correlation was found between the ability of a drug to inhibit contractions of the guinea pig ileum and its analgesic potency in intact animals. The system also permitted assessment of the antagonist potency of a drug. Kosterlitz and his collaborators (5) also discovered and developed a second extremely useful bioassay system, the vas deferens of the mouse. There was again excellent correlation between inhibition of contraction and the analgesic potency of a drug. Both systems seem to contain receptors with specificities much like those postulated to exist in the brain.

III. DISCOVERY OF OPIATE RECEPTORS

The direct demonstration of the existence of the putative opiate receptors proved difficult. Van Praag and Simon (6) were the first to try to detect opiate receptor binding in brain homogenate. It was relatively easy to demonstrate binding of an opiate ([^{3}H] dihydromorphine) but much more difficult to distinguish between specific and nonspecific binding. An attempt to detect specific binding by its sensitivity to the opiate antagonist nalorphine was unsuccessful.

Ingoglia and Dole (7) were the first to use the property of stereospecificity in the search for the opiate receptor. They injected l- and d-methadone into the lateral ventricle of rats, but found no difference in the rate of diffusion of the enantiomers into brain tissue.

Goldstein et al. (8) first used stereospecificity as the criterion for receptor binding in mouse brain homogenates. They incubated the homogenates with radioactive levorphanol in the presence of a large excess of either unlabeled dextrorphan or levorphanol. Free and bound radioactivity were separated by centrifugation. Stereospecific binding was defined as that portion of the binding that was prevented by excess levorphanol but not by an equally large excess of dextrorphan. In these experiments only 2% of total binding was found to be stereospecific. Moreover, in retrospect, this stereospecific binding had very different properties and distribution from what we now believe to be opiate receptors. Purification and characterization of the substance responsible for the stereospecific binding by the Goldstein group (9) showed it to be cerebroside sulfate, in agreement with results obtained in Horace Loh's laboratory (10).

Evidence for the existence in animal brain of stereospecific opiate binding that represents a major portion of the total binding came early in 1973, independently from three laboratories, in remarkably simultaneous reports* by Simon et al. (11), Pert and Snyder (12), and Terenius (13). These investigators all utilized very similar modifications of the procedure used by Goldstein et al. (8). Potent opiates, labeled with tritium at very high specific activity, permitted the use of the very low drug concentrations, minimizing nonspecific binding. The introduction of rapid washes with cold buffers of sediments after centrifugation or filters after filtration drastically reduced contamination by unbound or loosely bound radioactivity. In such experiments 50-90% of bound opiate was found to be bound stereospecifically (i.e., replaceable by unlabeled opiates but not by their inactive enantiomers).

Between 1973 and 1975 a great deal of work in the laboratories already mentioned, as well as in others, was devoted to a characterization of the stereospecific binding sites and accumulation of evidence as to their identity with the postulated and long-sought opiate receptors. Space does not permit a detailed discussion of these studies in a chapter on history (for a detailed review, see Ref. 14). Suffice it to say that the properties of the binding sites studied to date, their confinement to the nervous system, and their distribution within the nervous

*The first oral presentation on the "opiate receptor" was made by the author at the Symposium on Current Status of Pharmacological Receptors, at the annual spring meeting of the American Society for Pharmacology and Experimental Therapeutics (FASEB) in Atlantic City, N.J., on April 18, 1973.

system are all consistent with the hypothesis that they represent pharmacological receptors. Perhaps the most persuasive argument supporting this notion is the excellent correlation seen in several laboratories (15–17) between in vivo pharmacological potency and in vitro binding affinities of a large number of drugs that differ in analgesic potency over several orders of magnitude. Opiate receptors have been found in humans (18) and in all vertebrates but not in invertebrates (19). An interesting property of the receptors is their ability to undergo conformational changes (20–22). Attempts at solubilization and isolation of active opiate receptors have not yet been successful. However, what appears to be a receptor-drug complex has been solubilized (23).

IV. DISCOVERY OF ENDOGENOUS OPIOID PEPTIDES

The idea that the brain may possess its own analgesic system had been suggested even prior to the biochemical demonstration of opiate receptors, supported by the discovery that analgesia could be evoked by electrical stimulation of the brain. Reynolds (24) showed in 1969 that electrical stimulation of the central gray region of rat brain produced a profound and long-lasting analgesia. This finding was confirmed and thoroughly studied by Liebeskind and his collaborators (25). Analgesia by electrical stimulation of the central gray region of the brain has recently also been found effective in human patients with intractable pain (26). In work done subsequent to the discovery of the opioid peptides, the notion that electrical stimulation activates an endogenous system that produces analgesia, related in some way to that produced by opiates, was supported by the finding that naloxone partially reverses analgesia produced by electrical stimulation (27, 28). Moreover, it was shown that tolerance develops to this phenomenon and that opiate analgesia and analgesia produced by electrical stimulation exhibit cross-tolerance (29).

However, it was the discovery of stereospecific opiate receptors and the finding that they exist in every vertebrate from the hagfish to humans that triggered the active search for an endogenous opiatelike factor and ligand for the receptor. The rationale was the conviction that opiate receptors would not have survived evolution in so many species if their sole function was to bind substances derived from plants. A physiological function that resulted in a selective advantage to the organism seemed probable. Such a function demanded the existence of an endogenous ligand, the binding of which was the real reason for the existence of the receptor. The search for such endogenous ligands began with a survey of known neurotransmitters and hormones, but none was found that could bind to the receptor with high affinity. Thus began the search for a new substance or substances with high affinity for the receptor and opiatelike actions.

The first reports of such endogenous opioid activity again came simultaneously from two laboratories. John Hughes (30) in Hans Kosterlitz's laboratory at Aberdeen, Scotland, and Terenius and Wahlström (31) in Uppsala, Sweden, reported the presence of opioid activity in aqueous extracts of animal brain. The Aberdeen group made excellent use of the in vitro bioassays whose development they had pioneered. Terenius used competition for the opiate receptor as his criterion of opioid activity. At about this time Goldstein and his collaborators (32) reported the presence of opioid activity in extracts of bovine pituitary glands.

The work on the purification and characterization of opioid factors reached its zenith with the report in December 1975 by Hughes et al. (33) of the characterization of two pentapeptides that seemed to account for all of the opioid activity present in extracts of pig brain. The pentapeptides were identified as Tyr-Gly-Gly-Phe-Met and Tyr-Gly-Gly-Phe-Leu and were named by the authors methionine (Met)- and leucine (Leu)-enkephalin, respectively. The structures of the enkephalins were confirmed by Simantov and Snyder (34), who found and characterized peptides with the same structures, though present in a different ratio, in bovine brain.

The paper by Hughes et al. also presented the important and remarkable observation that the sequence of Met-enkephalin was present in the structure of β-lipotropin (residues 61-65). This is a peptide hormone containing 91 amino acids that was isolated by C. H. Li from pituitary glands in 1964 (35). Its name was derived from its rather weak lipid-mobilizing activity, but its real function was not known. The presence of the enkephalin sequence was shown to be an occurrence unique to this protein and stimulated interest in this problem among prominent scientists working on peptides of the hypothalamus and hypophysis. Guillemin et al. (36) isolated two peptides from extracts of sheep hypothalami and pituitaries which had remained in the freezer from Guillemin's Nobel prize-winning studies on hypothalamic releasing factors. When these peptides were sequenced they were found to represent sequences 61-76 and 61-77, respectively, of β-lipotropin (β-LPH). At about the same time Cox et al. (37) and Bradbury et al. (38) independently found potent opioid activity in the C-terminal fragment (61-91) of β-LPH, isolated in Li's laboratory from camel pituitary glands. These longer peptides have been named α (61-76)-, β (61-91)-, and γ (61-77)-endorphin, respectively, based on a suggestion by the author of this chapter (see Sec. V).

I shall stop my account there since clearly the rest of the history of this field is the subject of this entire book. Much is now known about the properties, distribution, and pharmacology of the opioid peptides. Several hundred analogs of the enkephalins and a number of analogs of the endorphins have been synthesized and a great deal is known about the relation between structure and activity. There is much speculation and a good deal of circumstantial evidence concerning the physiological function of opioid peptides, but it should be, and I am sure will be again and again, pointed out that proof of their functions is still lacking.

The discovery of opiate receptors and of endogenous opioid peptides, which are ligands of the receptors, have stimulated enormous excitement as well as intense research in laboratories all over the world, as should be evident from this timely book. The opiate receptor-endorphin system has been tentatively implicated in pain modulation, narcotic addiction, and even in some forms of mental illness. Whether or not these results hold up, the system shows great promise of increasing our understanding of behavior and brain function.

V. NOMENCLATURE

The editors have also asked me to say a few words about the history and present state of the nomenclature in this field. I shall therefore finish this chapter with a brief summary.

When evidence for the existence of opioid peptides was first obtained there was much confusion about nomenclature. Hughes and Kosterlitz called their active factors enkephalins, Goldstein referred to his substance as POP (for pituitary opioid peptide), and the laboratories of Terenius and Snyder spoke of MLF (for morphinelike factor). As evidence for a multiplicity of peptides increased there was more and more concern about the confusion of names. At the INRC (International Narcotics Research Conference) meeting in Airlie House, Virginia, in 1975, I suggested the name *endorphine*, a contraction of endo and morphine, as a general term for endogenous opioids. I had originally considered the term *endomorphine* but discarded it as too evocative of the multi-ring structure of morphine alkaloids.

My suggestion was enthusiastically received by a number of the participants, most notably Avram Goldstein, who suggested dropping the terminal "e" and then wrote a letter to the executive committee of INRC, suggesting adoption of the term *endorphin.* The term has since been widely accepted. The name *enkephalins* is applied specifically to the two pentapeptides isolated and characterized by Hughes and Kosterlitz. The present situation is the following: some investigators use endorphin as the generic term for all endogenous opioid peptides and the two enkephalins thus represent a subgroup. Others use *endorphin* strictly for the longer peptides (α-, β-, and γ-endorphin) and *enkephalin* for the pentapeptides, as though the two were separate groups, utilizing the phrase "endogenous opioid peptides" as the generic name. This appears to be the only, relatively minor, difference in usage that should be resolved. Resolution might perhaps best be delayed until the relationship between the enkephalins and longer-chain endorphins becomes clear. If the evidence for separate enkephalinergic and endorphinergic neurons holds up, restriction of the name *endorphin* to the longer peptides would be more appropriate. There is also the question as to whether endogenous materials with opiatelike properties that are *not* peptides should be classified as endorphins. None have so far been definitely identified, but several such factors have been reported.

REFERENCES

1. W. D. M. Paton, *Br. J. Pharmacol., 11*: 119 (1957).
2. W. Schaumann, *Br. J. Pharmacol., 12*: 115 (1957).
3. E. A. Gyang and H. W. Kosterlitz, *Br. J. Pharmacol., 27*: 514 (1966).
4. H. W. Kosterlitz and A. A. Waterfield, *Annu. Rev. Pharmacol. Toxicol., 15*: 29 (1975).
5. G. Henderson, J. Hughes, and H. W. Kosterlitz, *Br. J. Pharmacol., 46*: 764 (1972).
6. D. Van Praag and E. J. Simon, *Proc. Soc. Exp. Biol. Med., 122*: 6 (1966).
7. N. A. Ingoglia and V. P. Dole, *J. Pharmacol. Exp. Ther., 175*: 84 (1970).
8. A. Goldstein, L. I. Lowney, and B. K. Pal, *Proc. Natl. Aca. Sci. U.S.A., 68*: 1972 (1971).
9. L. I. Lowney, K. Schultz, P. J. Lowery, and A. Goldstein, *Science, 183*: 749 (1974).
10. H. H. Loh, T. M. Cho, Y. C. Wu, and E. L. Way, *Life Sci., 14*: 2231 (1974).
11. E. J. Simon, J. M. Hiller, and I. Edelmann, *Proc. Natl. Acad. Sci. U.S.A., 70*: 1947 (1973).
12. C. B. Pert and S. H. Snyder, *Science, 179*: 1011 (1973).
13. L. Terenius, *Acta Pharmacol. Toxicol., 32*: 317 (1973).
14. E. J. Simon and J. M. Hiller, *Annu. Rev. Pharmacol. Toxicol., 18*: 71 (1978).
15. K. D. Stahl, W. van Bever, P. Janssen and E. J. Simon, *Eur. J. Pharmacol., 46*: 199 (1977).
16. R. S. Wilson, M. E. Rogers, C. Pert, and S. H. Snyder, *J. Med. Chem., 18*: 240 (1975).
17. I. Creese, and S. H. Snyder, *J. Pharmacol. Exp. Ther., 194*: 205 (1975).
18. J. M Hiller, J. Pearson, and E. J. Simon, *Res. Commun. Chem. Pathol. Pharmacol., 6*: 1052 (1973).
19. C. B. Pert, D. Aposhian, and S. H. Snyder, *Brain Res., 75*: 356 (1974).
20. C. B. Pert and S. H. Snyder, *Mol. Pharmacol., 10*: 868 (1974).
21. E. J. Simon, J. M. Hiller, J. Groth and I. Edelman, *J. Pharmacol. Exp. Ther., 192*: 531 (1975).
22. E. J. Simon and J. Groth, *Proc. Natl. Acad. Sci. U.S.A., 72*: 2404 (1975).
23. E. J. Simon, J. M. Hiller and I. Edelman, *Science, 190*: 389 (1975).
24. D. V. Reynolds, *Science, 164*: 444 (1969).
25. D. J. Mayer, T. L. Wolfle, H. Akil, B. Carder and J. C. Liebeskind, *Science, 174*: 1351 (1971).
26. D. E. Richardson and H. Akil, *J. Neurosurg., 47*: 178 (1977).
27. H. Akil, D. J. Mayer and J. C. Liebeskind, *Science, 191*: 961 (1976).
28. Y. Hosobuchi, T. F. Adams, and R. Linchitz, *Science, 197*: 183 (1977).
29. D. J. Mayer and R. Hayes, *Science, 188*: 941 (1975).
30. J. Hughes, *Brain Res., 88*: 295 (1975).
31. L. Terenius and A. Wahlström, *Acta Pharmacol. Toxicol., 35* (Suppl. 1): 55 (1974).
32. H. Teschemacher, K. E. Opheim, B. M. Cox, and A. Goldstein, *Life Sci., 16*: 1771 (1975).

33. J. Hughes, T. W. Smith, H. W. Kosterlitz, L. A. Fothergill, B. A. Morgan, and H. R. Morris, *Nature*, *258*: 577 (1975).
34. R. Simantov and S. H. Snyder, *Life Sci.*, *18*: 781 (1976).
35. C. H. Li, *Nature*, *201*: 924 (1964).
36. N. Ling, R. Burgus, and R. Guillemin, *Proc. Natl. Acad. Sci, U.S.A.*, *73*: 3942 (1976).
37. B. M. Cox, A. Goldstein, and C. H. Li, *Proc. Natl. Acad. Sci. U.S.A.*, *73*: 1821 (1976).
38. A. F. Bradbury, D. G. Smyth, C. R. Snell, N. J. M. Birdsall and E. C. Hulme, *Nature*, *260*: 793 (1976).

chapter 2

Structural Relationships of the Potent Endorphins

Derek G. Smyth

National Institute for Medical Research
London, England

The study of peptides with opiate activity is one of the few fields of research that can be seen to have had its origin at a particular point in time. When it was found that brain contains receptors with a high affinity for opiate alkaloids, it became implicit that endogenous opiates must exist to react with those receptors, since these alkaloids do not occur in mammalian tissue. Thus in time and in concept it was the discovery of the opiate receptors that triggered the search for the natural ligands.

In this chapter the procedures that were employed for isolation of the two known potent endorphins are described. In addition, a hypothesis is presented that, apart from the enkephalins, which may serve as short-acting neurotransmitters, there are at least three functionally distinct endorphins.

I. NUMBER AND VARIETY OF OPIOID PEPTIDES

The first experiemental evidence for the existence of mammalian opiates appeared in 1974–1975, when several groups reported that brain or pituitary contain substances that have opiate activitly (1–4). There was general agreement that these substances were peptides (Table 1) and late in 1975 the first peptides with opiate-like properties, methionine-enkephalin (a) and leucine-enkephalin (b) were identified and their amino acid sequences determined (5):

(a) Tyr-Gly-Gly-Phe-Met
(b) Tyr-Gly-Gly-Phe-Leu

TABLE 1 Discovery of Endogenous Peptides with Opiate Activity

Tissue of origin	Assay	Approximate molecular weight	Reference
Brain	Receptor binding	1800	Terenius and Wahlström (1)
Brain	Guinea pig ileum; mouse deferens	700	Hughes et al. (2)
Brain	Receptor binding	1000	Pasternak et al. (3)
Pituitary	Guinea pig ileum; rat vas deferens; receptor binding	1750	Cox et al. (4)

Isolated in microgram quantities, the enkephalins were found to act like morphine in in vitro assays (guinea pig ileum and mouse vas deferens), but they appeared to possess only slight analgesic properties (6, 7).

phine in in vitro assays (guinea pig ileum and mouse vas deferens); but they ap-
pituitary prohormones, had already led to isolation of two related peptides (8, 9). Their sequences indicated that they were derived biosynthetically from *lipotropin*, a 91-residue polypeptide of known structure (10) but unknown function [it is now realized that lipotropin represents an intermediate formed from a 31,000-dalton prohormone which includes the sequences of both lipotropin and corticotropin (11, 12)] . One of the new peptides, which was obtained in milligram quantities from porcine pituitary, contained 31 amino acid residues and was provisionally named the *C-fragment* of lipotropin (9, 13). More recently the name *β-endorphin* has become accepted and the peptide has been shown to be present in camel (14), ox (15), sheep (16), and human pituitary (17, 18). Porcine β-endorphin (lipotropin C-fragment):

> Tyr-Gly-Gly-Phe-Met-Thr-Ser-Glu-Lys-Ser-Gln-Thr-Pro-Leu-Val-Thr-Leu-
> Phe-Lys-Asn-Ala-Ile-Val-Lys-Asn-Ala-His-Lys-Lys-Gly-Gln

The other new peptide found in porcine pituitary contained 27 residues and was named *C′-fragment* of lipotropin (8); it lacked the four C-terminal residues of the C-fragment but was present in similar quantity. Because the C- and C′-fragments were isolated from pituitary, it had been assumed that their potential biological activities would be expressed in the periphery rather than in brain, and accordingly various endocrine functions were being explored. With the identification of the enkephalins, however, it became clear that the methionine containing pentapeptide corresponds to the sequence of amino acids at the NH_2-terminus of lipotropin C-fragment and this suggested the possibility that the C-fragment might possess opiate activity. Further study then revealed that not only is the C-fragment a highly potent analgesic (19, 20) but it also occurs in brain (21, 22); with these findings the two fields of research converged.

Today, one of the most perplexing aspects of the opiate field is the number and variety of naturally occurring peptides that seem to have opiate properties. After the isolation of the enkephalins and the C- and C′-fragments of lipotropin, several other peptides with sequences corresponding to portions of the C-terminal region of lipotropin were reported to occur in pituitary and possess a degree of opiate activity (23, 24). With the exception of Leu-enkephalin, this series of peptides (endorphins and enkephalins) were thought to share a common origin and they are frequently described as a "family" of endogenous opiates (Fig. 1). Recent evidence, however, suggests that the enkephalins—despite the coincidence of sequence with the N-terminus of lipotropin C-fragment—do not originate biosynthetically from that peptide. The five residues of Leu-enkephalin have been shown to be present at the N-terminus of two recently discovered opioid peptides, α-neo-endorphin (25) and dynorphin (26, 46). Although the structures of these peptides have not been completely solved, their partial sequences diverge from the sequence of β-endorphin. Dynorphin:

Tyr-Gly-Gly-Phe-Leu-Arg-Arg-Ile-Arg-Pro-Lys-Leu-Lys-Trp-Asp-Asn-Gln

It is thereby clear that Leu-enkephalin (and the two "Leu-endorphins") originate from precursors that are different from the 31,000-dalton ACTH-lipotropin prohormone; and evidence is accumulating that Met-enkephalin, too, is formed from an independent biologically active precursor (27, 28).

Of the series of peptides shown in Fig. 1, only the C- and C′-fragments are generated from the 31,000-dalton prohormone by enzyme cleavage at sequences

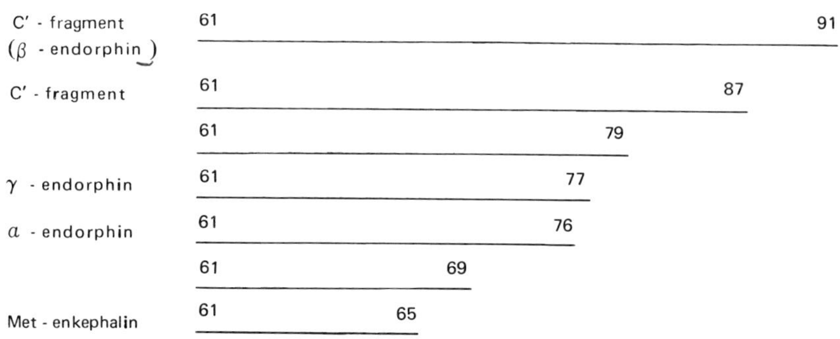

FIGURE 1 Naturally occurring fragments of lipotropin with opiate properties. The numbers represent residue positions in the sequence of lipotropin. The C- and C′-fragments have also been isolated in inert N-acetyl forms (43). Methionine-enkephalin appears to have an independent precursor.

of paired basic residues, with specificity similar to that involved in the activation of intracellular prohormones (29, 30). Thus the C- and C′-fragments bear a special relationship to each other and to their prohormone and seem likely to have physiological significance. It is notable that analogous pairs of peptides can be discerned in the Leu-endorphins (dynorphin and α-neo-endorphin) and their N-terminal fragment, Leu-enkephalin, and in Met-endorphin (the putative precursor of Met-enkephalin) and Met-enkephalin (Fig. 2). These pairs of peptides seem at present to be the major endogenous opiates in brain and pituitary; they are generated by similar enzymic mechanisms.

II. ISOLATING ENDORPHINS

It is perhaps surprising that the endorphins, whose most obvious activities are expressed in the brain, are in fact present in high concentration in the pituitary, and in practice pituitary tissue has proved to be a fertile source for isolation of the potent endorphins and their related fragments. Moreover, an additional factor in favor of pituitary extraction is the ready availability of pituitary glands, whereas brain, particularly that of a large animal, is less accessible.

The steps involved in the isolation of β-endorphin (and of lipotropin C′-fragment) are presented in Fig. 3. Acid acetone extracts of 500 g of porcine pituitary were freed from fatty material and from high molecular weight products by acetone and salt precipitations. After removal of the salts, stepwise elution of the peptide mixture on a column of carboxymethyl Sephadex led to the separation of three groups of peptides. The relatively neutral fraction which was eluted in 0.2 M sodium phosphate at pH 6.8 was resolved by gel filtration on

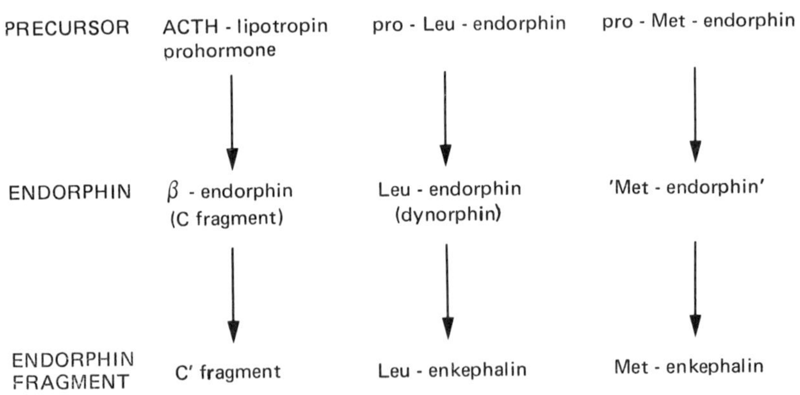

FIGURE 2 Proposed biosynthetic origins of opiate peptides. The precursor(s) of Met-enkephalin, Met-endorphin, are currently being identified. (From Ref. 27.)

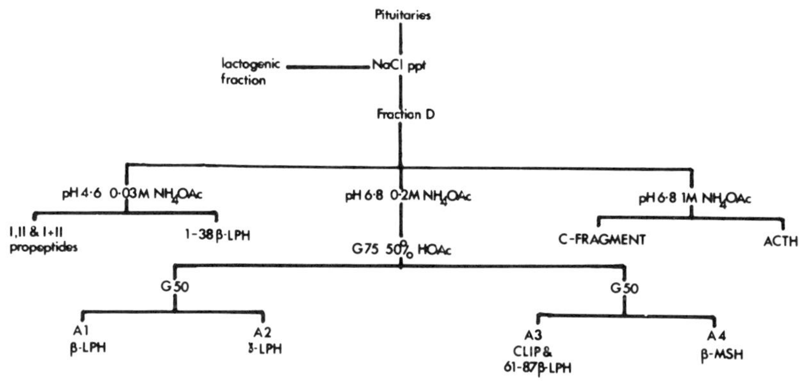

FIGURE 3 Protocol for fractionation of porcine pituitary glands.

Sephadex G50. The C′-fragment (LPH 61–87) emerged together with the C-terminal fragment of ACTH (corticotropinlike intermediary peptide) and the peptide was then obtained in homogeneous form by chromatography on SP-Sephadex C25 at neutral pH.

β-Endorphin (LPH 61–91), which is a very basic peptide, was present in the group of peptides that exhibited the most retention on the CM-Sephadex

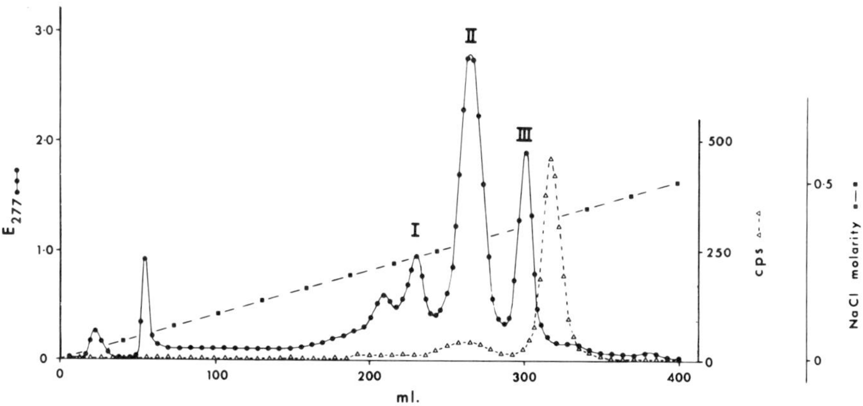

FIGURE 4 Chromatography of the basic peptides extracted from porcine pituitary. The peptides were eluted from a column (70 x 0.9 cm) of SP-Sephadex C25 in 0.02 M sodium phosphate at pH 7.0 with a linear gradient from 0 to 0.5 M sodium chloride. The mixer volume was 200 ml and the fraction size 3.2 ml. N-Acetyl C-fragment (I), corticotropin (II), and C-fragment (III) emerged in the positions indicated; [^{125}I] C-fragment (Δ) was eluted after the unlabeled peptide.

column, and after desalting it was obtained in substantial quantity by fractionation on a column of SP-Sephadex (Fig. 4). The amounts of β-endorphin and lipotropin C′-fragment obtained from 500 g of pig pituitaries were 10 μmol (33 mg) and 4 μmol (12 mg), respectively. Thus isolation of these peptides from the glands (rather than chemical synthesis) would at present appear to be the method of choice for their preparation.

At the present time dynorphin has not been isolated in pure form but sequence analysis of the impure peptide was feasible because the contaminating peptide(s) possessed a blocked NH_2-terminus and did not interfere. Although only a few micrograms of the peptide were obtained, sensitive techniques of sequence analysis permitted its complete structure to be determined (26, 45). Consequently, methods in the initial stages of purification involved extraction and back extraction with butanol, separation from β-endorphin on BioGel P6, then preparative reverse-phase high-performance liquid chromatography on C_{18} columns, first with a methanol gradient in trifluoroacetic acid and then with an acetonitrile gradient in neutral Tris buffers, followed by elution of the active product in trifluoroacetic acid. The steps were monitored with the aid of assay on the guinea pig ileum.

Pooled material from four batches was loaded on a BioGel column in 0.1 M ammonium carbonate at pH 8.7. The peak of slow reversing activity was lyophilized and further purified on CM-Sephadex in sodium borate at pH 11 with a gradient to pH 12. Desalting was carried out on BioGel P2 in butanol/acetic acid/water. The desalted material was finally purified by HPLC (C_{18} column) using a 10–50% acetonitrile gradient in 5 mM trifluoroacetic acid. This extensive purification provided a few micrograms of the biologically active peptide.

The isolation of β-endorphin (22) and dynorphin (26) has been hampered by the hydrophobic character of the two peptides, which caused major difficulties due to absorption to glass and the column supports used for chromatography. Such difficulties were particularly troublesome in the chromatography of small amounts of the peptides and became increasingly irksome as the peptides approached purity, when they were no longer accompanied by other adsorbable substances. With β-endorphin the problem was overcome when small quantities of peptide were involved by the use of a dissociating solvent (50% acetic acid) during gel filtration and ion exchange chromatography. With dynorphin, where the problem seems more acute, each step of purification led to severe losses of peptide. It appears that there is an urgent need for the development of improved techniques for the purification of hydrophobic peptides.

III. PHYSIOLOGY AND DIFFERENTIATION OF ENDORPHINS

The first steps toward elucidating the physiological roles of the significant opioid peptides has involved isolation and chemical identification of the potent endorphins and examination of their distribution in the various regions of the central nervous system (CNS) where opiate receptors occur. Recent studies conducted in the pituitary and brain of the rat have concentrated on the peptides that are generated from lipotropin by cleavage at paired basic residues, the C- and C′-fragments and their α, N-acetylated derivatives, all of which react with antisera to β-endorphin. The results have revealed that the proportions of these peptides differ greatly in different tissues, strongly suggesting that the processing mechanisms are under physiological control.

The distribution of the peptides with lipotropin C-terminal immunoreactivity has been investigated by the method of immunofluorescent staining using antibodies that were raised against β-endorphin or lipotropin (31–34). The results showed that in the rat all the cells of the pars intermedia gave intense staining, but in the anterior pituitary only isolated cells stained and in the posterior pituitary there was no staining at all. In the brain the regions that have been shown to contain peptides with lipotropin C-terminal immunoreactivity are the hypothalamus, midbrain, amygdala, hippocampus, colliculae, and the periaqueductal gray, but the majority of the fluorescence is seen in the hypothalamus. To identify the products visualized by the immunofluorescent technique, the peptides have been extracted from the tissues, resolved by gel filtration and ion exchange chromatography, and estimated by immunoassay (34). This extensive purification is necessary because the antibodies used in the fluorescence studies react with a number of peptides that occur naturally. These include the C′-fragment (LPH 61–87), the α, N-acetyl derivatives of the C- and C′-fragments, lipotropin, and the 31,000-dalton ACTH-endorphin prohormone, in addition to the C-fragment (β-endorphin); and it is important to note that of these peptides only β-endorphin has potent analgesic properties.

It was found by gel filtration of the tissue extracts that while the pars intermedia of rat and pig pituitary contains a negligible amount of the precursor polypeptides (31,000-dalton ACTH-endorphin prohormone and lipotropin), it contains a large quantity of peptides the size of β-endorphin; however, ion exchange chromatography of those peptides showed that β-endorphin itself (Fig. 5, peak 4) accounts for less than 10% of the total immunoreactive peptides. In the anterior pituitary, on the other hand, gel filtration shows that there is a substantial quantity of the 31,000-dalton prohormone and lipotropin as well as peptides similar in size to β-endorphin. Chromatography reveals that β-endorphin accounts for a high proportion (>50%) of the total immunoactive peptides. Thus in one region of rat pituitary, the potent opiate peptide β-endorphin is only a minor component, whereas in the other it is generated in relatively high yield from the prohormone. It will be of interest to learn whether the endorphins in the pars intermedia of other animals are also stored in inactivated forms.

In rat brain, as in the pars intermedia, there is a negligible concentration of lipotropin or 31,000-dalton prohormone. However, the nature of the peptides in the hypothalamus is in striking contrast to the peptides of the pars intermedia region of pituitary: in the hypothalamus the major immunoreactive peptide by

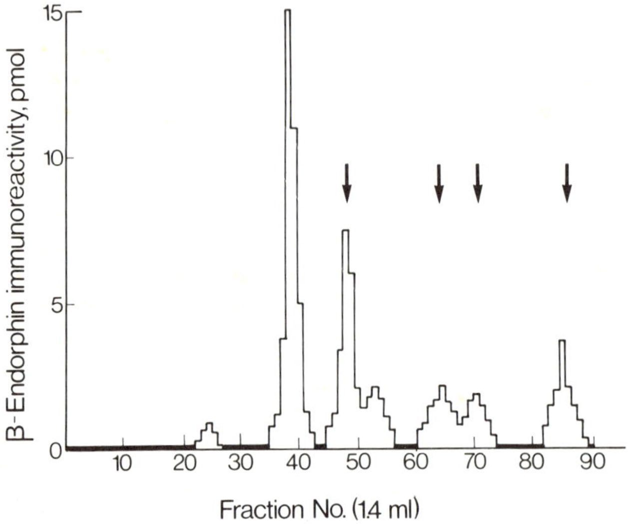

FIGURE 5 Resolution of peptides the size of β-endorphin, extracted from rat pars intermedia. Extraction was carried out on the freshly dissected pituitaries of eight Sprague-Dawley rats and the peptides were first separated by gel filtration. Ion exchange chromatography on the β-endorphin peak obtained from the Sephadex G75 column was on a column (0.60 x 0.6 cm) of SP-Sephadex C25 in 50% acetic acid with a linear gradient from 0 to 0.5 M sodium chloride; mixer volume 100 ml. The elution positions of the radiolabeled reference peptides (*α*, N-acetyl C′-fragment, C′-fragment, *α*, N-acetyl β-endorphin, and β-endorphin) are indicated respectively from left to right by arrows. Aliquots (20 μl) of each fraction were immunoassayed using β-endorphin antiserum. The most rapidly eluted immunoreactive peptides co-ran with products obtained by acetylation of bovine *α*, N-acetyl C′-fragment with acetic anhydride in vitro and therefore appear to be ϵ, N-acetyl derivatives of the *α*, N-acetyl C′-fragment.

far is β-endorphin (Fig. 6). On the other hand, the processing of lipotropin in the hippocampus generates the acetyl derivative of the C′-fragment as the principal "endorphin," while in the mid-brain the four peptides have been observed in more equal amounts (though acetyl C′-fragment still predominates). Thus it is only in the hypothalamus that efficient processing of the 31,000-dalton prohormone takes place to generate β-endorphin. This clearly implies that the potent opiate properties of β-endorphin are expressed most effectively in the brain, particularly in the hypothalamic region.

The production and storage of essentially inactive fragments, namely the C′-fragment and the N-acetyl derivatives of β-endorphin and the C′-fragments, seem to indicate that the "endorphins" present in certain regions of pituitary and brain are formed during physiological mechanisms for negating the activity of β-endorphin.

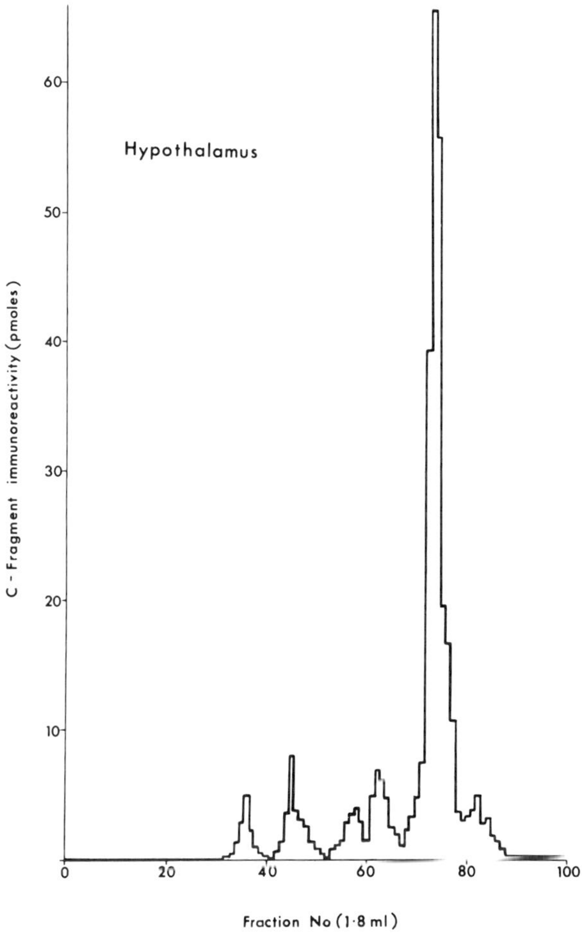

FIGURE 6 Resolution of peptides the size of β-endorphin extracted from rat hypothalamus on SP-Sephadex C25. (From Ref. 34.)

The evidence suggests that in the pars intermedia of the pituitary the potential for opiate activity associated with the C-terminal region of the ACTH-endorphin prohormone is not realized, either as a consequence of N-acetylation or because of proteolysis of β-endorphin at the C-terminus; the processing of the 31,000-dalton prohormone appears to be organized there for the production of α-melanotropin. At the molecular level, activation of the 31,000-dalton prohormone to release β-endorphin is initiated by cleavage between the lysylarginine and tyrosine residues at positions 59, 60, and 61 in the porcine lipotropin sequence and that further cleavage between the lysyllysine and glycine residues at positions 88, 89, and 90 leads to formation of the relatively inert C′-fragment; and with respect to analgesic activity the latter process may be regarded as a "switch-off" mechanism. The β-endorphin and C′-fragment thus appear to represent active and inactivated peptides, respectively; furthermore, an analogous relationship can be seen between dynorphin and Leu-enkephalin.

Each of the opiate peptides derived from lipotropin exhibits a similar potency in the guinea pig ileum assay (35) and on this basis each one could be capable of fulfilling a physiological role as an opiate, with a cental or peripheral function. In certain assays, however, β-endorphin exhibits a unique potency. For example, as an analgesic agent it is 500 times more active than the C′-fragment (36) and it is highly potent in displacing [^{3}H] naloxone from brain opiate receptors in vitro (37). This would seem to imply that it is β-endorphin and not the C′-fragment which is functionally important with respect to the receptors involved in the analgesic assays. In contrast, in the ileum assay only Leu-endorphin (dynorphin) exhibits a unique potency—the activity of a synthetic peptide corresponding to the 13 residues at its N-terminus is 700 times that of Leu-enkephalin (26). This suggests that the opiate receptors in the ileum interact with the structure of dynorphin much more efficiently than they do with the structure of Leu-enkephalin or the other peptides (including β-endorphin). It thus appears that different populations of opiate receptors respond preferentially to different opiate ligands, the analgesic receptors to β-endorphin and the ileum receptors to dynorphin; and by analogy it is anticipated that a further group of receptors will be found to react preferentially with *Met-endorphin*, the putative precursor of Met-enkephalin.

IV. ADDRESS SEQUENCES: A HYPOTHESIS

These observations may be rationalized in molecular terms by the following hypothesis: that the common N-terminal tetrapeptide of β-endorphin and dynorphin (Tyr-Gly-Gly-Phe) be regarded as the "active site" or "message" of the endorphins, while the contiguous sequence serves as an "address" component which directs each peptide toward the appropriate receptor (38, 39). Thus the specificity of an endorphin for its complementary receptor is governed by the sequence of amino acids that follows the N-terminal tetrapeptide. Inclusion of the full C-terminal sequence appears to be mandatory for the high potency and specificity of each endorphin, but it is notable that the tetrapeptide on its own has the capacity to elicit an opiate response (37, 40). In β-endorphin the address moiety (residues 5–31) contributes greatly to the analgesic potency, but it does not have a significant effect on activity in the ileum. In contrast, the address sequence that follows the N-terminal tetrapeptide in dynorphin strongly potentiates its action on the ileum but does not provide potent analgesia. These data demonstrate that the address sequences, which distinguish the endorphins, confer specificity and potency for different opiate receptors (Table 2).

TABLE 2 Proposed Relationship between Endogenous Opiate Peptides and Their Specific Receptors

Opiate ligand	Signal Sequence	Specificity sequence (potentiator)	Receptor
L_1: β-Endorphin (C-fragment)	Tyr-Gly-Gly-Phe-	Met address[1]	R_1
L_2: Leu-endorphin (dynorphin)	Tyr-Gly-Gly-Phe-	Leu address[2]	R_2
L_3: Met-endorphin	Tyr-Gly-Gly-Phe-	Met address[3]	R_3

In the potent endorphins the address sequence may also serve to stabilize the core tetrapeptide against degradation. The structures of β-endorphin and dynorphin are much more resistant than those of the smaller peptides to attack by aminopeptidases in brain (41, 42) and it is to be expected that they will have relatively long lasting central actions. Indeed, the effects of β-endorphin administered into the ventricles of the brain are known to persist for several hours.

Since β-endorphin is contained within the same single-chain prohormone as α-melanotropin, a physiological mechanism could be envisaged for ensuring that only one of the two bioactivities is generated at a given time. In this context β-endorphin contains within its sequence consecutive basic residues that invite the action of processing enzymes, and cleavage at the site seems to play a role in eliminating the activity of the potent opiate, converting β-endorphin to the much less active C′-fragment and dynorphin to Leu-enkephalin. This mechanism could thus permit the selective expression of activity of either β-endorphin or another biologically active peptide [such as α-MSH (melanocyte-stimulating hormone)] derived from the same percursor.

It is of interest that in the enkephalins the "core" tetrapeptide is linked to a single amino acid residue (methionine or leucine). These short peptides do not exhibit outstanding potencies in the conventional opiate assays and they are highly unstable in brain; in addition, it is possible that the lack of a major address component may render them relatively nonspecific in their interaction with opiate receptors. These properties, however, are appropriate to a neurotransmitter role.

V. CONCLUSIONS

The concept of "message" and "address" regions in the structures of β-endorphin and dynorphin not only supports the prediction that further potent endorphins will be found, but it implies that each endorphin will act with high efficiency at its complementary receptor to produce a different form of opiate activity. In addition, the hypothesis that the differing C-terminal regions impose specificity on the endogenous opiate ligands is consistent with data demonstrating the existence of multiple opiate receptors (44–47). It leads to the view that there must be at least three functionally significant endorphins which act independently as long-lasting neuromodulators in the central nervous system.

REFERENCES

1. L. Terenius and A. Wahlström, *Acta Pharmacol. Toxicol., 35* (Suppl. 1): 55 (1974).
2. J. Hughes, B. Smith, B. A. Morgan, and L. Fothergill, *Life Sci., 16*: 1753 (1975).
3. G. W. Pasternak, R. Goodman, and S. H. Snyder, *Life Sci., 16*: 1775 (1975).
4. B. M. Cox, K. E. Opheim, H. Teschemacher, and A. Goldstein, *Life Sci., 16*: 1777 (1975).
5. J. Hughes, T. W. Smith, H. W. Kosterlitz, L. A. Fothergill, B. A. Morgan, and H. R. Morris, *Nature, 258*: 577 (1975).
6. J. D. Belluzzi, N. Grant, V. Garsky, D. Sarantakis, C. D. Wise, and L. Stein, *Nature, 260*: 625 (1976).
7. W. S. Feldberg, and D. G. Smyth, *J. Physiol., 260*: 30 (1976).
8. A. F. Bradbury, D. G. Smyth, and C. R. Snell, in *Peptides: Chemistry, Structure and Biology* (J. Meienhofer and R. Walter, eds.) Ann Arbor Science Publishers, Ann Arbor Mich., 1975, p. 609.
9. A. F. Bradbury, D. G. Smyth, and C. R. Snell, in *The Polypeptide Hormones: Molecular and Cellular Aspects*, Ciba Foudnation Symp. No. 41, Churchill, London, 1976, p. 61.
10. C. H. Li, L. Barnafi, M. Chretien, and D. Chung, *Nature, 208*: 1093 (1965).
11. R. E. Mains, B. A. Eipper, and N. Ling, *Proc. Natl. Acad. Sci. U.S.A., 74*: 3014 (1977).
12. S. Nakanishi, A. Inove, T. Kita, M. Nakamura, A. C. Y. Chang, S. N. Cohen, and S. Numa, *Nature, 278*: 423 (1979).
13. A. F. Bradbury, D. G. Smyth, and C. R. Snell, *Biochem. Biophys. Res. Commun., 69*: 950 (1976).
14. C. H. Li and D. Chung, *Nature, 260*: 622 (1976).
15. C. H. Li, L. Tan, and D. Chung, *Biochem. Biophys. Res. Commun., 77*: 1088 (1977).
16. N. G. Seidah, N. Dragon, S. Benjannet, R. Routhier, and M. Chretien, *Biochem. Biophys. Res. Commun., 74*: 1528 (1977).
17. M. Chretien, S. Benjannet, N. Dragon, N. G. Seidah, and M. Lis, *Biochem. Biophys. Res. Commun., 72*: 472 (1976).
18. C. H. Li, D. Chung, and B. A. Doneen, *Biochem. Biophys. Res. Commun., 72*: 1542 (1976).
19. H. H. Loh, L. F. Tseng, E. Wei, and C. H. Li, *Proc. Natl. Acad. Sci, U.S.A., 73*: 2156 (1976).

20. W. F. Feldberg and D. G. Smyth, *Br. J. Pharmacol., 60:* 445(1977)
21. A. F. Bradbury, W. F. Feldberg, D. G. Smyth, and C. R. Snell, in *Opiates and Endogenous Opiate Peptides* (H. W. Kosterlitz, ed.), Elsevier/North-Holland, Amsterdam, 1976, p. 9.
22. D. G. Smyth, C. R. Snell, and D. E. Massey, *Biochem. J., 175*: 261 (1978).
23. N. Ling, R. Burgus, and R. Guillemin, *Proc. Natl. Acad. Sci. U.S.A., 73*: 3942 (1976).
24. L. Graf, E. Barat, and A. Patthy, *Acta Biochim. Biophys. Acad. Sci. Hung., 11* (2-3): 121 (1976).
25. K. Kangawa, H. Matsuo, and M. Igarishi, *Biochem. Biophys. Res. Commun., 86*: 153 (1979).
26. A. Goldstein, S. Tachibana, L. I. Lowney, M. Hunkapiller, and L. Hood, *Proc. Natl. Acad. Sci. U.S.A., 76*: 6666 (1979).
27. A. S. Stern, R. V. Lewis, S. Kimura, J. Rossier, L. D. Gerber, L. Brink, S. Stein, and S. Udenfriend, *Proc. Natl. Acad. Sci. U.S.A., 76*: 6680 (1979).
28. W. Y. Huang, R. C. C. Chang, A. J. Kastin, D. H. Coy, and A. V. Schally, *Proc. Natl. Acad. Sci. U.S.A., 76*: 6177 (1979).
29. D. F. Steiner, W. Kemmler, H. S. Tager, and J. D. Peterson, *Fed. Proc., 33*: 2105 (1974).
30. B. M. Austen and D. G. Smyth, in *Molecular Endocrinology* (I. MacIntyre and M. Szelke, eds.) Proc. 7th Inter. Congr. Endocrinol., Elsevier/North-Holland, Amsterdam, 1979, p. 99.
31. F. E. Bloom, E. Battenberg, J. Rossier, N. Ling, and R. Guillemin, *Proc. Natl. Acad. Sci. U.S.A., 75*: 1591 (1978).
32. S. J. Watson, J. D. Barchas, and C. H. Li, *Proc. Natl. Acad. Sci. U.S.A., 74*: 5155 (1977).
33. G. Pelletier, R. Leclerc, F. Labrie, J. Cote, M. Chretien, and M. Lis, *Endocrinology, 100*: 770 (1977).
34. S. Zakarian and D. G. Smyth, *Proc. Natl. Acad. Sci. U.S.A., 76*: 5972 (1979).
35. A. A. Waterfield, J. Smokcum, J. Hughes, H. W. Kosterlitz, and G. Henderson, *Eur. J. Pharmcol., 43*: 1017 (1977).
36. M. J. Geisow, J. F. W. Deakin, J. O. Dostrovsky, and D. G. Smyth, *Nature, 269*: 167 (1977).
37. A. F. Bradbury, D. G. Smyth, C. R. Snell, N. J. M. Birdsall, and E. C. Hulme, *Nature, 260*: 793 (1976).
38. D. G. Smyth in *Proceedings of the International Narcotics Research Conference*, N. Falmouth, Mass. (E. Leong Way, ed.), Elsevier/North-Holland, Amersterdam, 1979, in press.
39. D. G. Smyth and S. Zakarian, in *Proceedings of the Sixth American Peptide Symposium*, (E. Gross and J. Meienhöffer, eds.), Ann Arbor Science Publishing, Ann Arbor, Mich., 1979, in press.
40. B. A. Morgan, J. D. Hower, K. P. Guest, B. K. Handa, G. Metcalfe, and C. F. C. Smith, in *Peptides: Proceedings of the Fifth American Peptide Symposium* (M. Goodman and J. Meienhöffer, eds.), Wiley, New York, 1977, p. 111.
41. B. M. Austen and D. G. Smyth, *Biochem. Biophys. Res. Commun., 76*: 477 (1977).

42. B. M. Austen, C. J. Evans, and D. G. Smyth, *Biochem. Biophys. Res. Commun.*, *91*: 1211 (1979).
43. D. G. Smyth, D. E. Massey, S. Zakarian, and M. D. A. Finnie, *Nature*, *279*: 252 (1979).
44. J. Lord, A. A. Waterfield, J. Hughes, and H. W. Kosterlitz, *Nature*, *267*: 495–498 (1977).
45. L. Terenius and A. Wahlström, *Eur. J. Pharmacol.*, *40*: 241–248 (1976).
46. A. Goldstein, W. Fischli, L. I. Lowney, M. Hunkapiller, and L. Hood, *Proc. Natl. Acad. Sci. U.S.A.*, in press (1981).
47. D. G. Smyth and S. Zakarian, *Nature*, *288*: 613-615 (1980).

chapter 3

Structure-Activity Relationships

William L. Dewey

Medical College of Virginia
Richmond, Virginia

I. INTRODUCTION

The discovery of opioid activity for a number of endogenous peptides has lead to the synthesis of a large number of analogs in an attempt to identify a more stable, potent, and specific-acting compound. The pharmacological properties of the endogenous opiate peptides are discussed in detail in other chapters and included here only as standards of comparison for the synthetic compounds. Some selectivity is made among the various activities demonstrated for the peptides. The major emphasis is placed on those responses most generally regarded as an indication of opiate effect. Finally, an attempt is made to present a thorough overview of this rapidly expanding field and the author apologizes to those investigators whose compounds have inadvertently been overlooked. A number of peptides have been synthesized and tested by a number of pharmaceutical firms. The publication of these results will add to our knowledge in this area. The reader is referred to an excellent review by Morley on the same subject which appeared during the preparation of this chapter (1). No attempt is made to duplicate that material in this chapter.

The first peptides isolated and identified with opiate effects were reported by Hughes and his colleagues in December 1975 (2). They reported that two pentapeptides, H-Tyr-Gly-Gly-Phe-Met-OH and H-Tyr-Gly-Gly-Phe-Leu-OH, existed in a 4:1 ratio in porcine brain. In the following year Simantov and Snyder (3) reported that the same two pentapeptides existed in bovine brain, but the ratio of their concentration was reversed. That is, there was four times as much Leu-enkephalin as Met-enkephalin extractable from bovine brain. Additional experiments demonstrated the presence of these peptides in other species.

TABLE 1 β-Lipotropin Fragments with Morphinelike Activities

Amino acid sequence of β-lipotropin	Name	References
60–65	Arginine-enkephalin	5
61–65	Methionine-enkephalin	2
61–68	Octapeptide	6
61–69	Nonapeptide	7
61–76	α-Endorphin	6
61–77	γ-Endorphin	6
61–78	δ-Endorphin	7
61–79	δ-Endorphin	6
61–87	C′-fragment	7
61–91	β-Endorphin (C-fragment)	7, 8

The amino acid sequence of Met-enkephalin is exactly the same as the amino acids numbered 61-65 in β-lipotropin (β-LPH), a 91-amino acid peptide isolated from the pituitary of a number of species, including humans (4). This observation has lead to the hypothesis that β-LPH is a precursor for Met-enkephalin and prompted the search for other fragments of β-LPH with opioid characteristics. Fragments of β-LPH have been isolated and identified as having acttivities similar to morphine, as shown in Table 1.

Feldberg and Smyth (7) investigated the antinociceptive properties of a number of the endogenous peptides isolated from porcine lipotropin following their infusion into the third ventricle of cats. C-Fragment (i.e., amino acids 61-91) was found to be 90–180 times as potent as morphine in this preparation. LPH 61-78, LPH 61-69, or LPH 61-65 (Met-enkephalin) had at best weak and short-lasting antinociceptive activity in this system. C-Fragment or β-endorphin was found to be 17–48 times as potent as morphine in the mouse tail flick, hot plate, and writhing tests when given centrally, and 3.4 times as potent as morphine by the intravenous route of administration (8).

The data presented in Tables 2 through 9 are presented so that one can compare the potencies of the peptides with the prototype alkaloidal opiate, morphine, and Met-enkephalin as the prototype peptide. In a number of studies normorphine was used rather than morphine. This is most often true in the guinea pig ileum assay. The compounds are listed in what the author perceives to be a logical fashion. Various studies on the same peptide are presented in succession so that one can determine the extent of consistency in potency among different procedures. There are instances of inconsistencies among laboratories when the same assay system has been used.

This can be attributed to the different supplies of the compounds, slight variations in the biological procedures, normal animal variation, and many other factors.

An attempt has been made to present as much material as possible in this tabular format. Therefore, each assay system has not been described. It is suggested that the reader consult the primary reference for the details. Unless otherwise indicated, the peptides given were intracerebroventricularly for the in vivo studies such as the tail flick test. Opiate binding is used in these tables to include opiate receptor affinity studies and radioreceptor assays using any one of a number of radiolabeled ligands. At times, more specific information is given since there are great differences in the affinity for various ligands. One trend that exists throughout these tables is the marked differences in potency of morphine and Met-enkephalin in a number of these test procedures. This causes a large discrepancy between the relative potency of the new compounds to morphine and to Met-enkephalin. In a few bioassays, particularly in vivo tests, Met-enkephalin was inactive and a potency comparison with the synthetic analog could not be made. In Tables 2 through 9 the word "inactive" appears when either the new peptide or the prototype was inactive. If a potency ratio is given for the new compound and one prototype opiate, the word "inactive" indicates that the other prototype is inactive and not the new analog. If the word "inactive" is present in both columns, the new peptide is inactive. Investigators did not always include the potency of both morphine and Met-enkephalin in their papers. These instances are designated in the appropriate column as not tested (N.T.).

II. PEPTIDES WITH FEWER THAN FIVE AMINO ACIDS

It is clear from the data presented in Table 2 that a number of peptides with fewer than five amino acids have been synthetized and tested for their opiatelike activity. Many of these are fragments of the naturally occurring Met-enkephalin. The majority of these compounds were found to be either inactive or much less potent than the naturally occurring enkephalins. One clear exception is the interesting dipeptide called kyotorphin, the activity of which was reported by Takagi and his colleagues (9). Most of the other di- and tri-peptides tested were found to be inactive in the guinea pig ileum, myenteric plexus, and adenylate cyclase test systems. Generally, peptides with four amino acids were more active than the smaller peptides but still were shown to have only minimal potency. Some of the tetrapeptides with D-Ala at position 2 and a rather large moiety on the Phe in position 4 were more potent than Met-enkephalin in the guinea pig ileum assay. Most of these compounds, reported on by Bower and colleagues, are repeated here to make the point that some specificity existed since all tetrapeptides with a large substitution on the 4-phenylalanine were not active. Certain tripeptides with D-Ala at position 2 and a large substitution on the carboxy terminus amino acid also were more potent than the prototype compounds. It is interesting that D-Ala-Gly-Leu-O-Me was essentially inactive in the opiate binding, suggesting that at least for these compounds the substitution on the carboxy terminus is just as important for opiate activity as the D-Ala in position 2.

TABLE 2 Comparison of the Opioid Effects of Peptides with Fewer Than Five Amino Acids

Peptide	Test system	Relative potency to: Morphine	Met-Enk	Ref.
Tyr-Arg	Tail pinch	N.T.[a]	4.2	9
Tyr-Gly	Myenteric plexus	Inactive	Inactive	10
Phe-Leu	Adenylate cyclase	Inactive	Inactive	11
D-Ala-Gly-Leu-O-Me	Opiate binding	N.T.	<0.001	12
Tyr-Gly-Gly	Guinea pig ileum	Inactive	Inactive	13
Tyr-Gly-Gly	Myenteric plexus	Inactive	Inactive	10
Tyr-Gly-Gly	Tail flick	Inactive	Inactive	14
Tyr-Gly-Gly	Naloxone binding	Inactive	Inactive	14
Tyr-Gly-Gly	Adenylate cyclase	Inactive	Inactive	11
Tyr-Gly-Gly	Vas deferens	0.05	0.001	15
Gly-Gly-Phe	Guinea pig ileum	Inactive	Inactive	13
Gly-Gly-Phe	Adenylate cyclase	Inactive	Inactive	11
Tyr-D-Ala-Gly-NMeCH_2CH_2-Ph	Guinea pig ileum	5.3	5.3	16
Tyr-D-Ala Gly-NMeCH_2CH_2-Ph	Tail flick	1.0	10.0	16
Tyr-D-Ala-Gly-NMeCH_2CH_2-Ph	Vas deferens	2.5	0.075	16
Tyr-D-Ala-Gly-NHCH_2CH_2-Ph	Guinea pig ileum	4.4	4.4	16
Tyr-D-Ala-Gly-NHCH_2CH_2Ph	Tail flick	1.0	10.0	16
Tyr-D-Ala-Gly-NHCH_2CH_2-Ph	Vas deferens	0.77	0.02	16
Tyr-Gly-Gly-Phe	Adenylate cyclase	0.05	0.0003	17
Tyr-Gly-Gly-Phe	Opiate binding	0.0003	0.0003	17
Tyr-Gly-Gly-Phe	Guinea pig ileum	0.005	0.001	13
Tyr-Gly-Gly-Phe	Opiate binding	0.045	0.09	18
Tyr-Gly-Gly-Phe	Opiate binding	N.T.	0.02	19
Tyr-Gly-Gly-Phe	Opiate binding	<0.001	<0.001	20
Tyr-Gly-Gly-Phe	Vas deferens	N.T.	0.01	21
Tyr-Gly-Gly-Phe	Guinea pig ileum	N.T.	0.01	21
Tyr-Gly-Gly-Phe	Myenteric plexus	N.T.	0.001	10
Tyr-Gly-Gly-Phe	Vas deferens	0.2	0.006	15

TABLE 2 (Continued)

Peptide	Test system	Relative potency to: Morphine	Met-Enk	Ref.
Tyr-Gly-Gly-Phe-NH_2	Vas deferens	0.1	0.007	22
Tyr-Gly-Gly-Phe-$CONH_2$	Opiate binding	~0.075	~0.15	18
Tyr-Gly-Phe-Leu	Adenylate cyclase	0.23	0.002	23
Tyr-Gly-Gly-Trp	Opiate binding	N.T.[a]	0.02	19
Gly-Gly-Phe-Met	Vas deferens	N.T.	0.001	24
Gly-Gly-Phe-Leu	Vas deferens	N.T.	0.001	24
Tyr-D-Ala-Gly-Phe	Opiate binding	N.T.	0.28	12
Tyr-D-Ala-Gly-Phe-NH_2	Guinea pig ileum	5.15	5.15	16
Tyr-D-Ala-Gly-Phe-NH_2	Vas deferens	2.0	0.06	16
Tyr-D-Ala-Gly-Phe-$NHCH_2CH_2CH$-Me_2	Vas deferens	N.T.	0.44	25
Tyr-D-Ala-Gly-Phe-$NHCH_2CH_2CH$-Me_2	Guinea pig iluem	N.T.	9.4	25
Me-Tyr-D-Ala-Gly-Phe-N-(Me)-CH_2CH_2CH-Me_2	Vas deferens	N.T.	0.26	25
Me-Tyr-D-Ala-Gly-Phe-N-(Me)-CH_2CH_2CH-Me_2	Guinea pig ileum	N.T.	10	25
Tyr-D-Ala-Gly-Phe-N-(Me)-CH_2CH_2CH-Me_2	Vas deferens	N.T.	0.15	25
Tyr-D-Ala-Gly-Phe-N-(Me)-CH_2CH_2CH-Me_2	Guinea pig ileum	N.T.	8	25
Me-Tyr-D-Ala-Gly-Phe-$NHCH_2CH_2CH$-Me_2	Vas deferens	N.T.	0.35	25
Me-Tyr-D-Ala-Gly-Phe-$NHCH_2CH_2CH$-Me_2	Guinea pig ileum	N.T.	5.2	25
Tyr-D-Ala-Gly-Me-Phe-$NHCH_2CH_2CH$-Me_2	Vas deferens	N.T.	0.14	25
Tyr-D-Ala-Gly-Me-Phe-$NHCH_2CH_2CH$-Me_2	Guinea pig ileum	N.T.	5	25
Me-Tyr-D-Ala-Gly-Me-Phe-$NHCH_2CH_2CH$-Me_2	Vas deferens	N.T.	0.05	25
Me-Tyr-D-Ala-Gly-Me-Phe-$NHCH_2CH_2CH$-Me_2	Guinea pig ileum	N.T.	2.35	25
Tyr-D-Ala-Gly-Me-Phe-$NCH_3CH_2CH_2CH$-Me_2	Vas deferens	N.T.	0.03	25
Tyr-D-Ala-Gly-Me-Phe-$NCH_3CH_2CH_2CH$-Me_2	Guinea pig iluem	N.T.	0.65	25

TABLE 2 (Continued)

Peptide	Test system	Relative potency to: Morphine	Met-Enk	Ref.
Me-Tyr-D-Ala-Gly-Me-Phe-$NCH_3CH_2CH_2CH$-Me_2	Vas deferens	N.T.[a]	0.04	25
Me-Tyr-D-Ala-Gly-Me-Phe-$NCH_3CH_2CH_2CH$-Me_2	Guinea pig ileum	N.T.	0.71	25
Tyr-D-Ala-Gly-Me-Phe-$NHCH_2CH_2N$-(O)-Me	Vas deferens	N.T.	0.018	25
Tyr-D-Ala-Gly-Me-Phe-$NHCH_2CH_2N$-(O)-Me	Guinea pig ileum	N.T.	8.5	25
Me-Tyr-D-Ala-Gly-Me-Phe-$NHCH_2CH_2N$-(O)-Me	Vas deferens	N.T.	0.04	25
Me-Tyr-D-Ala-Gly-Me-Phe-$NHCH_2CH_2N$-(O)-Me	Guinea pig ileum	N.T.	4.53	25
Tyr-D-Ala-Gly-Me-Phe-$NHCH_2CH_2N$-(O)-Me-(O)	Vas deferens	N.T.	0.18	25
Tyr-D-Ala-Gly-Me-Phe-$NHCH_2CH_2N$-(O)-Me-(O)	Guinea pig ileum	N.T.	6.50	25
Me-Tyr-D-Ala-Gly-Me-Phe-$NHCH_2CH_2N$-(O)-Me-(O)	Vas deferens	N.T.	0.03	25
Me-Tyr-D-Ala-Gly-Me-Phe-$NHCH_2CH_2N$-(O)-Me-(O)	Guinea pig ileum	N.T.	7.9	25

[a]N.T., not tested.

III. SUBSTITUTIONS FOR AMINO ACID 61 IN LPH 61-65

The data presented in Table 3 show that a number of Met-enkephalin analogs have been synthesized with alterations in the tyrosine at position 61 of LPH. Many of these are an alteration in tyrosine itself, whereas others are substitutions of another amino acid. These data and those presented in Tables 8 and 9 indicate that tyrosine is important for opiate activity. The majority of the new peptides were much less potent than Met-enkephalin. However, the addition of a methyl on the tyrosyl nitrogen gave a compound that showed an increase in activity in a number of assay systems. The removal of the amino group on the tyrosine gave a compound that was less active than either morphine or Met-enkephalin in most experiments. The substitution of other amino acids for tyrosine caused a significant decrease in activity in each test system. The substitution of D-Tyr for L-Tyr caused a loss of opiate activity, suggesting certain conformational requirements at this position. It is evident from the data presented in Table 3 as well as the data in other tables in this series that although there are many exceptions, often there is a good agreement for the potency of the new peptides in various opiate assay systems and that there is good agreement between the potency of analogs determined in different laboratories. Often the major differences are between the potency of the prototype alkaloid and the peptide in the assay. This led Kosterlitz and his colleagues to propose the existance of μ- and δ-receptors to classify those preparations most sensitive to each of the two types of opiates.

The data presented in Table 3 and summarized above suggest a similarity between tryosine at position 1 and the phenethylamine moiety of morphine. Although a number of the analogs synthesized support this expected comparison, it is interesting to note that the substitution of N-allyltyrosine for tyrosine did not yield a compound with opiate antagonistic activity. It has been known for many years that N-allyl alkaloid opiates are narcotic antagonists.

TABLE 3 Effect of Substitution for Amino Acid 61 of LPH 61–65, Methionine-Enkephalin, on Opiate Activity

		Relative potency to:		
Substitution	Test system	Morphine	Met-Enk	Reference
des-NH_2-Tyr	Guinea pig ileum	Inactive	Inactive	13
des-NH_2-Tyr	Guinea pig ileum	N.T.[a]	Inactive	21
des-NH_2-Tyr	Vas deferens	N.T.	Inactive	21
Tyr-Me	Guinea pig ileum	0.007	0.002	13
Tyr-Me	Guinea pig ileum	1.0	1.0	16
Tyr-Me	Opiate binding	~2.25	9	18
Tyr-Me	Vas deferens	6.67	0.2	16
Me-Tyr-(O-B_3)	Opiate binding	<0.045	<0.09	18
N-Me-Tyr	[^{3}H]Leu-Enk binding	100	0.3	26
N-Me-Tyr	Opiate binding	1.6	0.38	26
N-Me-Tyr	Vas deferens	0.28	0.24	26
N-Me-Tyr	Guinea pig ileum	1.08	1.47	26
Tyr-N-carbamyl	Opiate binding	<0.045	<0.09	18
cPr-Me-Tyr	Guinea pig ileum	0.015	0.015	16
cPr-Me-Tyr	Vas deferens	0.26	0.008	16
(O-Me)-Tyr	Myenteric plexus	N.T.	0.17	10
Phe	Guinea pig ileum	0.017	0.004	13
Phe	Opiate binding	0.0005	0.001	27

TABLE 3 (Continued)

Substitution	Test system	Relative potency to: Morphine	Met-Enk	Reference
Phe	Opiate binding	0.001	0.002	5
Phe	Opiate binding	0.0002	0.0002	17
Phe	Guinea pig ileum	N.T.[a]	0.002	21
Phe	Adenylate cyclase	0.25	0.0015	17
Phe	Vas deferens	N.T.	0.0003	21
Phe	Myenteric plexus	N.T.	0.002	10
Ala	Myenteric plexus	N.T.	0.002	10
D-Ala	Myenteric plexus	N.T.	Inactive	28
Gly	Myenteric plexus	N.T.	Inactive	28
Sar	Opiate binding	0.003	0.005	27
His	Opiate binding	$<$0.0002	$<$0.0004	27
L-Dopa	Opiate binding	0.001	0.002	27
L-Dopa	Opiate binding	0.002	0.004	5
Trp	Opiate binding	0.0002	0.0004	27
Trp	Opiate binding	0.0004	0.0008	5

[a]N.T., not tested.

IV. SUBSTITUTIONS FOR AMINO ACID 62 OR 63 IN LPH 61-65

The data presented in Table 4 show that few analogs have been synthesized with only alterations in amino acid 62 of LPH 61-65. However, some of the most interesting results have occurred by substituting D-alanine for glycine at this position. This substitution did not increase potency in opiate binding assays but inhibits the rapid metabolic breakdown that occurs in biological tissues with Met-enkephalin. In some assay systems this has increased the potency of the analogs several hundredfold. L-Alanine substitution was found to yield a peptide that was generally less active than the naturally occurring peptide. The substitution of other D-amino acids at this position was found not to increase potency. The substitution of D-alanine for glycine at amino acid 63 of LPH in the enkephalin pentapeptide produced a peptide with a marked decrease rather than an increase in potency in the opiate assays. The potencies of some of these compounds are presented in Table 5. The resultant peptide was also inactive when L-alanine was substituted for glycine at the amino acid 63 position of LPH.

TABLE 4 Effect of Substitution for Amino Acid 62 of LPH 61-65, Methionine-Enkephalin, on Opiate Activity

Substitution	Test system	Relative potency to: Morphine	Relative potency to: Met-Enk	References
Me-Gly	Opiate binding	0.45	0.9	18
Pro	Opiate binding	<0.045	<0.09	18
Ala	Adenylate cyclase	1.0	0.008	23
Ala	Myenteric plexus	N.T.[a]	0.06	28
Ala	Naloxone binding	N.T.	0.05	19
Ala	Opiate binding	<0.045	<0.09	18
D-Ala	Vas deferens	2.21	5.6	26
D-Ala	Vas deferens	7.16	5.26	15
D-Ala	Vas deferens	6.25	6.25	16
D-Ala	Myenteric plexus	N.T.	3.16	28
D-Ala	Guinea pig ileum	166	5.00	16
D-Ala	Guinea pig ileum	4.42	6.02	26
D-Ala	Opiate binding	0.25	0.5	27
D-Ala	Naloxone binding	N.T.	0.54	19
D-Ala	Naloxone binding	1.77	0.58	26
D-Ala	Leu-Enk binding	379	1.18	26
D-Ala	Opiate binding	0.2	2.5	29
D-Ala	Opiate binding	1.2	6.8	30
D-Ala	Tail flick	1.4	97	30
D-Ala	Tail flick	2.5	4.0	16

TABLE 5 Effect of Substitution for Amino Acid 63 of LPH 61-65, Methionine-Enkephalin, on Opiate Activity

Substitution	Test system	Relative potency to: Morphine	Relative potency to: Met-Enk	References
D-Ala	Myenteric plexus	N.T.[a]	0.4	10
D-Ala	Myenteric plexus	N.T.	0.4	28
D-Ala	Vas deferens	0.05	0.002	15
D-Ala	Opiate binding	<0.0004	0.002	15
Ala	Myenteric plexus	N.T.	<0.01	28

[a]N.T., not tested.

TABLE 6 Effect of Substitution for Amino Acid 64 of LPH 61–65, Methionine-Enkephalin, on Opiate Activity

Substitution	Test system	Relative potency to: Morphine	Met-Enk	Reference
Tyr	Guinea pig ileum	N.T.[a]	0.003	21
Tyr	Vas deferens	N.T.	0.001	21
Ala	Myenteric plexus	N.T.	Inactive	28
D-Ala	Myenteric plexus	N.T.	<0.01	29
D-Phe	Opiate binding	N.T.	<0.01	19
D-Phe	Myenteric plexus	N.T.	<0.01	28
Gly	Myenteric plexus	N.T.	Inactive	28
Trp	Opiate binding	N.T.	1.29	19
D-Trp	Opiate binding	N.T.	<0.01	19

[a]N.T., not tested.

V. SUBSTITUTIONS FOR AMINO ACID 64 IN LPH 61–65

Few alterations to or substitutions for Phe in position 64 of LPH 61–65 have appeared. Those included in Table 6 indicate that all but Trp caused a decrease in potency relative to Met-enkephalin. The substitution of D-Trp caused a decrease rather than an increase in potency. Substitutions at most other positions of LPH 61–65 have been more fruitful.

VI. SUBSTITUTIONS FOR AMINO ACID 65 IN LPH 61–65

The data presented in Table 7 show that considerable interest has emerged in the synthesis of enkephalin analogs with a substitution for amino acid 65 of LPH 61–65. The apparent large number of compounds in this table may be somewhat misleading since Leu-enkephalin is included. Leu-enkephalin, which is the other naturally occurring pentapeptide reported by Hughes et al. (2), is obviously of considerable interest. In some systems, Leu-enkephalin is more potent than Met-enkephalin, whereas in other systems Leu-enkephalin has less potency. D-Leu substitution at position 65 of LPH 61–65 yielded a compound less potent in most test systems. One exception was the mouse vas deferens assay, where is was slightly more potent than Met-enkephalin and approximately equally potent with L-Leu-enkephalin.

The substitution of D-Met for L-Met in LPH 61–65 caused a significant reduction in potency in the guinea pig myenteric preparation and in the opiate receptor binding assays by a number of different investigators. This amide is also more potent in both isolated organ studies and in vivo assays since it also has the advantage over Met-enkephalin of being less susceptible to enzymatic breakdown. Substitutions of methyl or ethyl on the amide nitrogen of methionine yielded pentapeptides which were less potent than Met-enkephalin. Oxidation of the methionine yielded compounds that had variable potencies compared to Met-enkephalin. Leu-enkephalin or O-methyl-Leu-enkephalin were found consistently to be less potent than either Met- or Leu-enkephalin. The substitution of other amino acids in position 65 yielded enkephalins less potent than Met-enkephalin, one exception being Nle, which was three times more potent than Met-enkephalin in the adenylate cyclase assay. As can be seen in Table 8, descarboxy Nle at position 65 and D-Ala at 62 yielded a peptide with considerable in vivo activity.

TABLE 7 Effect of Substitution for Amino Acid 65 of LPH 61–65, Methionine-Enkephalin, on Opiate Activity

		Relative potency to:		
Substitution	Test system	Morphine	Met-Enk	Reference
D-Met	Myenteric plexus	N.T.[a]	0.105	28
Met-NH_2	Opiate binding	1.0	2.0	27
Met-NH_2	Opiate binding	1	?	5
Met-NH_2	Myenteric plexus	N.T.	3.02	10
Met-NH_2	Longitudinal strip	0.9	0.7	22
Met-NH_2	Guinea pig ileum	2.77	1.52	31
Met-NH_2	Vas deferens	11	0.5	22
Met-NH_2	Vas deferens	2.7	0.08	15
Met-NH_2	Hot plate	0.008	1	22
Met-$NHCH_3$	Vas deferens	5	0.24	22
Met-NH-Et	Vas deferens	10	0.3	15
Met-NH-Et	Myenteric plexus	N.T.	2.46	10
Met-(O)	Myenteric plexus	N.T.	0.2	10
Met-(O)	Vas deferens	11.3	0.35	15
Met-O-Me	Vas deferens	5	0.15	15
Met-ol	Tail flick	0.02	1.6	30
Met-ol	Opiate binding	8.24	1.46	30
Met-$CONH_2$	Opiate binding	1.5	3	18
(des-carboxy)-Met	Vas deferens	1.5	0.07	22
Leu	Opiate binding	0.14	0.29	5
Leu	Opiate binding	0.27	1.8	32
Leu	Opiate binding	215	0.67	26
Leu	Opiate binding	0.61	0.2	26
Leu	Opiate binding	N.T.	0.38	19

TABLE 7 (Continued)

Substitution	Test system	Relative potency to: Morphine	Met-Enk	Reference
Leu	Opiate binding	0.42	0.42	17
Leu	Opiate binding	0.32	1.82	15
Leu	Opiate binding	0.14	0.29	27
Leu	Opiate binding	N.T.	1.8	12
Leu	Naloxone binding	0.02	0.25	14
Leu	In vivo binding	Inactive	Inactive	20
Leu	Adenylate cyclase	37.5	0.3	11
Leu	Adenylate cyclase	50	0.5	23
Leu	Adenylate cyclase	167	1.0	17
Leu	Myenteric plexus	N.T.[a]	0.37	10
Leu	Guinea pig ileum	0.15	0.21	26
Leu	Guinea pig ileum	0.7	0.17	13
Leu	Guinea pig ileum	0.30	0.17	31
Leu	Vas deferens	38	1.19	15
Leu	Vas deferens	64.5	1.64	26
Leu	Tail flick	0.005	0.31	14
D-Leu	Tail flick	0.006	Inactive	33
D-Leu	Myenteric plexus	N.T.	0.15	28
D-Leu	Vas deferens	45	1.41	15
D-Leu	Opiate binding	0.14	0.8	15
Leu-NH_2	Opiate binding	0.05	0.1	5
Leu-NH_2	Opiate binding	0.03	0.07	27
Leu-NH_2	Adenylate cyclase	10	0.08	23
Leu-O-Me	Vas deferens	8.9	0.28	15
Leu-O-Me	Opiate binding	0.058	0.001	15
Leu-O-Me	Adenylate cyclase	15	0.12	23
Leu-O-Me	Guinea pig ileum	0.2	1.0	34
Ile	Vas deferens	25	0.78	15
Nle	Opiate binding	0.56	0.56	17
Nle	Opiate binding	0.04	0.23	15
Nle	Opiate binding	800	0.2	20
Nle	In vivo binding	Inactive	0.38	20
Nle	Adenylate cyclase	500	3.0	17
Nle	Guinea pig ileum	1.8	0.45	13
Nle	Guinea pig ileum	N.T.	0.5	35

TABLE 7 (Continued)

Substitution	Test system	Relative potency to: Morphine	Met-Enk	Reference
Nle	Vas deferens	5.1	0.16	15
Nle-methyl ester	Guinea pig ileum	N.T.	0.9	35
Ala	Opiate binding	0.0006	0.003	15
Ala	Myenteric plexus	N.T.[a]	0.029	28
Ala	Vas deferens	0.1	0.003	15
D-Ala	Myenteric plexus	N.T.	0.065	28
Thr	Opiate binding	0.01	0.02	5
Gly	Opiate binding	0.0004	0.002	15
Gly	Myenteric plexus	N.T.	<0.01	28
Gly	Guinea pig ileum	N.T.	0.02	21
Gly	Vas deferens	0.01	0.003	15
Gly	Vas deferens	N.T.	0.03	21
Val	Vas deferens	1.3	0.04	15
Val	Opiate binding	0.04	0.23	15
Leucinol	Vas deferens	4	0.13	15

[a]N.T., not tested.

TABLE 8 Effect of Substitution for More Than One Amino Acid of LPH 61–65, Methionine-Enkephalin, on Opiate Activity

Substitution	Test system	Relative potency to: Morphine	Met-Enk	Ref.
(D-Tyr)^1-(Thr)^4	Myenteric plexus	N.T.[a]	<0.01	28
(D-Tyr)^1-(Leu)^5	Vas deferens	0.16	0.005	15
(des-NH_2-Tyr)^1-(Leu)^5	Opiate binding	Inactive	Inactive	14
(des-NH_2-Tyr)^1-(Leu)^5	Tail flick	Inactive and toxic		14
(des-NH_2-Tyr)^1-(Met-NH_2)^5	Longitudinal strip	<0.03	<0.002	22
(Me-Tyr)^1-(Met-$CONH_2$)^5	Opiate binding	1.5	3	18
(N-Me_3-Tyr)^1-(Met-NH_2)^5	Guinea pig ileum	5.25	5.25	16
(N-Me_3-Tyr)^1-(Met-NH_2)^5	Vas deferens	3.3	0.1	16
(N-Me_3-Tyr)^1-(Met-NH_2)^5	Tail flick (i.v.t.)	2.00	5.0	16
(N-Me_3-Tyr)^1-(Met-NH_2)^5	[^{3}H]Leu-Enk binding	34	0.11	26
(N-Me_3-Tyr)^1-(Met-NH_2)^5	Naloxone binding	4.35	1.42	26
(N-Me_3-Tyr)^1-(Met-NH_2)^5	Vas deferens	12.86	9.33	26
(N-Me_3-Tyr)^1-(Met-NH_2)^5	Guinea pig ileum	2.75	3.76	26

TABLE 8 (Continued)

Substitution	Test system	Relative potency to: Morphine	Relative potency to: Met-Enk	Ref.
(N-Me-Tyr)^1-(Leu)^5	Vas deferens	24	0.75	15
(N-Me-Tyr)^1-(Leu)^5	Opiate binding	0.005	0.03	15
(O-Me-Tyr)^1-(Leu)^5	Vas deferens	0.75	0.023	15
(O-Me-Tyr)^1-(Leu)^5	Opiate binding	0.0008	0.005	15
(Me-Tyr)^1-(Leu-NH_2)^5	Guinea pig ileum	2.23	4.85	36
(Me-Tyr)^1-(Leu-NH_2)^5	Vas deferens	3.4	0.85	36
(N-Me-Tyr)^1-(Leu-O-Me)^5	Vas deferens	6.7	0.21	15
(N-Me-Tyr)^1-(Leu-O-Me)^5	Opiate binding	0.007	0.04	15
(N-Me_2-Tyr)^1-(Leu)^5	Vas deferens	0.4	0.0125	15
(N-Me_2-Tyr)^1-(Leu)^5	Opiate binding	0.001	0.006	15
(N-Me_2-Tyr)^1-(Leu-O-Me)^5	Vas deferens	0.7	0.02	15
(N-Me_2-Tyr)^1-(Leu-O-Me)^5	Opiate binding	0.0004	0.002	15
(BOC-Tyr)^1-(Leu)^5	Vas deferens	0.01	0.0003	15
(Me-Tyr-(O-B_3)^1-(Met-$CONH_2$)^5	Opiate binding	<0.045	<0.09	18
(β-homo-Tyr)^1-(Leu)^5	Vas deferens	1.2	0.038	15
(β-homo-Tyr)^1-(Leu)^5	Opiate binding	<0.0004	<0.002	15
(N-Me-Tyr)^1-(Met-NH-Pr)^5	Tail flick	1.0	10.0	16
(N-Me-Tyr)^1-(Met-NH-Pr)^5	Vas deferens	8.3	0.25	16
(AC-Tyr)^1-(Met-NH_2)^5	Opiate binding	N.T.[a]	0.001	37
(N-Me-Tyr)^1-(Met-NH-Pr)^5	Guinea pig ileum	4.7	4.7	16
(N^{α}-Me-Tyr)^1-(des-COOH-Nle)^5	Guinea pig ileum	1.55	1.2	38
(N^{α}-Me-Tyr)^1-(des-COOH-Nle)^5	Tail flick	0.09	8	38
(Phe)^1-(Met-NH_2)^5	Vas deferens	<0.03	<0.002	22
(Phe)^1-(Met-NH_2)^5	Longitudinal strip	<0.03	<0.002	22
(Phe)^1-(Met-NH_2)^5	Hot plate	<0.003	<0.04	22
(D-Ala)^2-(D-Met)^5	Vas deferens	228	7.12	15
(D-Ala)^2-(Trp)^4	Opiate binding	N.T.	0.34	19
(D-Ala)^2-(D-Met)^5	Opiate binding	0.438	0.15	15
(D-Ala)^2-(D-Met)^5	Opiate binding	N.T.	2.0	12
(D-Ala)^2-(D-Met)^5	Myenteric plexus	N.T.	4.19	28
(D-Ala)^2-(Met-NH_2)^5	Tail flick	1.0	10.0	16

TABLE 8 (Continued)

Substitution	Test system	Relative potency to: Morphine	Relative potency to: Met-Enk	Ref.
(D-Ala)^2-(Met-NH_2)^5	Guinea pig ileum	8.0	8.0	16
(D-Ala)^2-(Met-NH_2)^5	Opiate binding	0.25	0.5	27
(D-Ala)^2-(Met-NH_2)^5	Vas deferens	63.3	1.9	16
(D-Ala)^2-(Met-NH_2)^5	Tail flick	0.5	Inactive	33
(D-Ala)^2-(Met-ol)^5	Tail flick	25	1,700	30
(D-Ala)^2-(Met-ol)^5	Opiate binding	3.65	20.6	30
(D-Ala)^2-(Met-(O)-ol)^5	Tail flick	100	6,800	30
(D-Ala)^2-(Met-(O)-ol)^5	Opiate binding	1.22	5.64	30
(D-Ala)^2-(Met-NH-Pr)^5	Tail flick	1.0	10.0	16
(D-Ala)^2-(Met-NH-Pr)^5	Vas deferens	173.3	5.2	16
(D-Ala)^2-(Met-NH-Pr)^5	Guinea pig ileum	4.8	4.8	16
(D-Ala)^2-(D-Met-O-Me)^5	Vas deferens	148	4.62	15
(D-Ala)^2-(D-Met-O-Me)^5	Opiate binding	0.234	1.34	15
(D-Ala)^2-(Met-O-Me)^5	Vas deferens	94	2.94	15
(D-Ala)^2-(Met-O-Me)^5	Opiate binding	0.70	4	15
(D-Ala)^2-(D-Met-NH_2)^5	Myenteric plexus	N.T.[a]	2.46	28
(D-Ala)^2-(Met-NH_2)^5	Vas deferens	31	7.75	36
(D-Ala)^2-(Met-NH_2)^5	Guinea pig ileum	1.67	3.63	36
(D-Ala)^2-(Leu)^5	Opiate binding	1.094	6.25	15
(D-Ala)^2-(Leu)^5	Opiate binding	0.9	6.25	32
(D-Ala)^2-(Leu)^5	Vas deferens	267	8.34	15
(D-Ala)^2-(Leu)^5	Myenteric plexus	N.T.	5.28	28
(D-Ala)^2-(Leu)^5	Myenteric plexus	N.T.	2.3	28
(D-Ala)^2-(D-Leu)^5	Opiate binding	1.346	7.7	15
(D-Ala)^2-(D-Leu)^5	Opiate binding	N.T.	7.69	12
(D-Ala)^2-(D-Leu)^5	Opiate binding	1.1	7.8	32
(D-Ala)^2-(D-Leu)^5	Opiate binding	1.346	7.69	15
(D-Ala)^2-(D-Leu)^5	Vas deferens	1,227	38.3	15
(D-Ala)^2-(D-Leu)^5	Myenteric plexus	N.T.	6.84	28
(D-Ala)^2-(D-Leu)^5	Tail flick	31.7	Inactive	33
(D-Ala)^2-(D-Leu-NH-Et)^5	Opiate binding	N.T.	0.2	12
(D-Ala)^2-(Leu-NH_2)^5	Tail flick	31.7	Inactive	39
(D-Ala)^2-(Leu-NH_2)^5	Vas deferens	N.T.	1.6	24

TABLE 8 (Continued)

Substitution	Test system	Relative potency to: Morphine	Met-Enk	Ref.
(D-Ala)^2-(Leu-NH_2)^5	Guinea pig ileum	N.T.[a]	5.0	24
(D-Ala)^2-(Leu-NH_2)^5	Tail flick (i.v.)	0.4	Inactive	39
(D-Ala)^2-(D-Leu-NH_2)^5	Myenteric plexus	N.T.	4.06	39
(D-Ala)^2-(Leu-NH_2)^5	Guinea pig ileum	5.0	5.0	16
(D-Ala)^2-(Leu-NH_2)^5	Vas deferens	53.3	1.6	16
(D-Ala)^2-(Leu-NH_2)^5	Tail flick	1.0	10.0	16
(D-Ala)^2-(Az-Leu-NH_2)^5	Guinea pig ileum	1.5	7.5	33
(D-Ala)^2-(D-Leu-O-Me)^5	Opiate binding	0.389	2.22	15
(D-Ala)^2-(D-Leu-O-Me)^5	Vas deferens	74	2.3	15
(D-Ala)^2-(Leu-O-Me)^5	Opiate binding	0.389	2.22	15
(D-Ala)^2-(Leu-O-Me)^5	Vas deferens	95	2.97	15
(D-Ala)^2-(N^{α}-Me)-Leu)^5	Myenteric plexus	N.T.	3.87	28
(D-Ala)^2-(N^{α}-Me)-Leu-NH_2)^5	Myenteric plexus	N.T.	7.11	28
(D-Ala)^2-(Leu-NH_2-CH_2-CH_2-NH-Me)^5	Guinea pig ileum	4.7	23.5	34
(D-Ala)^2-(Leu-NH-CH_2-CH_2-N-Me_2)^5	Guinea pig ileum	3.8	19	34
(D-Ala)^2-(Leu-O-CH_2-CH_2-OH)^5	Guinea pig ileum	2.7	13.5	34
(D-Ala)^2-(Leu-NH-CH_2-CH_2-OH)^5	Guinea pig ileum	1.7	8.5	34
(D-Ala)^2-(D-β-homo-Leu)^5	Vas deferens	44	1.4	15
(D-Ala)^2-(Nle)^5	Guinea pig ileum	N.T.	3.0	35
(D-Ala)^2-(Nle)^5	Vas deferens	209	6.53	15
(D-Ala)^2-(Nle)^5	Opiate binding	0.389	2.22	15
(D-Ala)^2-(des-COOH-Nle)^5	Guinea pig ileum	5.1	3.93	38
(D-Ala)^2-(des-COOH-Nle)^5	Tail flick	0.16	Inactive	38
(D-Ala)^2-(Thr)^5	Vas deferens	9	0.28	15
(D-Ala)^2-(Thr)^5	Opiate binding	0.039	0.22	15
(D-Ala)^2-($NHCH_2$-CH_2-CH-Me_2)	Guinea pig ileum	9.4	9.4	16
(D-Ala)^2-($NHCH_2$-CH_2-CH-Me_2)	Vas deferens	14.6	0.44	16
(D-Ala)^2-($NHCH_2$-CH_2-CH-Me_2)	Tail flick	1.0	10.0	16

TABLE 8 (Continued)

Substitution	Test system	Relative potency to: Morphine	Met-Enk	Ref.
(D-Ala)^2-(Pro)^5	Vas deferens	4	0.125	15
(D-Ala)^2-(Pro)^5	Opiate binding	0.0006	0.003	15
(D-Ala)^2-(Pro)^5	Tail flick	N.T.[a]	167	38
(D-Ala)^2-(Pro)^5	Guinea pig ileum	N.T.	0.4	35
(D-Ala)^2-(Pro-NH$_2$)^5	Tail flick	N.T.	1025	40
(D-Ala)^2-(Pro-NH-Et)^5	Guinea pig ileum	1.25	2.72	36
(D-Ala)^2-(Pro-NH-Et)^5	Vas deferens	2.12	0.53	36
(D-Ala)^2-(Pro-NH)^5	Tail flick	3.9	Inactive	41
(D-Ala)^2-(Pro-NH)^5	Tail flick (i.v.)	0.22	Inactive	41
(D-Ala)^2-(Pro-NH$_2$)^5	Guinea pig ileum	2.53	5.49	36
(D-Ala)^2-(Pro-NH$_2$)^5	Vas deferens	1.96	0.49	36
(D-Ala)^2-(Pro-NH-Et)^5	Tail flick	16.9	Inactive	37
(D-Ala)^2-(Pro-NH-Et)^5	Tail flick (i.v.)	0.19	Inactive	41
(D-Ala)^2-(Pro-NH-Amyl)^5	Tail flick	0.08	Inactive	41
(D-Ala)^2-(NH-Amyl)^5	Tail flick (i.v.)	0.1	Inactive	41
(D-Ala)^2-(D-Ala)^5	Myenteric plexus	N.T.	2.05	28
(D-Ala)^2-(D-Lys)^5	Myenteric plexus	N.T.	3.28	28
(D-Ala)^2-(D-Phe)^5	Myenteric plexus	N.T.	5.22	28
(D-Ala)^2-(D-Phe)^5	Myenteric plexus	N.T.	0.32	28
(Ala)^2-(Trp)^4	Opiate binding	N.T.	0.02	19
(Ala)^2-(Met-NH$_2$)^5	Opiate binding	0.025	0.05	27
(Ala)^2-(Leu)^5	Opiate binding	0.014	0.014	17
(Ala)^2-(Leu)^5	Vas deferens	0.3	0.009	15
(Ala)^2-(Leu)^5	Adenylate cyclase	10.0	0.06	17
(Ala)^2-(Leu)^5	Opiate binding	0.0007	0.004	15
(D-N-Me-Ala)^2-(D-Leu-O-Me)^5	Opiate binding	N.T.	0.22	12
(α-Me-Ala)^2-(D-Leu-O-Me)^5	Opiate binding	<0.0004	0.002	15
(α-Me-Ala)^2-(D-Leu-O-Me)^5	Vas deferens	0.3	0.009	15
(α-Me-Ala)^2-(D-Leu)^5	Opiate binding	<0.0004	0.002	15
(α-Me-Ala)^2-(D-Leu)^5	Vas deferens	1.5	0.05	15
(Pro)^2-(Met-NH$_2$)^5	Opiate binding	0.001	0.002	27
(Sar)^2-(Met-NH$_2$)^5	Opiate binding	0.013	0.025	27
(Sar)^2-(Leu)^5	Vas deferens	0.12	0.004	15

TABLE 8 (Continued)

Substitution	Test system	Relative potency to: Morphine	Met-Enk	Ref.
$(Sar)^2$-$(Leu)^5$	Opiate binding	0.0004	0.002	15
$(D\text{-}Val)^2$-$(Met\text{-}NH_2)^5$	Opiate binding	0.025	0.05	27
$(D\text{-}Phe)^2$-$(Met\text{-}NH_2)^5$	Opiate binding	0.05	0.1	27
$(D\text{-}Phe)^2$-$(Met\text{-}NH_2)^5$	Opiate binding	0.05	0.1	27
$(D\text{-}Leu)^2$-$(Leu)^5$	Vas deferens	6.4	0.2	15
$(D\text{-}Trp)^2$-$(Leu)^5$	Vas deferens	1.6	0.05	15
$(D\text{-}Trp)^2$-$(D\text{-}Leu)^5$	Opiate binding	N.T.[a]	0.0025	12
$(D\text{-}Trp)^2$-$(Leu)^5$	Opiate binding	0.44	2.5	15
$(D\text{-}Trp)^2$-$(Leu)^5$	Opiate binding	N.T.	2.2	12
$(Pro)^2$-$(Leu)^5$	Vas deferens	<0.01	<0.0003	15
$(Pro)^2$-$(Leu)^5$	Opiate binding	<0.0004	<0.002	15
$(GABA)^2$-$(Leu)^5$	Adenylate cyclase	0.3	0.002	23
$(D\text{-}Met)^2$-$(Nle)^5$	Guinea pig ileum	N.T.	3.5	35
$(D\text{-}Met)^2$-$(Leu\text{-}NH_2)^5$	Guinea pig ileum	12.7	27.5	36
$(D\text{-}Met)^2$-$(Leu\text{-}NH_2)^5$	Vas deferens	14.7	3.68	36
$(D\text{-}Met)^2$-$(Pro\text{-}NH_2)^5$	Guinea ileum	13.5	29.2	36
$(D\text{-}Met)^2$-$(Pro\text{-}NH_2)^5$	Vas deferens	3.88	0.97	36
$(D\text{-}Met)^2$-$(Leu\text{-}O\text{-}Me)^5$	Vas deferens	11.96	2.99	36
$(D\text{-}Met)^2$-$(Leu\text{-}O\text{-}Me)^5$	Guinea pig ileum	29	63	36
$(D\text{-}Met)^2$-$(Pro\text{-}NH_2)^5$	Hot plate	25.0	N.T.	37
$(D\text{-}Met)^2$-$(Pro\text{-}NH_2)^5$	Tail flick	N.T.	16,161	40
$(D\text{-}Met)^2$-$(Pro\text{-}NH_2)^5$	Tail flick	78.5	N.T.	37
$(D\text{-}Met)^2$-$(Pro\text{-}NH\text{-}Et)^5$	Tail flick (i.v.)	0.55	Inactive	41
$(D\text{-}Met)^2$-$(Pro\text{-}NH\text{-}Et)^5$	Tail flick	16.9	Inactive	41
$(D\text{-}Met)^2$-$(Pro\text{-}NH_2)^5$	Vas deferens	7.96	N.T.	37
$(D\text{-}Met)^2$-$(Pro\text{-}NH_2)^5$	Tail flick (i.v.)	5.5	Inactive	41
$(D\text{-}Met)^2$-$(Pro\text{-}NH_2)^5$	Tail flick	49.8	Inactive	41
$(D\text{-}Met)^2$-$(Pro\text{-}NH_2)^5$	Guinea pig ileum	7.86	N.T.	37
$(D\text{-}Met)^2$-$(Thz\text{-}NH_2)^5$	Tail flick (i.v.)	4.2	Inactive	39
$(D\text{-}Met)^2$-$(Thz\text{-}NH_2)^5$	Tail flick	7.7	Inactive	39
$(D\text{-}Thr)^2$-$(Thz\text{-}NH_2)^5$	Tail flick	27.1	Inactive	39
$(D\text{-}Thr)^2$-$(Thz\text{-}NH_2)^5$	Tail flick (i.v.)	4.8	Inactive	39
$(D\text{-}Ser)^2$-$(Pro\text{-}NH\text{-}Et)^5$	Guinea pig ileum	0.97	2.11	36

TABLE 8 (Continued)

Substitution	Test system	Relative potency to: Morphine	Met-Enk	Ref.
(D-Ser)^2-(Pro-NH-Et)^5	Vas deferens	1.24	0.31	36
(D-Ser)^2-(Pro-NH$_2$)^5	Guinea pig ileum	1.01	2.2	36
(D-Ser)^2-(Pro-NH$_2$)^5	Vas deferens	0.76	0.19	36
(D-Ser)^2-(Met-O-Me)^5	Guinea pig ileum	6.59	14.3	36
(D-Ser)^2-(Met-O-Me)^5	Vas deferens	118	29.5	36
(D-Eth)^2-(Pro-NH$_2$)^5	Tail flick	N.T.[a]	3,809	40
(D-Nle)^2-(Pro-NH$_2$)^5	Tail flick	N.T.	5,291	40
(D-Phe)^2-(Pro-NH$_2$)^5	Tail flick	N.T.	167	40
(Ala)^3-(Leu)^5	Vas deferens	0.8	0.025	15
(Ala)^3-(Leu)^5	Opiate binding	N.T.	0.0025	12
(Ala)^3-(Leu)^5	Opiate binding	0.0004	0.002	15
(Ser)^3-(Leu)^5	Vas deferens	0.1	0.003	15
(Ser)^3-(Leu)^5	Opiate binding	0.004	0.02	15
(Ser)^3-(Leu)^5	Adenylate cyclase	0.05	0.0004	23
(Tyr)^4-(Leu)^5	Opiate binding	0.0002	0.001	15
(Tyr)^4-(Leu)^5	Vas deferens	0.05	0.002	15
(D-Ala)^3-(Leu)^5	Opiate binding	0.00007	0.0004	15
(D-Ala)^3-(Leu)^5	Vas deferens	0.1	0.0003	15
(D-Ala)^3-(Nle)^5	Guinea pig ileum	N.T.	<0.05	35
(Pro)^3-(Leu)^5	Vas deferens	0.01	0.003	15
(Pro)^3-(Leu)^5	Opiate binding	0.0001	0.0006	15
(Car)^4-(Leu)^5	Opiate binding	N.T.	1.16	42
(Cl-Phe)^4-(Nle)^5	Guinea pig ileum	1.2	0.3	13
(D-Phe)^4-(Leu)^5	Vas deferens	0.01	0.0003	15
(D-Phe)^4-(Leu)^5	Opiate binding	<0.0004	<0.002	15
(O-Me-Tyr)^4-(Leu-O-Me)^5	Opiate binding	N.T.	0.0004	12
(Tyr)^4-(Leu)^5	Opiate binding	N.T.	0.32	19
(Me-Tyr)^1-(D-Ala)^2-(Leu-NH$_2$)^5	Vas deferens	43	10.78	36
(Me-Tyr)^1-(D-Ala)^2-(Leu-NH$_2$)^5	Guinea pig ileum	2.95	6.4	36
(N-Me$_2$-Tyr)^1-(D-Ala)^2-(D-Leu-O-Me)	Vas deferens	3	0.09	15

TABLE 8 (Continued)

Substitution	Test system	Relative potency to: Morphine	Met-Enk	Ref.
(N-Me_2-Tyr)^1-(D-Ala)^2-(D-Leu-O-Me)	Opiate binding	0.0005	0.003	15
(N-Me-Tyr)^1-(D-Ala)^2-(Leu)^5	Vas deferens	66	2.06	15
(N-Me-Tyr)^1-(D-Ala)^2-(Leu)^5	Opiate binding	0.018	0.1	15
(N-Me-Tyr)^1-(D-Ala)^2-(Leu-O-Me)^5	Vas deferens	21.5	0.67	15
(N-Me-Tyr)^1-(D-Ala)^2-(Leu-O-Me)^5	Opiate binding	0.005	0.03	15
(N-Me-Tyr)^1-(D-Ala)^2-(D-Leu)^5	Vas deferens	229	7.15	15
(N-Me-Tyr)^1-(D-Ala)^2-(D-Leu-O-Me)^5	Vas deferens	18.3	0.57	15
(N-Me_2-Tyr)^1-(D-Ala)^2-(Leu)^5	Vas deferens	12	0.38	15
(N-Me_2-Tyr)^1-(D-Ala)^2-(Leu)^5	Opiate binding	0.002	0.01	15
(N-Me_2-Tyr)^1-D-Ala)^2-(Leu-O-Me)^5	Vas deferens	9.7	0.3	15
(N-Me_2-Tyr)^1-(D-Ala)^2-(Leu-O-Me)^5	Opiate binding	0.007	0.004	15
(N-Me_2-Tyr)^1-(D-Ala)^2-(D-Leu)^5	Vas deferens	33.6	1.05	15
(N-Me_2-Tyr)^1-(D-Ala)^2-(D-Leu)^5	Opiate binding	0.001	0.007	15
(O-Ac-Tyr)^1-(D-Ala)^2-(Leu)^5	Vas deferens	28	0.9	15
(O-Ac-Tyr)^1-(D-Ala)^2-(Leu)^5	Opiate binding	0.004	0.3	15
(3, 5-I_2-Tyr)^1-(D-Ala)^2-(Leu)^5	Vas deferens	0.4	0.013	15
(O-Me-Tyr)^1-(O-Me-Tyr)^4-(Leu)^5	Vas deferens	0.03	0.0009	15
(O-Me-Tyr)^1-(O-Me-Tyr)^4-(Leu)^5	Opiate binding	0.004	0.022	15
(D-Tyr)^1-(D-Ala)^2-(Leu)^5	Vas deferens	0.7	0.002	15

TABLE 8 (Continued)

Substitution	Test system	Relative potency to: Morphine	Met-Enk	Ref.
(D-Tyr)^1-(D-Ala)^2-(Leu)^5	Opiate binding	N.T.[a]	0.00007	12
(D-Tyr)^1-(D-Ala)^2-(Leu)^5	Opiate binding	0.002	0.01	15
(D-Tyr)^1-(D-Ala)^2-(D-Leu)^5	Vas deferens	0.3	0.009	15
(D-Tyr)^1-(D-Ala)^2-(D-Leu)^5	Opiate binding	<0.0004	0.002	15
(N-Me-Tyr)^1-(D-Ala)^2-(D-Leu-NH_2)^5	Opiate binding	N.T.	1.0	12
(N-Me-Tyr)^1-(D-Ala)^2-(D-Met-NH_2)^5	Opiate binding	N.T.	0.06	12
(Phe)^1-(D-Ala)^2-(Leu)^5	Vas deferens	2.5	0.08	15
(Phe)^1-(D-Ala)^2-(Leu)^5	Opiate binding	N.T.	0.2	12
(Phe)^1-(D-Ala)^2-(Leu)^5	Opiate binding	0.005	0.03	15
(Phe)^1-(Tyr)^4-(Leu)^5	Vas deferens	0.01	0.0003	15
(Phe)^1-(Tyr)^4-(Leu)^5	Opiate binding	0.0004	0.002	15
(D-Ala)^2-(D-Ala)^3-(Leu)^5	Vas deferens	0.35	0.01	15
(D-Ala)^2-(D-Ala)^3-(Leu)^5	Vas deferens	0.35	0.01	15
(D-Ala)^2-(D-Ala)^3-(Leu)^5	Opiate binding	0.0009	0.005	15
(D-Ala)^2-(D-Ala)^3-(Nle)^5	Guinea pig ileum	N.T.	0.05	15
(D-Ala)^2-(Ala)^3-(Leu)^5	Vas deferens	12	0.375	15
(D-Ala)^2-(Ala)^3-(Leu)^5	Opiate binding	0.04	0.25	15
(D-Ala)^2-(D-Pro)^3-(Leu)^5	Vas deferens	0.02	0.0006	15
(D-Ala)^2-(D-Pro)^3-(Leu)^5	Opiate binding	<0.0004	0.002	15
(D-Ala)^2-(Asn)^3-(Leu)^5	Vas deferens	0.9	0.03	15
(D-Ala)^2-(Asn)^3-(Leu)^5	Opiate binding	0.005	0.03	15
(D-Ala)^2-(Sar)^3-(Leu)^5	Vas deferens	18	0.56	15
(D-Ala)^2-(Sar)^3-(Leu)^5	Opiate binding	<0.0004	0.002	15
(D-Ala)^2-(D-Phe)^4-(Leu)^5	Vas deferens	0.2	0.006	15
(D-Ala)^2-(Leu)^4-(Leu)^5	Vas deferens	0.01	0.0003	15
(D-Ala)^2-(Leu)^4-(Leu)^5	Opiate binding	<0.0004	0.002	15
(D-Ala)^2-(His)^4-(Leu)^5	Vas deferens	0.08	0.003	15
(D-Ala)^2-(His)^4-(Leu)^5	Opiate binding	0.0008	0.005	15
(D-Ala)^2-(c-Ph-Gly)^4-(Leu)^5	Vas deferens	0.04	0.001	15
(D-Ala)^2-(c-Ph-Gly)^4-(Leu)^5	Opiate binding	0.0008	0.005	15
(D-Ala)^2-(D-Phe)^4-(Leu)^5	Opiate binding	0.0004	0.002	15

TABLE 8 (Continued)

Substitution	Test system	Relative potency to: Morphine	Met-Enk	Ref.
(D-Ala)^2-(Me-Phe)^4-(Met-(O)-ol)^5	Tail flick	500	34,000	30
(D-Ala)^2-(Me-Phe)^4-(Met-(O)-ol)^5	Opiate binding	6.1	34.3	30
(D-Ala)^2-(Cl-Phe)^4-(D-Leu-(O)-Me)^5	Opiate binding	N.T.[a]	10	12
(D-Ala)^2-(pCl-Phe)^4-(D-Leu-NH-Et)^5	Opiate binding	N.T.	0.25	12
(D-Ala)^2-(Ala)^3-(Leu)^5	Vas deferens	0.04	0.001	15
(Ala)^2-(Ala)^3-(Leu)^5	Opiate binding	<0.0004	0.002	15
(Ala)^2-(D-Ala)^3-(Leu)^5	Vas deferens	0.04	0.001	15
(Ala)^2-(D-Ala)^3-(Leu)^5	Opiate binding	<0.0001	0.002	15
(Ala)^2-(D-Ala)^3-(Met)^5	Vas deferens	0.01	0.0003	15
(Ala)^2-(D-Ala)^3-(Met)^5	Opiate binding	<0.0004	0.002	15
(Me-Tyr)^1-(D-Ala)^2-(Me-Phe)^4-(Met-(O)-ol)^5	Tail flick	1,000	68,000	43

[a]N.T., not tested.

VII. SUBSTITUTIONS FOR MORE THAN ONE AMINO ACID IN LPH 61-65

Hundreds of pentapeptides with more than one substitution for the amino acids in LPH 61-65 have been synthetized and studied in a number of biological assay systems. The effects of many of these are presented in Table 8. The most potent analogs that have appeared are presented in this table. The last compound listed in Table 8, (Me-Tyr)^1-(D-Ala)^2-(Me-Phe)^4-(Met-(O)-ol)^5, is the most potent. Many of the substitutions referred to above that increased potency when made individually apparently were additive in this compound. The most significant observation is that this compound is 1000 times as potent as morphine when administered into the cerebral ventricle and the mice tested in the tail flick test. The 68,000 increase in potency over Met-enkephalin in part reflects the lack of potency of the endogenous peptide in this test system. The tyrosyl analog of this potent analog was approximately one-half as potent, that is, 50 times the potency of morphine and 34,000 times the potency of Met-enkephalin. When only (D-Ala)^2 and (Met-(O)-ol)^5 were substituted in LPH 61-65 the potency was still 100 times that of morphine and 6800 times that of Met-enkephalin in the tail flick test. However, this same analog was only 1.22 times as potent as morphine and 5.64 times as potent as Met-enkephalin in the opiate binding assay. These results suggest that these two changes protected each end of the pentapeptide from enzymatic breakdown but also increased affinity for the opiate receptor. Many analogs with a D-Ala substitution at position 62 of LPH 61-65 and an alteration or substitution at position 65 which interferes with inactivation at the carboxy terminus have been shown to increase potency in most opioid bioassays.

Many other analogs, most notably those which have a D-Ala substitution in position 62 of LPH 61-65 and another D-amino acid substituted at position 65 have shown marked increases in potency over Met-enkephalin in a number of opiate assays. Substitution of other D-amino acids at position 62 together with substitutions at position 65 also increased the potency over that of Met-enkephalin. The most potent of these resulted from the substitution of D-Ser, D-Eth, D-Nle, and D-Phe at position 62. A number of analogs have been synthesized with D-Met at position 62 and a substitution for methionine at position 65. Most of these new pentapeptides were more potent than morphine or Met-enkephalin. D-Val, D-Phe, D-Leu, and D-Trp substituted at position 62 and another substitution at position 65 yielded compounds with less potency than Met-enkephalin. The substitution of another L-amino acid for L-Gly at position 62 generally yielded a compound with decreased potency regardless of other substitutions in the pentapeptide.

Dramatic changes in potency were not observed in pentapeptides with an alteration at position 61 and another change in the amino acid sequence of LPH 61-65. The substitution of either D- or L-amino acids for Gly at position 63 together with another change in the pentapeptide also did not yield compounds with increased potency in the in vitro and in vivo bioassays. The pentapeptides were less potent than Met-enkephalin, with alterations only at positions 64 and 65. Generally, substitution of leucine for methionine at position 65 and the alteration of the amino acid at another position in LPH 61-65 decreased rather than increased the potency. The enormous range of potencies of the pentapeptides in Table 8 is striking.

VIII. PEPTIDES WITH MORE THAN FIVE AMINO ACIDS

The data presented in Table 9 show that a number of fragments of LPH larger than the pentapeptide Met-enkephalin have been tested for their potency in a number of opiate test systems. The majority of the peptides included in this table are fragments of LPH close to amino acids 61-65 (Met-enkephalin) in the 91-amino acid peptide. LPH 60-65 and 61-66 were less potent than morphine or Met-enkephalin. A preliminary report suggested narcotic antagonistic activity for LPH 60-65, but further experimentation yielded weak agonistic properties for this hexapeptide. The higher potency for LPH 61-66 compared to morphine in the vas deferens preparation is another indication of the weaker activity of the alkaloid than the peptides in this assay. LPH 61-66 was slighty less potent than Met-enkephalin in this test and considerably less potent than either Met-enkephalin or morphine in the opiate binding assay.

LPH 59–65 was found to be considerably less potent than morphine or Met-enkephalin in the opiate binding assay. Generally, LPH 61–68 and LPH 61–69 were found to be less potent than either morphine or Met-enkephalin. Some clear exceptions to this are presented in Table 9. LPH 61–75 was less potent than the prototype compounds in all but the adenylate cyclase assay, which happens to be the same assay in which LPH 61–69 was significantly more potent than morphine. Like the vas deferens preparation, the adenylate cyclase assay appears to be less sensitive to the alkaloids than the peptides. The majority of the studies of LPH 61–76, LPH 61–77, and LPH 61–79 yielded potencies less than that of Met-enkephalin.

TABLE 9 Comparison of the Opioid Effects of Peptides with More Than Five Amino Acids

		Relative potency to:		
Peptide	Test system	Morphine	Met-Enk	Reference
LPH 60–65	Guinea pig ileum	1.66	0.42	13
LPH 60–65	Opiate binding	0.15	0.00004	14
LPH 60–65	Opiate binding	0.2	0.4	5
LPH 61–66	Opiate binding	0.1	0.2	5
LPH 61–66	Vas deferens	22	0.69	15
LPH 59–65	Opiate binding	0.1	0.2	5
LPH 61–68	Guinea pig ileum	N.T.[a]	0.66	40
LPH 61–68	Myenteric plexus	N.T.	0.67	28
LPH 61–69	Opiate binding	1.3	1.3	17
LPH 61–69	Opiate binding	Inactive	Inactive	20
LPH 61–69	Guinea pig ileum	N.T.	0.6	40
LPH 61–69	Guinea pig ileum	1.43	0.36	13
LPH 61–69	Myenteric plexus	N.T.	0.6	10
LPH 61–69	Myenteric plexus	N.T.	0.6	28
LPH 61–69	Adenylate cyclase	50.0	0.3	17
LPH 61–69	Guinea pig ileum	N.T.	0.51	47
LPH 61–75	Adenylate cyclase	8.33	0.05	17
LPH 61–75	Opiate binding	0.17	0.17	17
LPH 61–75	Opiate binding	N.T.	0.7	45
LPH 61–76	Myenteric plexus	N.T.	0.36	10

TABLE 9 (Continued)

Peptide	Test system	Relative potency to: Morphine	Met-Enk	Reference
LPH 61–76	Myenteric plexus	N.T.[a]	0.36	28
LPH 61–76	Guinea pig ileum	N.T.	0.36	44
LPH 61–76	Opiate binding	0.33	N.T.	44
LPH 61–77	Opiate binding	4.0	N.T.	44
LPH 61–77	Myenteric plexus	N.T.	0.23	10
LPH 61–77	Myenteric plexus	N.T.	0.23	28
LPH 61–77	Guinea pig ileum	N.T.	0.23	44
LPH 61–79	Guinea pig ileum	N.T.	0.37	45
LPH 61–79	Guinea pig ileum	N.T.	0.37	44
LPH 61–79	Guinea pig ileum	N.T.	0.42	47
LPH 61–79	Myenteric plexus	N.T.	0.37	28
LPH 61–81	Opiate binding	N.T.	1.85	45
LPH 61–86	Opiate binding	N.T.	1.92	45
LPH 61–87	Guinea pig ileum	N.T.	0.48	44
LPH 61–87	Opiate binding	2.0	N.T.	44
LPH 61–87	Myenteric plexus	N.T.	0.48	28
LPH 61–88	Opiate binding	N.T.	3.57	45
LPH 61–89	Opiate binding	N.T.	4.17	45
LPH 61–91	Opiate binding	0.13	1.67	29
LPH 61–91	Opiate binding	3.5	N.T.	44
LPH 61–91	Myenteric plexus	N.T.	4.5	28
LPH 61–91	Myenteric plexus	N.T.	4.5	10
LPH 61–91	Guinea pig ileum	2.0	N.T.	37
LPH 61–91	Guinea pig ileum	N.T.	1.37	47
LPH 61–91	Vas deferens	2.54	N.T.	37
LPH 61–91	Tail flick	5.32	N.T.	37
LPH 61–91	Tail flick	34.7	Inactive	39
LPH 61–91	Tail flick (i.v.)	4.2	Inactive	39
LPH 61–91	Hot plate	10.3	N.T.	37
LPH 62–91	Guinea pig ileum	N.T.	Inactive	44
LPH 62–91	Myenteric plexus	N.T.	Inactive	28
LPH 66–91	Myenteric plexus	N.T.	Inactive	28

TABLE 9 (Continued)

Peptide	Test system	Relative potency to: Morphine	Met-Enk	Ref.
LPH 66–91	Guinea pig ileum	N.T.[a]	Inactive	44
LPH 61–76 NH_2	Myenteric plexus	N.T.	0.72	28
LPH 61–76 NH_2	Guinea pig ileum	N.T.	0.72	44
LPH 61–77 NH_2	Guinea pig ileum	N.T.	0.5	44
LPH 61–77 NH_2	Myenteric plexus	N.T.	0.41	28
$(Leu)^{65}$ LPH 60–65	Opiate binding	0.007	0.04	15
$(Leu)^{65}$ LPH 60–65	Vas deferens	2.5	0.08	15
$(Leu)^{65}$ LPH 61–66 $(Gly)^{67}$	Opiate binding	0.0035	0.02	15
$(Leu)^{65}$ LPH 61–66 $(Gly)^{67}$	Vas deferens	9	0.28	15
$(D\text{-}Ala)^{62}$-$(D\text{-}Leu)^{65}$-$(D\text{-}Thr)^{66}$ LPH 61–66	Vas deferens	11.1	0.35	15
$(D\text{-}Ala)^{62}$-$(D\text{-}Thr)^{66}$ LPH 61–66	Guinea pig ileum	1.0	5.0	34
$(D\text{-}Ala)^{62}$-$(Trp)^{64}$ LPH 61–66	Opiate binding	N.T.	0.59	19
$(D\text{-}Ala)^{62}$ LPH 61–66	Opiate binding	1.625	3.57	15
$(D\text{-}Ala)^{62}$ LPH 61–66	Opiate binding	N.T.	3.57	12
$(D\text{-}Ala)^{62}$ LPH 61–66	Vas deferens	229	7.16	15
$(D\text{-}Ala)^{62}$-$(Leu)^{65}$ LPH 61–66	Opiate binding	0.438	2.5	15
$(D\text{-}Ala)^{62}$-$(Leu)^{65}$ LPH 61–66	Vas deferens	461	14.4	15
$(D\text{-}Ala)^{62}$-$(D\text{-}Leu)^{65}$ LPH 61–66	Opiate binding	0.1	0.7	15
$(D\text{-}Ala)^{62}$-$(D\text{-}Leu)^{65}$ LPH 61–66	Vas deferens	19	0.6	15
$(D\text{-}Ala)^{62}$-$(D\text{-}Met)^{65}$ LPH 61–66	Opiate binding	0.05	0.28	15
$(D\text{-}Ala)^{62}$-$(D\text{-}Met)^{65}$ LPH 61–66	Vas deferens	4	0.1	15
LPH-$(Sar)^{59}$ LPH 60–65	Opiate binding	0.005	0.01	5

TABLE 9 (Continued)

Peptide	Test system	Relative potency to: Morphine	Met-Enk	Ref.
$(Lys)^{60}$-$(D\text{-}Ala)^{62}$-$(Az\text{-}Leu\text{-}NH)^{65}$ LPH 60–65	Guinea pig ileum	1.0	5.0	34
$(Lys)^{60}$-$(D\text{-}Ala)^{62}$-$(Met\text{-}O\text{-}Me)^{65}$ LPH 60–65	Guinea pig ileum	2.7	13.5	34
$(Lys)^{60}$-$(D\text{-}Ser)^{62}$-$(Met\text{-}O\text{-}Me)^{65}$ LPH 60–65	Guinea pig ileum	14	70	34
$(Leu)^{65}$ LPH 60–66	Opiate binding	0.02	0.13	15
$(Leu)^{65}$ LPH 60–66	Vas deferens	10	0.31	15
$(D\text{-}Ala)^{62}$-$(D\text{-}Leu)^{65}$-$(Phe)^{66}$-$(Gly)^{67}$ LPH 61–67	Opiate binding	0.004	0.03	15
$(Leu)^{65}$ LPH 61–76	Guinea pig ileum	N.T.[a]	0.17	44
$(Leu)^{65}$ LPH 61–76	Opiate binding	0.01	N.T.	44
$(D\text{-}Ala)^{62}$-$(D\text{-}Leu)^{65}$-$(PHe)^{66}$-$(Gly)^{67}$ LPH 61–67	Vas deferens	6.3	0.2	15
$(D\text{-}Ala)^{62}$-$(D\text{-}Leu)^{65}$-$(Lys)^{66}$-$(Lys)^{67}$ LPH 61–67	Opiate binding	0.004	0.02	15
$(D\text{-}Ala)^{62}$-$(D\text{-}Leu)^{65}$-$(Lys)^{66}$-$(Lys)^{67}$ LPH 61–67	Vas deferens	1.6	0.05	15
$(D\text{-}Ala)^{62}$-$(D\text{-}Leu)^{65}$-$(Lys)^{66}$-$(Lys)^{67}$ LPH 61–67	Vas deferens	1.6	0.05	15
$(D\text{-}Ala)^{62}$ LPH 61–76	Myenteric plexus	N.T.	0.37	28
$(Leu)^{65}$ LPH 61–76	Myenteric plexus	N.T.	0.10	28
$(D\text{-}Ala)^{62}$-$(D\text{-}Leu)^{65}$ LPH 61–76	Myenteric plexus	N.T.	0.017	28
$(D\text{-}Ala)^{62}$-$(D\text{-}Leu)^{65}$ LPH 61–77	Myenteric plexus	N.T.	0.03	28
$(D\text{-}Ala)^{62}$ LPH 61–77	Myenteric plexus	N.T.	0.37	28

TABLE 9 (Continued)

Peptide	Test system	Relative potency to: Morphine	Met-Enk	Reference
$(Leu)^{65}$ LPH 61-77	Myenteric plexus	N.T.[a]	0.08	28
$(Leu)^{5}$ LPH 61-77	Guinea pig ileum	N.T.	0.09	44
$(Leu)^{5}$ LPH 61-77	Opiate binding	5.4	N.T.	44
$(D\text{-}Tyr)^{61}$ LPH 61-91	Tail flick	0.005	N.T.	46
$(D\text{-}Ala)^{62}$ LPH 61-91	Tail flick	1.0	N.T.	46
$(Leu)^{65}$ LPH 61-91	Myenteric plexus	N.T.	0.75	28
$(D\text{-}Phe)^{64}$ LPH 61-91	Tail flick	<0.003	N.T.	46
$(D\text{-}Met)^{65}$ LPH 61-91	Tail flick	0.01	N.T.	46
$(Leu)^{5}$ LPH 61-91	Opiate binding	9.5	N.T.	44
$(Leu)^{5}$ LPH 61-91	Guinea pig ileum	N.T.	0.75	44

[a]N.T., not tested.

Many of the longer peptides were more potent than the endogenous pentapeptides. The extent of the increase is not striking in most cases. LPH 61-81, LPH 61-86, LPH 61-88, and LPH 61-89 but not LPH 61-87 were approximately two to four times as potent as Met-enkephalin. Interestingly, LPH 61-87 was found to be more potent than morphine in the opiate binding assay but less potent than Met-enkephalin in the guinea pig ileum.

As pointed out earlier in this chapter LPH 61-91 β-endorphin is more potent than Met-enkephalin in most assay systems. This is particularly true in the tail flick and other in vivo test procedures. It is generally accepted that the biological half-life of β-endorphin far exceeds that of Met-enkephalin. The slight increase in potency of β-endorphin over Met-enkephalin in the opiate binding assay supports the contention that the decreased enzymatic breakdown of β-endorphin contributes to its increased potency. The lack of activity of LPH 62-91 indicates that the tyrosyl moiety at position 61 is necessary for the opiate activitiy of β-endorphin. In light of this, it is not surprising that LPH 66-91 is without opiate activity.

The potency of LPH fragments larger than a pentapeptide with substitutions for one or more amino acids have been synthesized and tested in various biological assays. LPH 61-76 amide and LPH 61-77 amide were slightly more potent than LPH 61-76 and LPH 61-77, respectively. These amides were still less potent than Met-enkephalin. The substitution of Leu for Met at position 65 in LPH 60-65 caused a decrease in potency.

A number of peptides with more than five amino acids and D-Ala substituted for Gly at position 62 have been tested. Generally, as was the case with the pentapeptides, the D-Ala substitution at LPH 62 increased potency. LPH 61-66 with a

D-Ala substitution at position 62 was seven times as potent as Met-enkephalin in the vas deferens preparation. Substituting Leu at position 65 in the same molecule (i.e., LPH 61-66 with D-Ala at 62 and Leu at 65) was 14 times as potent as Met-enkephalin. However, the substitution of D-Leu at position 65 in this molecule caused a reduction in potency lower than that of Met-enkephalin. This suggests that conformational changes at position 65 in LPH 61-66 are important for opiate potency. This observation has been confirmed in that the substitution of D-Met for L-Met at position 65 in LPH 61-66 also caused a marked reduction in opiate potency.

None of the substituted longer peptides were found to be much more potent than Met-enkephalin or β-endorphin. Substitution of D-Tyr for L-Tyr at position 61 in LPH 61-69 caused a significant reduction in potency in the tail flick test. Interestingly, the substitution of D-Ala for Gly at position 62 of LPH 61-91 also caused a reduction in tail flick potency. Similarly, D-Phe substitution at position 64 and D-Met at position 65 each caused a decrease in the tail flick potency of β-endorphin.

IX. SUMMARY AND CONCLUSIONS

The information presented in Tables 3 through 8 shows that many synthetic analogs of Met-enkephalin have been synthesized and tested in a number of bioassay systems for their opiate potency. A very wide range of potencies has emerged. Obviously, many of the peptides are inactive as opiate agonists, while one was 68,000 times more potent than Met-enkephalin. It seems somewhat useless to try and synthesize yet more potent pentapeptides. Considerable information has been obtained as a result of this enormous synthetic effort. The importance of the tyrosyl moiety in position 61; the increased potency due to the substitution of D-Ala in position 62, which retards enzymatic degradation at the N terminus; the value of the bulk on Phe in position 64; and the resistance to enzymatic breakdown at the carboxy terminus by the amide form of the peptides are examples of ways to increase the potency of the pentapeptides. Multiple changes are additive, as shown in Table 8. Unfortunately, as expected, this information has not given us much insight into the nature of the opiate receptor. As a matter of fact, the data presented in these tables support the multiple opiate receptor hypothesis of Martin (48) and Kosterlitz (49) and their colleagues.

The peptides that have been tested for opiate activity have all shown a very similar profile of pharamcological activity. However, the principal objective of structure-activity studies should be to determine which portion of the molecule is responsible for certain actions and then to synthesize analogs with greater specificity and potency. Thus far, changes in the naturally occurring peptides have not caused changes is specificity of action. The question still remains: Can alterations and substitutions of amino acids in the naturally occurring substances alter the profile of activity in such a way as to cause a lessening of side effects of a potential therapeutic agent among the opiate peptides?

Although the expense of the peptides and their limited availability have hindered work in this area, Wei (50, 51) has shown that β-endorphin and other opiate peptides produce physical dependence of the opiate type when infused into the cerebroventricle of rodents. Similarly, isolated guinea pig ileum incubated in buffer containing a stable opiate peptide contracts on exposure to naloxone, as does a segment of ileum incubated in morphine (52). This has been interpreted as an assay for naloxone-induced withdrawal in this isolated organ preparation. Burks and his colleagues (53) have shown that the stable opiate peptides also resemble the alkaloids with respect to their effects on the gastrointestinal tract.

Des-tyrosyl-γ-endorphin (LPH 62–77) is relatively devoid of opiate activity but has been shown by De Wied, Van Ree, and their colleagues to be very potent in altering the behavioral patters of the rat (54). These results were interpreted by these investigators to suggest that des-tyrosyl-γ-endorphin or a closely related peptide was an endogenous neuroleptic. These results were supported by other work from their laboratory showing behavioral changes induced by other fragments of LPH, including β-endorphin and Met-enkephalin.

Finally, the activity of three opiate peptides is worthy of additional comment. First, kyotorphin is particularly interesting since it is by far the smallest peptide (Tyr-Arg) with opiate effects. Also, its profile of opiate activity differs somewhat from that of morphine. Second, the pentapeptide with substitutions at all positions in LPH 61–65 but position 63 (see the last peptide in Table 8) is one of the most potent synthetic peptides tested to date. An alteration in position 63 has not emerged that caused an increase in opiate activity. Third, a new endogenous peptide has been isolated from the pituitary gland and identified by Goldstein and his colleagues (55). This compound is the most potent endogenous opiate identified to date and therefore has been named "dynorphin." The amino acid sequence of 1–13 dynorphin is Tyr-Gly-Gly-Phe-Leu-Arg-Arg-Ile-Arg-Pro-Lys-Leu-Lys. It can easily be seen that this tridecapeptide contains Leu-enkephalin as its first five amino acids. There are no striking resemblences between the rest of the amino acid sequence of Dynorphin and another portion of LPH. Scientists working in this exciting field of research anxiously anticipate the elucidation of the pharmacology of Dynorphin and the probable discovery of other endogenous opiates. Possibly one for each type of opiate receptor.

ACKNOWLEDGMENT

The preparation of this manuscript and the work from the author's laboratory were supported in part by USPHS Grant DA 01647.

REFERENCES

1. J. S. Morley, Structure-activity relationships of enkephalin-like peptides. *Annu. Rev. Pharmacol.*, *20*: 81–110 (1980).
2. J. Hughes, T. W. Smith, H. W. Kosterlitz, L. A. Fothergill, B. A. Morgan, and H.R. Morris, Identification of two related pentapeptides from the brain with potent opiate agonist activity. *Nature*, *258*: 577–579 (1975).
3. R. Simantov and S. H. Snyder, Isolation and structure identification of a morphine-like peptide "enkephalin" in bovine brain. *Life Sci.*, *18*: 781–788 (1976).
4. C. H. Li, L. Barnafi, M. Chretion, and D. Chung, Isolation and amino acid sequence of β-LPH from sheep pituitary glands. *Nature*, *208*: 1093–1094 (1965).
5. J. K. Chang, T. W. Fong, A. Pert, and C. B. Pert, Opiate receptor affinities and behavioral effects of enkephalin: structure-activity relationships of ten synthetic peptide analogues. *Life Sci.*, *18*: 1473–1482 (1976).
6. A. F. Bradbury, D. G. Smyth, C. R. Snell, N. J. M. Birdsall, and E. C. Hulme, C-fragment of lipotropin has a high affinity for brain opiate receptors. *Nature*, *260*: 793–795 (1976).
7. W. Feldberg and D. G. Smyth, C-fragment of lipotropin—an endogenous potent analgesic peptide. *Br. J. Pharmacol.*, *60*: 445–453 (1977).
8. C. H. Li, D. Yamashiro, L. F. Tseng, and H. H. Loh, Synthesis and analgesic activity of human β-endorphin. *J. Med. Chem.*, *20*: 325–328 (1977).
9. H. Takagi, M. Satoh, H. Shiomi, A. Akaike, H. Ueda, S. Kawajiri, M. Yamamoto, and H. Amano, Identification of a new opioid peptide from the bovine brain and its mechanism of action. In *Endogenous and Exogenous Opiate Agonists and Antagonists* (E. L. Way, ed.), Pergamon Press, Elmsford, N.Y., 1980, pp. 201–204.
10. N. Ling and R. Guillemin, Morphinomimetic activity of synthetic fragments of β-lipotropin and analogs. *Proc. Natl. Acad. Sci. U.S.A.*, *73*: 3308–3310 (1976).
11. W. A. Klee and M. Nirenberg, Mode of action of endogenous opiate peptides. *Nature*, *263*: 609–612 (1976).
12. H. Y. Meltzer, R. J. Miller, R. G. Fessler, M. Simonovic, and V. S. Fang, Effects of enkephalin analogues on prolactin release in the rat. *Life Sci.*, *22*(21): 1931–1938 (1978).
13. A. R. Day, M. Lujan, W. L. Dewey, L. S. Harris, J. A. Radding, and R. J. Freer, Structure activity relationships of enkephalins in the stimulated guinea pig ileum. *Res. Commun. Chem. Pathol. Pharmacol.*, *14*: 597–603 (1976).
14. H. H. Buscher, R. C. Hill, D. Romer, F. Cardinaux, A. Closse, D. Hauser, and J. Pless, Evidence for analgesic activity of enkephalin in the mouse. *Nature*, *261*: 423–425 (1976).
15. F. R. Beddell, R. B. Clark, G. W. Hardy, L. A. Lowe, F. B. Ubatuba, J. R. Vane, and S. Wilkinson, Structural requirements for opioid activity of analogues of the enkephalins. *Proc. R. Soc. Lond. B*, *198*: 249–265 (1977).

16. B. A. Morgan, J. D. Bower, K. P. Guest, B. K. Handa, G. Metcalf, and C. F. C. Smith, Structure-activity relationships of enkephalin analogs. In *Peptides: Proceedings of the Fifth American Peptide Symposium* (M. Goodman and J. Meienhofer, eds.), Wiley, New York, 1977, pp. 111–114.
17. A. Wahlstrom, M. Brandt, L. Moroder, E. Wunsch, G. Lindeberg, U. Ragnarsson, L. Terenius, and B. Hemprecht, Peptides related to β-lipotropin with opioid activity. *FEBS Lett.*, *77*: 28–32 (1977).
18. A. F. Bradbury, W. F. Feldberg, D. G. Smyth, and C. R. Snell, Lipotropin C-fragment: an endogenous peptide with potent analgesic activity. In *Opiates and Endogenous Opioid Peptides* (H. Kosterlitz, ed.), Elsevier/North-Holland, Amsterdam, 1976, pp. 9–17.
19. P. W. Schiller, C. F. Yam, and J. Prosmanne, Synthesis, opiate receptor affinity and conformational parameters of [4-tryptophan]-enkephalin analogs. *J. Med. Chem.*, *21*: 1110–1116 (1978).
20. W. L. Dewey, T. T. Chau-Pham, A. R. Day, M. Lujan, L. S. Harris, and R. J. Freer, The effects of enkephalins on the isolated guinea pig ileum, stereospecific binding of dihydromorphine and antinociception in mice. In *Opiates and Endogenous Opioid Peptides* (H. Kosterlitz, ed.), Elsevier/North-Holland, Amsterdam, 1976, pp. 103–110.
21. B. A. Morgan, C. F. C. Smith, A. A. Waterfield, J. Hughes, and H. W. Kosterlitz, Structure-activity relationships of methionine enkephalin. *J. Pharm. Pharmacol.*, *28*: 660–661 (1976).
22. R. C. A. Frederickson, R. Nickander, E. L. Smithwick, R. Schuman, and F. H. Norris, Pharamcological activity of Met-enkephalin and analogues in vitro and in vivo—depression of single neuronal activity in specified brain regions. In *Opiates and Endogenous Opioid Peptides* (H. Kosterlitz, ed.), Elsevier/North-Holland, Amsterdam, 1976, pp. 239–246.
23. N.S. Agarwal, V. J. Hurby, R. Katz, W. Klee, and M. Nirenberg, Synthesis of leucine enkephalin derivatives: structure function studies. *Biochem. Biophys. Res. Commun.*, *76*: 129–135 (1977).
24. J. M. Hambrook, B. A. Morgan, M. J. Rance, and C. F. C. Smith, Mode of deactivation of the enkephalins by rat and human plasma and rat brain homogenates. *Nature*, *262*: 782–783 (1976).
25. J. D. Bower, B. K. Handa, A. C. Lane, J. A. H. Lord, G. Metcalf, B. A. Morgan, M. J. Rance, P. M. Richards, and C. F. C. Smith, Structure function studies in peptides related to the β-LPH 61–64 sequence. In *Endogenous and Exogenous Opiates Agonists and Antagonists* (E. L. Way, ed.), Pergamon Press, Elmsford, N.Y., 1980, pp. 29–32.
26. H. W. Kosterlitz, J. Hughes, A. H. Lord, and A. A. Waterfield, Enkephalins endorphins and opiate receptors. *Neurosci. Symp.*, *2*: 291–307 (1977).
27. C. B. Pert, D. L. Bowie, B. T. W. Fong, and J. K. Chang, Synthetic analogues of Met-enkephalin which resist enzymatic destruction. In *Opiates and Endogenous Opioid Peptides* (H. Kosterlitz, ed.), Elsevier/North-Holland, Amsterdam, 1976, pp. 79–85.
28. N. Ling, S. Minick, L. Lazarus, J. Rivier, and R. Guillemin, Structure-activity relationships of enkephalin and endorphin analogs. In *Peptides: Proceedings of*

the Fifth American Peptide Symposium (M. Goodman and J. Meienhofer, eds.), Wiley, New York, 1977, pp. 96–99.
29. C. B. Pert, D. L. Bowie, J. L. Morell, and E. Gross, Agonist-antagonist properties of N-allyl-[D-Ala]2-Met-enkephalin. *Nature*, *269*: 73–75 (1977).
30 D. Romer, H. H. Buscher, R. C. Hill, J. Pless, W. Bauer, F. Cardinaux, A. Closse, D. Hauser, and R. Huguenin, A synthetic enkephalin analogue with prolonged parenteral and oral analgesic activity. *Nature*, *268*: 547–549 (1977).
31. M. M. Puig, P. Gascon, G. L. Craviso, R. A. Bjur, G. Natsueda, J. M. Stewart, and J. M. Musacchio, *Arch. Int. Pharmacodyn. Ther.*, *226*: 69–80 (1977).
32. J. K. Chang, R. J. Miller, and P. Cuatreacasas, Interaction of enkephalin with opiate receptors in intact cultured cells. *Mol. Pharmacol.*, *14*: 961–970 (1978).
33. E. T. Wei, L. F. Tseng, H. H. Loh, and C. H. Li, Comparison of the behavioral effects of β-endorphin and enkephalin analogs. *Life Sci.*, *21*: 321–328 (1977).
34. A. S. Dutta, J. J. Gormley, E. F. Hayward, J. S. Morley, J. S. Shaw, C. J. Stacey, and M. T. Turnbull, Enkephalin analogues eliciting analgesia after intravenous injection. *Life Sci.*, *21*: 559–562 (1977).
35. S. Bajusz, A. Z. Ronai, J. I. Szekely, Z. Dunai-Kovacs, I. Berzetri, and L. Graf, Enkephalin analogs with enhanced opiate activity (preliminary communication). *Acta Biochem. Biophys. Acad. Sci. Hung.*, *11*: 305–309 (1976).
36. J. S. Shaw and M. J. Turnbull, In vitro profile of some opioid pentapeptide analogues. *Eur. J. Pharmacol.*, *49*: 313–317 (1978).
37. J. I. Szekely, A. Z. Ronai, Z. Dunai-Kovacs, E. Miglecz, I. Berzetri, S. Bajusz, and L. Graf, (D-Met^2-Pro^5)-enkephalinamide: a potent morphine-like analgesic. *Eur. J. Pharmacol.*, *43*: 293–294 (1977).
38. A. R. Day, J. M. Carney, J. A. Rosecrans, W. L. Dewey, and R. J. Freer, Synthesis of two enzyme resistant enkephalin analogs possessing enhanced analgesic activity. *Res. Commun. Chem. Pathol. Pharmacol.*, *20*: 59–68 (1978).
39. D. Yamashiro, L. Tseng, and C. H. Li, [D-Thr^2, Thz^5]- and [D-Met^2, Thz^5]-Enkephalinamides: potent analgesics by intravenous injection. *Biochem. Biophys. Res. Commun.*, *78*: 1124–1129 (1977).
40. S. Bajusz, A. Patthy, A. Kenessey, L. Graf, J. I. Szekely, and A. Z. Ronai, Is there correlation between analgesic potency and biodegradation of enkephalin analogs? *Biochem. Biophys. Res. Commun.*, *84*(4): 1045–1053 (1978).
41. S. Bajusz, A. Z. Ronai, J. I. Szekely, L. Graf, Z. Dunai-Kovacs, and I. Berzetri, A superactive antinociceptive pentapeptide (D-Met^2, Pro)^5 enkephalinamide, *FEBS Lett.*, *76*: 91–92 (1977).
42. A. Eberle, O. Leukart, P. Schiller, J. Fauchere, and R. Schwyzer, Hormone-receptor interations: [4-carboranylalanine, 5-leucine]-enkephalin as a structural probe for the opiate receptor. *FEBS Lett.*, *82*: 325–328 (1977).
43. J. Pless, W. Bauer, F. Cardinaux, A. Closse, D. Hauser, and R. Huguenin, Structure-activity relationship of enkephalin analogs. In *Molecular Endocrineology* (I. MacIntyre and M. Szelke, eds.), Elsevier/North-Holland, Amsterdam, 1977, pp. 279–285.
44. R. Guillemin, N. Ling, L. Lazarus, R. Burgus, S. Minick, F. Bloom, R. Nicoll, G. Siggins, and D. Segal, The endorphins, novel peptides of brain and hypophysial

origin with opiate-like activity: biochemical and biologic effects. *Ann. N.Y. Acad. Sci., 297*: 131–157 (1977).

45. H. W. Yeung, D. Yamashiro, W. C. Chang, and C. H. Li, Synthesis and opiate activity of human β-endorphin analogs with various chain lengths. *Int. J. Peptide Protein Res., 12*: 42–46 (1978).
46. D. Yamashiro, L. F. Tseng, B. A. Doneen, H. H. Loh, and C. H. Li, β-Endorphin synthesis and morphine-like activity of analogs with D-amino acid residues in positions 1, 2, 4, and 5. *Int. J. Peptide Protein Res., 10*: 159–166 (1977).
47. L. Graf, J. I. Szekely, A. Z. Ronai, Z. Dunai-Kovacs, and S. Bajusz, Comparative study on analgesic effect of Met^5-enkephalin and related lipotropin fragments. *Nature, 263*: 240–241 (1976).
48. W. R. Martin, G. Eades, J. A. Thompson, R. E. Huppler, and P. Gilbert, The effects of morphine and nalorphine-like drugs in the nondependent and morphine-dependent chronic dog. *J. Pharmacol. Exp. Ther., 197*: 517–532 (1976).
49. J. A. Lord, A. F. Waterfield, J. Hughes, and H. W. Kosterlitz, Endogenous opioid peptides: multiple agonists and receptors. *Nature, 267*: 495–499 (1977).
50. E. Wei, Enkephalin analogs: correlation of potencies for analgesia and physical dependence. In *Charactertistics and Function of Opioids* (J. M. van Ree and L. Terenius, eds.), Elsevier/North-Holland, Amsterdam, 1978, pp. 445–446.
51. E. Wei, Enkephalin analogs and physical dependence. In *Endogenous and exogenous opiate agonists and antagonists* (E. L. Way, ed.), Pergamon Press, Elmsford, N.Y., 1980, pp. 33–36.
52. R. Shulz and A. Herz, Dependence liability of enkephalin in the myenteric plexus of the guinea pig. *Eur. J. Pharmacol., 39*: 429–432 (1976).
53. T. F. Burks, Central effects of β-endorphin on intestinal transit. In *Endogenous and Exogenous Opiate Agonists and Antagonists* (E. L. Way, ed.), Pergamon Press, Elmsford, N.Y., 1980, pp. 147–149.
54. D. De Wied, G. L. Kovacs, B. Bohers, J. M. van Ree, and H. M. Greven, Neuroleptic activity of the neuropeptide βLPH 62–77 [Des-Tyr]^1 γ endorphin. *Eur. J. Pharmacol., 49*: 427–436 (1978).
55. A. Goldstein, S. Tachibana, L. T. Lowney, M. Hunkapiller, and L. Hood, Dynorphin-(1–13), an extraordinarily potent opioid peptide. *Proc. Natl. Acad. Sci. U.S.A., 76*: 6666–6670 (1979).

chapter 4

Assay of the Endorphins and Related Analogs

John A. H. Lord, Michael J. Rance, and Colin F. C. Smith

Reckitt and Colman Ltd.
Hull, England

I. INTRODUCTION

The isolation and identification of opioid peptides was made possible only by the development of assays capable of the detection and quantification of such compounds. By the very nature of the problem, bioassay techniques were the only methods available in the early phase of the study of the endorphins, and the problems presented by the use of such techniques have been known for some time. Gaddum (1) in his classic text on pharmacology stated that the qualitative identification of a natural substance depends entirely on the development of quantitative methods of assay. Such quantitative methods are of little use, however, unless something is known of the nature of the substance or substances producing the measured biological effect. This is due to the fact that the measured response, such as inhibition of electrically stimulated contractions of smooth muscle preparations, will not in general be a specific one. In the case of the opioids, the problem was simplified by the availability of very specific antagonists, such as naloxone, and it was this fact that enabled Hughes and his collaborators (2, 3) to use the sensitive mouse vas deferens preparation in a specific manner during the isolation of the enkephalins.

Application of sophisticated chromatographic techniques to the problem soon demonstrated that the enkephalins were only two of a series of peptides having broadly similar agonist effects at opiate receptors. As a consequence, the criterion of naloxone reversibility of a bioassay response ceased to be adequate to define the qualitative identity of endogenous opioid substances. Further methods, such as radioimmunoassay, had to be used in conjunction with chromatographic methods in order to distinguish between closely related compounds.

It is our intention to review the methodology of assay techniques that can be utilized in the study of opioid peptides and to show how the application of a variety of these techniques can yield useful qualitative and quantitative results in the study of opioid peptides. In addition, we hope to demonstrate that by the application of bioassay techniques to the study of peptide analogs of the natural materials, data can be generated which can be used to predict in vivo pharmacological profiles. Such approaches have been used to support and exploit the existence of differing populations of pharmacological receptors for compounds such as adrenergic agonists and antagonists (4) and histamine antagonists (5) with the subsequent development of drugs with selective action at these populations of receptors.

The idea that pharmacologically differentiable populations of opiate receptors might exist was proposed (6) prior to the discovery of the endogenous opioid peptides and has been supported by evidence obtained using bioassay techniques (7). We also attempt, therefore, to review the ways in which the assay systems developed in the study of the endorphins might be applied to the identification of opioid drugs with selective action at differing receptor populations.

II. ISOLATED TISSUE ASSAYS

The use of isolated tissue preparations for the assay and evaluation of the structure-activity relationships of opioid substances was pioneered to Kosterlitz and his collaborators in the 1960s. The two tissues most widely used are the guinea pig ileum as a segment or as the myenteric plexus-longitudinal muscle preparation (9). In the former tissue, narcotic agonists depress the output of the acetylcholine produced by electrical stimulation of the intramural nerves (10), whereas in the latter, it is the output of noradrenaline that is depressed (9). Other isolated tissue preparations that have been reported to contain opiate receptors, and hence are responsive to opioids, are the cat nictitating membrane (11), the rabbit heart (12), and the rabbit ear artery (13).

Studies have concentrated on the guinea pig ileum and mouse vas deferens systems, as these preparations are simple to set up and use, remain stable for long periods (> 6 hr), and produce reproducible results. With certain exceptions, such as codeine, correlations of in vitro agonist potency with in vivo analgesic potency was good for both tissues (14) for a range of drugs with widely differing structures. These systems have been applied to the assay of the endorphins and their analogs with great success and, together with the more recently described rabbit ear artery preparation (13), form the basis for discussion in this chapter.

Prior to a discussion of methodology it is appropriate to define some parameters which can be readily determined in in vitro systems and which can be used to define both narcotic agonist and antagonist character.

Agonist activity is readily defined by the concentration of the test substance required to inhibit by 50% the tissue response (ID_{50}). Antagonist activity can be defined by the equilibrium constant K_e (15), derived from the mass action equation

$$K_e = \frac{a(1 - x)}{x}$$

where a is the molar concentration of the antagonist and x is the fraction of receptors occupied. The parameter x can be determined from the dose ratio (DR), which is the ratio of concentrations of the test agonist required to obtain the same depression of the tissue response in the presence or absence of a given concentration of antagonist:

$$x = \frac{DR - 1}{DR}$$

so that

$$K_e = \frac{a}{DR - 1}$$

When a is the concentration of antagonist required to produce a dose ratio of 2, K_e = a, and hence the negative logarithm of K_e is equivalent to the parameter pA_2 first used by Arunlakshana and Schild (16) to characterize antagonist activity.

The guinea pig ileum, mouse vas deferens, and rabbit ear artery preparations have been used in the author's laboratory to characterize the pharmacological profile of a series of peptide analogs of the enkephalins. The methods described below are modifications of the basic techniques reported by Kosterlitz and his collaborators (8, 9) and by Knoll (13).

A. Guinea Pig Ileum Preparation

Guinea pigs were killed by a blow on the head, the abdomen opened, and the terminal portion of the ileum removed. The 10 cm nearest to the ileo-cecal junction was discarded and the remaining tissued placed in warm (30-36°) oxygenated (95% O_2, 5% CO_2) Krebs solution. The contents were washed from the lumen using Krebs solution. A length of ileum (ca. 3 cm) was set up for electrical transmural stimulation in an organ bath (40 ml) containing warm oxygenated Krebs solution, as shown in Fig. 1. Contractions of the ileum were produced by 0.5 msec square-wave pulses at supramaximal voltage delivered at a rate of 0.1 Hz. The contractions were measured by an isometric transducer connected to a flat-bed recorder. Hexamethonium bromide or mepyramine maleate were not added routinly to the bath fluid, as these agents have rarely been found to be effective in reducing the spontaneous activity that sometimes occurs with this preparation. The bath fluid was automatically changed at a set time period (normally 20 min) by a pair of pericyclic pumps connected to a timer. A manual override allowed the bath fluid to be changed when it was required to break the time cycle.

The agonist activity of test peptides can be determined by the addition of increasing concentrations of the test substance to the bath. Log (dose) response lines can be plotted from the cumulative dose-response traces in the normal way. Con-

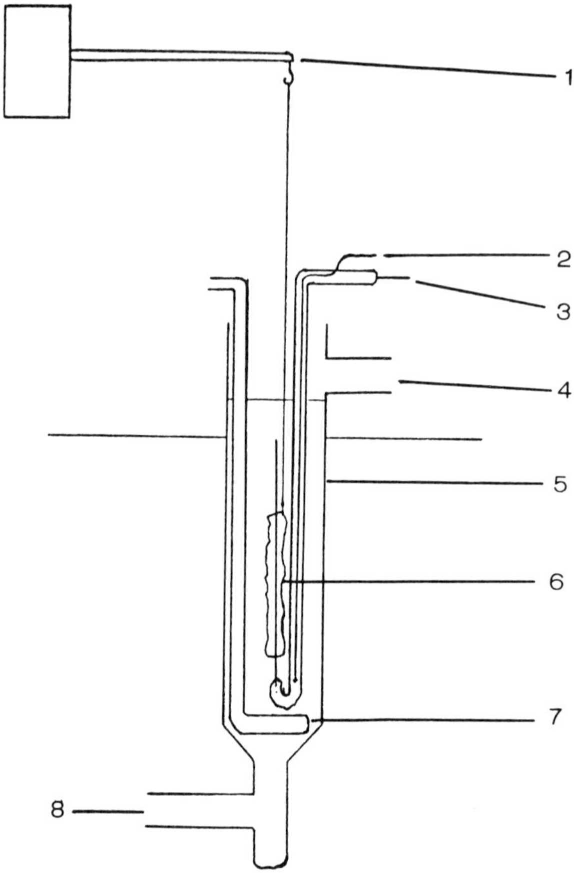

FIGURE 1 Isolated organ bath system used for the guinea pig ileum preparation. 1, Isometric transduer; 2, external platinum electrode; 3, internal platinum electrode; 4, Krebs inlet; 5, glass organ bath (50 ml); 6, ileum; 7, sintered glass oxygenator; 8, Krebs outlet.

struction of cumulative dose-response curves to a standard opioid (Met-enkephalin or normorphine) both before and after the test substance allows relative potency estimations to be made and gives a guide as to the stability and reproductibility of the preparation.

It has been reported (8, 15) that tachyphylaxis to opioids develops rapidly in the ileum preparation, making it difficult to use cumulative dose-response curves as described above. To overcome this problem, Gyang and Kosterlitz (8) showed that reproducible results could be obtained using a single-dose method in which doses of the test agonist (morphine) were added at intervals of 15–20 min to generate

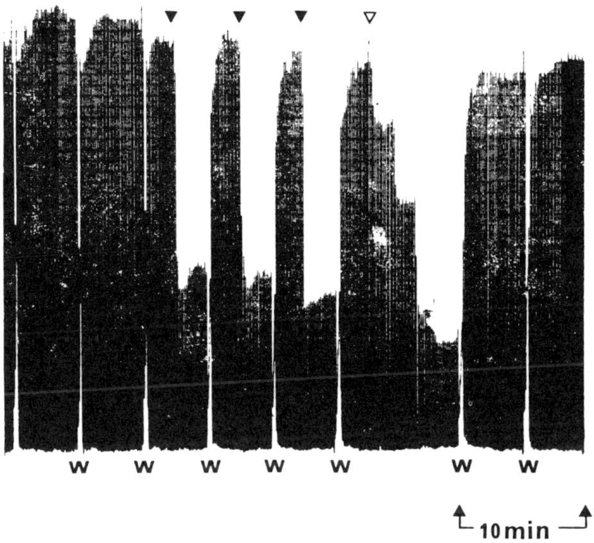

FIGURE 2 Responses of the guinea pig ileum to Met-enkephalin, demonstrating the absence of tachyphylaxis. ▼, Met-enkephalin injected to produce a final concentration of 250 ng/ml; ▽, cumulative dose-response curve to Met-enkephalin—25, 75, 250, 750 ng/ml; W, washout.

dose-response curves. In our hands the onset and offset of action of the enkephalins and their analogs has been rapid, with the result that tachyphylaxis has not been a problem with the ileum preparation (Fig. 2) and results obtained by cumulative-dose methods have been very similar to those obtained in single-dose studies (Table 1). Normorphine has been reported to possess a similar rapid onset and offset of action (17). Antagonist activity of test substances in the ileum preparation is readily demonstrated by the method of Kosterlitz and Watt (15). Both single-

TABLE 1 Comparison of ID_{50} Values for Met-Enkephalin on the Guinea Pig Ileum Determined Using Cumulative- and Single-Dose Response Curves[a]

Preparation number	Single-dose ID_{50} (μmol)	Cumulative-dose ID_{50} (μmol)
1	0.225 ± 0.0093	0.245 ± 0.0078
2	0.081 ± 0.0038	0.0779 ± 0.0078
3	0.111 ± 0.010	0.105 ± 0.0054

[a]Results are means ± S.E. (n = 4).

and multiple-dose methods appear to give similar values for the K_e of naloxone against agonists with rapid onset of action (7).

B. Mouse Vas Deferens Preparation

Choice of the strain of mouse used for this assay appears to be of some importance, as it has recently been demonstrated that normorphine is much less potent on the vasa defentia of C57/BL mice than on those of TO mice, although no significant difference in potency was seen between the strains with the enkephalins (Table 2) (18). For routine assay, male albino TO mice weighing 30 g were killed by a blow on the head, and the vasa deferentia removed. The assay was carried out in one of two ways.

Static Bath Technique The vas deferens was set up in an organ bath (40 ml) containing warm oxygenated modified Krebs solution and stimulated, via two platinum electrodes placed above and below the vas deferens, with 3 msec square-wave pulses at a frequency of 0.1 Hz. The voltage was varied (5-40 V as measured with an oscilloscope across the electrodes) to obtain the optimal balance between twitch height and sensitivity to the test agonist (Met-enkephalin). In some tissues it was found that the use of high voltages, although yielding large contractions, results in decreased sensitivity to the inhibitory effects of opioids. The tissue contractions were measured using an isometric transducer connected to a pen recorder. Measurement of agonist potency of test peptides can be carried out as described above for the guinea pig ileum preparation. A large (40 ml) organ bath is used in place of the smaller (3 ml) bath described by Hughes et al (19), as it has been found (C. F. C. Smith, unpublished observations) that the contractions in many preparations decline rapidly due to the build-up of metabolites in the small organ bath. In the larger volume of buffer the tissue response remains stable for periods greater than 20 min without change of the Krebs solution.

TABLE 2 Relative Agonist Potencies of Opioid Peptides in Vasa Deferentia of TO and C57/BL Mice

	Relative potency[a]	
Agonist	TO	C57/BL
Met-enkephalin	1	1
Leu-enkephalin	1.48 ± 0.13 (7)	1.51 ± 0.25 (4)
β-Endorphin	0.32 ± 0.05 (4)	0.17 ± 0.02 (3)
Normorphine	0.072 ± 0.009 (27)	0.0083 ± 0.0012 (17)

[a]IC_{50} values of internal standard, Met-enkephalin, were 19.0 ± 1.7 nM (27) in TO mice, 13.2 ± 1.4 nM (17) in C57/BL mice. Results are means ± S.E.; the number of determinations is shown in parentheses.

Source: Data from Ref. 18.

Perfusion Technique For perfusion studies the vas deferens was set up in a small (4 ml) organ bath through which warm oxygenated Krebs solution was constantly perfused at a rate of 3 ml/min using a small peripump. This system enables a stable preparation to be maintained for several hours. Test compounds were introduced by bolus injection into the buffer flowing through a side arm at the bottom of the bath (Fig. 3). Owing to the constant flow of buffer solution through the bath, the exact concentration of test compound at any time was not known, but as it was possible to compare each test compound with a standard (Met-enkephalin) in the same tissue, relative agonist potency estimates can be made on the basis of equiactive weights of test substance and standard. Culmulative dose-response curves can be obtained by sequential bolus injection of increasing amounts of test compound which can be removed rapidly from the bath by means of a second peripump, which delivers buffer at 20 ml/min, operating in parallel with the first pump.

The perfusion system relies largely on the fact that opioid peptides have a rapid onset of action in this in vitro system; a compound with a slow onset of action

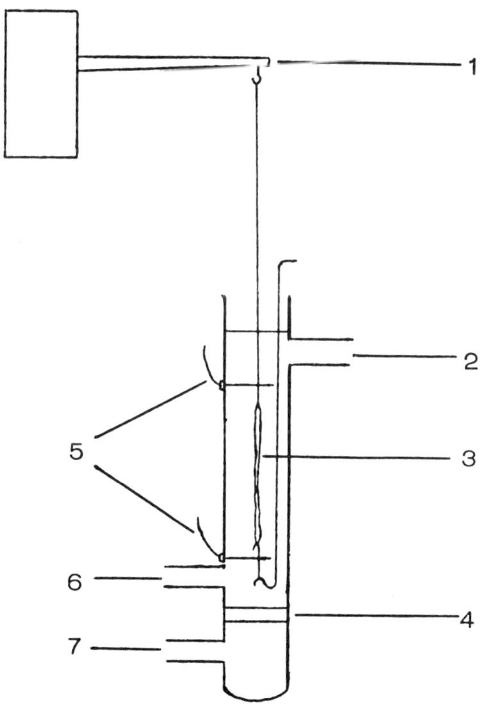

FIGURE 3 Isolated organ bath system used for the mouse vas deferens preparation. 1, Isometric transduer; 2, Krebs outlet; 3, vas deferens; 4, sintered glass disk; 5, platinum electrodes; 6, Krebs inlet; 7, O_2/CO_2 inlet.

would be washed from the bath before maximum effect was reached, with the result that its potency would be underestimated. Table 3 shows relative potency estimates made by static and perfusion techniques for a series of enkephalin-related peptides. It is clear that results from the perfusion system are in agreement with those obtained using the more standard technique, and hence the former method represents a powerful system for the primary screening of opioid peptide analogs.

Antagonist potency can also be assessed using the mouse vas deferens. It has been reported that the dose-response curves obtained in the mouse vas deferens to compounds with dual agonist-antagonist properties are much shallower than those obtained in the guinea pig ileum (14). This factor enables higher concentrations of partial agonists to be used in the vas deferens preparation without complete suppression of the twitch response. Thus assessment of the antagonist potency of compounds with relatively high intrinsic activity (such as cyclorphan) can be made. It is interesting to note that the enkephalin analog Tyr^1-N-cyclopropylmethyl, D-Ala^2-Met^5 enkephalin showed no antagonist activity in this sensitive assay despite reports that the related Tyr^1-N-allyl derivative possessed in vivo antagonist properties as determined by behavioral and binding assay methods (20).

C. Rabbit Ear Artery Preparation

The rabbit ear artery preparation described by Knoll (13) is of considerable interest, as the opiate receptors in this tissue appear to differ significantly from guinea pig ileum receptors in their structural requirements for activity; enkephalin and etorphine are agonists in this assay, but the tissue is unaffected by morphine and normorphine. The assay system described below is a modification of the method reported by Knoll (13).

New Zealand white rabbits (approx. 2.5 kg) were killed with pentobarbitone (intravenously), and then the central portion of the ear artery was removed and stripped of connective tissue, cannulated, and mounted in a small organ bath. Warm (30°C)

TABLE 3 Relative Potencies of Several Peptides Determined by the Static and Perfused Assay Methods on the Mouse Vas Deferens[a]

	Potency (Met-enkephalin = 1)	
Compound	Perfusion method	Static method
Leu-enkephalin	1.85 ± 0.2	1.86 ± 0.3
D-Ala^2-Met-enkephalin	4.25 ± 0.6	4.05 ± 0.9
Tyr-D-Ala-Gly-Phe-Pro-NH_2	0.12 ± 0.02	0.15 ± 0.07
Tyr-D-Ala-Gly-Me-Phe-Met-(O)-ol	0.36 ± 0.11	0.33 ± 0.13

[a]Results are means ± S.E. (n = 3).

oxygenated Krebs solution was perfused through the artery at a rate of 3 ml/min. The tissue was stimulated via platinum electrodes with trains of two to five square-wave pulses (1 msec in duration) delivered every minute at a frequency of 5 Hz. The vasoconstriction elicted in this way resulted in an increase in pressure which was measured and recorded. As continuous infusion of test peptides resulted in the rapid development of tachyphylaxis, making the construction of dose-response curves difficult, a bolus injection technique was used routinely. Test compounds were injected into the organ bath 30 sec after the previous stimulus response. The compound was in contact with the tissue for a short period, thus avoiding tachyphylaxis. Maximum depression of response occurred 1-2 min after injection of the compound and was followed by a rapid washout of drug effect. Dose-response curves are readily obtained using this method and relative potency values with respect to a standard agent (Met-enkephalin) can be calculated. A typical record is shown in Fig. 4, which demonstrates the lack of activity of normorphine on this tissue.

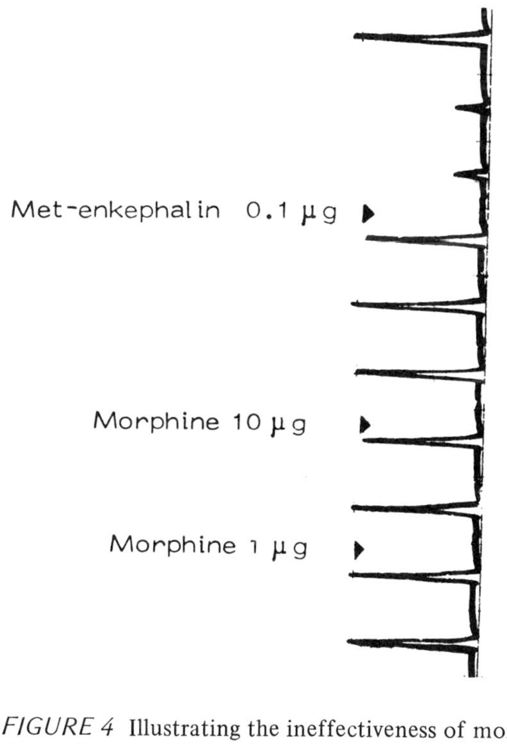

FIGURE 4 Illustrating the ineffectiveness of morphine in depressing the contractions of the rabbit ear artery. Experimental details as described in the text.

III. BINDING ASSAYS

Attempts to identify stereospecific binding sites for opiates were initiated by Goldstein and his collaborators (21, 22). These early studies, using a relatively low specific radioactivity ligand [^{14}C] levorphanol, were largely thwarted by high levels of nonspecific binding. Rapid progress was made following the introduction of techniques pioneered by Pert and Snyder (23, 24), Terenius (25), and Simon et al. (26). Stereospecific, saturable binding of opiates in rat brain was successfully demonstrated by the use of tritium-labeled ligands of high specific activity and high receptor affinity. Since that time many tritiated alkaloid-derived opioids have been utilized as ligands in receptor binding studies, including naloxone (23, 24), etorphine (26), dihydromorphine (25), oxymorphone, levorphanol, nalorphine, levallorphan (27), naltrexone (28), and buprenorphine (29).

Following the discovery of the endogenous opioid peptides, stereospecific opiate receptor binding has been used both as an assay system for the quantitative determination of the opioid peptides and as a means of investigating the complexity of the opioid peptides/opiate receptor system. The relative instability of the smaller peptides in biological systems has, however, required certain adaptions of technique routinely applied to alkaloid-derived ligands.

Most binding studies have been carried out with homogenate preparations from rat brain (23, 24), mouse brain (21, 30, 31), and guinea pig brain (32). Opiate receptor binding has also been detected in homogenate preparations of monkey and human brain (33) and in brains from a wide range of vertebrates (34) as well as in guinea pig ileum (35). Relatively few studies have been performed with mince preparations of guinea pig brain (35) and brain slices (36). Binding to neuroblastoma x glioma cells (37) and cerebrosides (38) has also been demonstrated.

A. Preparation of Brain Homogenates

In routine studies with rodent brain the animal is decapitated and the brain rapidly removed. The cerebellum may be discarded and the remainder homogenized in approximately 100 volumes of ice-cold Tris buffer (0.05 M; pH 7.4 at 25°C). After centrifugation at 18,000g for 20 min at 0°C, the supernatant is discarded and the pellet reconstituted to obtain a standard washed homogenate preparation (39). In other studies, a twice-washed preparation has been used with resuspension in fresh buffer solution of the pellets obtained from two centrifugations at 49,000g (32).

Because of the temperature dependence of Tris buffer (an 0.05 M solution has pH values of 9.5, 8.9, and 8.6 at 5, 25, and 37°C, respectively) the pH must be corrected at room temperature for the temperature conditions of the binding assay. Opiate binding shows a pH optimum of 7.4 (23), the binding sharply declining at more alkaline and acid pH values. Alternative buffer systems have been employed in some studies. In their work on the influence of temperature on opiate receptor binding of agonists and antagonists, Creese et al. (40) used ammonium phosphate buffer, and Terenius has adopted a HEPES buffer routinely (41).

B. The Binding Assay

Opiate receptor binding assays are carried out by incubation of a low concentration (often 1 nM) of high-specific-radioactivity tritiated ligand with the membrane preparation from brain in the presence or absence of a competing opioid species. The methodology of this basically simple experiment and the ways by which stereospecifically bound and nonreceptor bound material can be separated have been the subject of intense study, as results appear to be very sensitive to changes in technique.

It is essential that the stereospecific and saturable binding characteristics of the labeled ligand be established under equilibrium conditions prior to commencement of competitive binding studies. Binding of [^{3}H] naloxone and [^{3}H] dihydromorphine approaches equilibrium in brain homogenates in 5 min at 37°C, in 10 min at 25°C, and in 120 min at 0°C (42). [^{3}H] Leu-enkephalin appears to equilibrate with receptors at a similar rate to naloxone at 0°C (H. W. Kosterlitz and J. A. H. Lord, unpublished observations).

Incubations may be terminated by filtration of the contents under vacuum through glass fiber filters (Whatman GF-B). The filters are then washed with 2–4 volumes (5 ml) of cold buffer to remove readily eluted radioactivity. Considerable attention needs to be devoted to the conditions of incubation and filtration since these procedures can have marked effects on the characteristics of the measured opiate receptor binding (40). Incubations may also be terminated by centrifugation (41, 43, 44). Material retained by filters or obtained as pellets following centrifugation may be digested by suitable solublizers within liquid scintillation counting vials. Problems with chemiluminescence sometimes occur and can be overcome by heating or acidification with glacial acetic acid in toluene (1:3). Addition of appropriate scintillant allows the bound radioactivity to be determined by liquid scintillation counting techniques.

Specific binding is calculated routinely from the difference between the binding determined in the absence and presence of an excess of D(–) opiate [e.g., levorphanol, levallorphan, or (–)2-(3-furyl-methyl)-5, 9-dimethyl-2′-hydroxy-6, 7-benzomorphan (Mr 2266; Boehringer)]. Stereospecificity may be checked by the ineffectiveness of the pharmacologically inert enantiomer to reduce total binding at concentrations that would be saturating for the D(–) isomer. The use of a fixed concentration of 0.1 μM levorphanol (23) in determining nonspecific binding has been criticized (45) since it was found that higher concentrations of levorphanol were often necessary to suppress the stereospecific binding completely. In more recent studies, concentrations of at least 1 μM levallorphan have been used to suppress stereospecific binding (35, 46). As an alternative it has been suggested that the stereospecific binding of, for instance, [^{3}H] dihydromorphine should be determined in the presence and absence of excess unlabeled dihydromorphine (45).

Preliminary incubation of a homogenate at 37°C has been shown to enhance the stereospecific binding of both [^{3}H] naloxone and [^{3}H] dihydromorphine (40). This has been confirmed for the binding of [^{3}H] naltrexone and [^{3}H] Leu-enkephalin (H. W. Kosterlitz and J. A. H. Lord, unpublished observations), and it has been suggested that this enhancement may be due to removal of endogenous enkephalin (47). Thus preincubation of homogenate preparations at 37°C is a useful means of increasing the amount of stereospecific binding of labeled compounds. It has been found, however, that preincubation reduces the enhancement by sodium of [^{3}H] naloxone binding (40).

C. Effect of Temperature

In competitive binding assay experiments, incubations are normally continued until equilibrium has been reached and assays are frequently performed for 15 min at 37°C, 30 min at 25°C, and 120-150 min at 0°C. It has been reported that for incubations carried out at 0°C, sodium increases [^{3}H] naloxone binding by an increase in affinity without a change in the number of binding sites, in contrast to findings at higher temperatures (42). This observation might indicate a change in the membrane characteristics at 0°C and suggests caution in the interpretation of results from experiments at this temperature.

The influence of Met- and Leu-enkephalin on [^{3}H] opiate receptor binding at different temperatures has been studied by Simantov and Snyder (42) using [^{3}H] naloxone and [^{3}H] dihydromorphine. They found that the enkephalins were degraded by 65-85% at 25 and 37°C with incubation times greater than 10 min; this degradation has been ascribed to the action of hydrolyzing enzymes in brain tissue (48, 49). Degradation may be minimized by carrying out incubations at 0°C, in which case equilibrium of the labeled opiate of enkephalin with their binding sites is reached in approximately 2 hr (32, 42). Binding experiments with enkephalins have been carried out at 25 and 37°C in the presence of the enzyme inhibitor bacitracin (42). At a concentration of 50 μg/ml, bacitracin was reported to provide protection at 25°C for 60 min, but at 37°C Met-enkephalin was substantially degraded. It has been observed, however, that bacitracin at concentrations high enough to provide protection from peptidase enzymes causes some inhibition of receptor binding (H. W. Kosterlitz and J. A. H. Lord, unpublished observations).

Simantov and Snyder (50) have recently reported that the rates of association and dissociation of [^{3}H] Met-enkephalin with and from the opiate receptor are slow and show marked temperature dependence, observations consisitent with a requirement for conformation changes during the binding process.

The observations outlined above suggest that neither the use of protease inhibitors (e.g., bacitracin) nor the use of low temperatures offer the ideal answer to the study of the opiate receptor binding of labile peptides.

β-Endorphin does not appear to undergo proteolytic cleavage in the incubation medium, and the inhibition of [^{3}H] dihydromorphine binding by the peptide at 37°C remained constant for 2 hr (51, 52).

D. Effect of Ions

The effect of sodium on the stereospecific binding of alkaloid-derived opiate agonists and antagonists has been suggested as a means of determining the agonist-antagonist character of opioid species (27), as the binding of antagonists is relatively unaffected or slightly enhanced by inclusion of sodium (100 mM) in the incubation medium, whereas the affinity of agonists is greatly reduced. Compounds with mixed agonist-antagonist properties demonstrate intermediate sodium shifts.

Both Leu- and Met-enkephalin show reduced potency in competing for [^{3}H] naloxone binding in the presence of sodium (100 μM), suggesting that the peptides have agonist properties (7, 42). Biphasic Scatchard plots have been obtained for [^{3}H] Leu-enkephalin and there is a loss of the high-affinity site in the presence of 100 μM sodium (7). Manganese, previously demonstrated to enhance the binding of alkaloid-derived agonists at 25°C but not at 0°C, also enhances the inhibition by Met- and Leu-enkephalin of [^{3}H] naloxone at the higher temperature, with lesser effects elicited by magnesium and calcium; magnesium but not calcium also enhances the potencies of the enkephalins in competing for [^{3}H] dihydromorphine (42). Potassium, cesium, and rubidium have negligible effects. The sodium sensitivity of the displacement of [^{3}H] naloxone by several opioid peptides has been studied by Pert et al. (20). They found that β-endorphin, Met-enkephalin, and D-Ala^2-Met^5-enkephalinamide exhibited large sodium shifts which were characteristic of agonists. However, Tyr^1-N-allyl D-Ala^2-Met^5-enkephalin had a sodium shift of 2.5, which would indicate the presence of antagonist properties, although these could not be confirmed in the mouse vas deferens assay with this compound or with the related Tyr^1-N-cyclopropylmethyl derivative (C. F. C. Smith, unpublished results). A sodium shift of 1.3 has been reported for β-endorphin (43, 53), which would suggest an antagonist character, but this has again not been shown in isolated tissue studies (54, 55).

It appears, therefore, that, although the sodium shift technique is reasonably predictive of agonist-antagonist character with the alkaloid opiates, the same is not true of the opioid peptides. Substitution of the tyrosine nitrogen with classical antagonist functions, such as allyl or cyclopropylmethyl, does not appear to produce compounds with true antagonist character.

E. Use of Different Ligands

The labeled ligands that have been most frequently used for binding studies are the agonist [^{3}H] dihydromorphine and the antagonist [^{3}H] naloxone. Scatchard analysis has revealed that both these compounds show high- and low-affinity binding sites. Naloxone and dihydromorphine have mutual displacement abilities, but there is a component of naloxone binding which cannot be easily displaced by dihydromorphine (56). In general, agonists have a higher affinity for sites occupied by dihydromorphine than for those occupied by naloxone, and thus agonists are less effective in inhibiting antagonist binding. This difference has been exploited by Terenius and Wahlström (41) with the introduction of a parallel technique using two identical solutions containing both an agonist and antagonist ligand, one of which is labeled in each case. The differential binding of agonists and antagonists enables a determination of agonist-antagonist character to be made and results have been compared with the sodium shift technique (41).

TABLE 4 Inhibition (IC_{50}, nM) of Binding of [^{3}H]Opiates by Lipotropin Fragments in Brain Homogenates

β-LPH residue numbers	[^{3}H] naloxone[a]	[^{3}H] naltrexone[b]	[^{3}H] dihydromorphine[a]	[^{3}H] Leu-enkephalin[b]
1-91 (β-LPH)	1000	–	1000	–
61-91 (β-endorphin)	2.6	2.8	2.2	1.51
61-89	5	–	2.2	–
61-87	100	24.3	42	17.8
61-79	–	62.9	57.6	37.2
61-77	–	165	140	56.7
61-76 (α-endorphin)	–	71.8	88.2	16.8
61-69	60	–	21	–
61-68	160	–	45	–
61-65 (Met-Enk)	90	10.2	8	1.19
61-64	1000	–	300	–
Morphine	25	27.2	4.1	227
Naloxone	1.8	2.26	2.4	50.9

[a]Binding assays with homogenate preparation from whole rat brain minus cerebellum. Samples are incubated for 15 min at 30° in 50 mM Tris buffer (pH 7.4) and incubated with 1.0 nM [^{3}H] naloxone or 0.35 nM [^{3}H] dihydromorphine for 15 min at 30°C. Incubations terminated by centriguation and the bound radioactivity in the pellets counted by liquid scintillation techniques. Data from Ref. 43.

[b]Binding assays with homogenate preparation from whole guinea pig brain minus cerebellum. Samples incubated for 150 min at 0°C in 50 nM Tris buffer (pH 7.4) with 0.4 nM [^{3}H] naltrexone or 0.86 nM [^{3}H] Leu-enkephalin. Incubations terminated by filtration and the bound radioactivity assayed by liquid scintillation techniques. (H. W. Kosterlitz et al., reported to the Committee on Problems of Drug Dependence, 1977.)

More recently, Squires and Braestrup (57) have characterized two distinct binding sites for naloxone in rat brain, only one of which appears to interact with the potent oripavine derivatives etorphine and diprenorphine. The same authors also found differences in the regional distribution of these sites.

The evidence cited above indicates that, perhaps not surprisingly, the population of receptors with which opiates interact in brain is heterogeneous. The most dramatic differences have been seen with the use of labeled peptides as ligands; morphine appears to have a low affinity for [^{3}H] Leu-enkephalin binding sites (7). The physiological and pharmacological significance of opiate receptor heterogeneity is discussed in Sec. VI, but in methodological terms the result is that the sensitivity of assays for opiates differs significantly depending on the nature of the radioligand. Some results obtained for fragments of β-lipotropin (β-LPH) are shown in Table 4 to illustrate this point.

IV. RADIOIMMUNOASSAY

The technique of radioimmunoassay (RIA) was first applied to insulin in 1958 (58) and since that time immunoassay techniques have become major tools of the research scientist and clinical biochemist for the quantitation of drugs, neurotransmitters, hormones, and proteins in biological samples. It was not surprising, therefore, that following the discovery of the endorphins, many groups of workers have used immunoassay techniques for the quantification of these peptides. Antisera to the opioid peptides have in fact been utilized in two principal ways. Much work has been carried out using immunohistological techniques, but as these studies are reviewed elsewhere in this volume, discussion here is limited to the application of antisera to the direct RIA of the peptides.

In principle, radioimmunoassay is a competitive binding technique very similar to the opiate receptor based systems described in Sec. III. The basis of such assay systems can be readily understood from the following set of reactions:

$$\underset{\text{Labeled Ligand}}{L^*} + \underset{\text{Antibody}}{A} \rightleftharpoons \underset{\text{Labeled Complex}}{L^*-A}$$

$$+$$

$$\underset{\text{Unlabeled Ligand}}{L} \rightleftharpoons \underset{\text{Unlabeled Complex}}{L-A}$$

The binding of a radiolabeled ligand is competitively inhibited by the addition of the unlabeled ligand, and the degree of displacement of bound labeled ligand produced by an unknown concentration of unlabeled material can be compared to standards and used as a measure of the unknown concentration. The general principles of RIA have been extensively reviewed notably by Yalow and Berson (59), the originators of the technique, who describe in detail factors affecting the sensitivity and selectivity of the assay technique.

The difference between receptor binding studies and RIA lies in the nature of the binding species, and this difference is of the greatest importance in determining the specificity of assay systems. A problem with receptor binding studies is that all opioid peptides have an affinity for the receptor population and cannot be readily distinguished by this technique. The binding proteins in RIA are immunoglobulins generated with some degree of specificity against individual peptides, which provides the possibility of greater assay specificity.

Immunoassay techniques were first applied to large peptides and proteins that had antigenic properties in their own right. Smaller molecules did not have inherent antigenic properties, but it was discovered that if such small molecules (or *haptens*) were covalently bound to large carrier proteins, antisera with specific capacity to bind the haptens were generated. This system has been generally adopted for the RIA of small molecules, including alkaloid-derived opioid drugs (60) and, in fact, has certain advantages over the direct technique. Haptens can be coupled directly with the carrier protein using standard reagents. Alternatively, small bifunctional linking molecules or spacer groups (e.g., succinic acid) can be employed. The coupling of a hapten to a carrier protein, via a spacer group, has two advantages. First, the spacer group appears to make the hapten more sterically available for antigen formation, with the result that better quality antisera are obtained. Second, by appropriate use of spacer groups it is possible to control the area of the hapten that is responsible for the antigenic response; C-terminal specific antisera would be expected from an N-terminally coupled hapten. Many different methods of antigen preparation have been applied to the endorphins, and these are summarized in Table 5.

Several techniques also exist for the separation of protein-bound radiolabeled tracer from the free material displaced by the addition of unlabeled ligand, and again a variety of these methods have been applied to the RIA of the endorphins.

It can also be seen from Table 5 that the antisera obtained to date vary considerably in their specificity, although many assays have been reported only in a preliminary manner and information concerning specificity is not always complete. In a situation as complex as that with the β-LPH fractions, rigorous determination of cross-reactivity with related peptides is essential before in-depth interpretation of results is possible. The relationships between measured immunoreactivity and absolute levels of a particular peptide are difficult to define in such a situation, and problems of this kind are well illustrated by the work that has been reported concerning the gastrin-related peptides (69) and the parathyroid hormones (70).

Of the several assays reported to date for the enkephalins (61–65), none has succeeded in reducing cross-reactivity of the two pentapeptides to an insignificant level, although the antisera generated by Wesche et al. (64) showed $<1\%$ cross-reactivity. Similar specificity has been reported (66) for an antiserum generated at Burroughs Wellcome by Miller, which has been used both for RIA and immunofluorescence studies (71).

In a series as complex as the endorphins, the availability of pure peptides for use as analytical standards is a major problem. Synthesis of the short-chain analogs by solution methods is relatively straightforward, but the synthesis of the longer peptides (e.g., β-endorphin), even using solid-phase synthetic techniques, respresents a major task. Isolation of the natural materials is also complex and the problems of absolute purification and identification are daunting. It is perhaps not surprising, therefore, that the most complete RIA studies reported to date have come from laboratories with in-depth peptide synthesis and purification experience.

The specificity of β-endorphin antiserum, RB 100–10/27, reported by Guilleman and coworkers, has been throughly investigated (67). The results illustrate well the problems associated with the use of RIA in the assay of the endorphins and related compounds. It was concluded in these studies that the antiserum recognized an area of the β-endorphin molecule (Asn^{20}-His^{27}) near the C-terminus of the peptides and hence it does not bind the shortest peptides, the enkephalins, α- and γ-endorphin. The antiserum did, however, recognize both β-LPH itself and the proposed common β-LPH, ACTH precursor protein (31,000-dalton precursor) recently isolated by Mains et al. (72). It appears that the β-LPH terminal region is exposed in both these larger molecules and is hence available to interact with the antibody. It is apparent, therefore, that until further antisera become available toward the larger molecules with different sites of recognition, absolute quantification and identification of endorphin immunoreactivity will depend largely on concurrent use of RIA and chromatographic separation techniques.

V. NEUROBLASTOMA X GLIOMA HYBRID CELLS

Morphine and other alkaloid-related opiates have been shown to inhibit adenylate cyclase activity in homogenates of neuroblastoma x glioma cells (73, 74) and to inhibit cAMP accumulation in intact cells (75) by opiate receptor-mediated mechanisms. Endorphins have been shown to have similar effects to morphine in both intact cells and homogenates (76–81). The effect of the enkephalins on both basal and PGE_1- stimulated adenylate cyclase activity in the homogenate system is illustrated in Fig. 5. The concentration of opioids required to inhibit adenylate cyclase in this system are very similar to those required in opiate receptor binding studies (74), and measurement of this postreceptor effect represents an effective means of bioassay of opioid agonists. The utility of such a system for routine bioassay is limited by the relative complexity of technique required, but the hybrid cell system does offer some advantages over brain homogenates for both binding studies (73) and adenylate cyclase/cAMP assay, in that problems of enzymatic degradation of the shorter peptides do not appear to be as acute in the cell culture system (79, 81, 82).

TABLE 5 Antisera Raised against the Endorphins Used for Radioimmunoassay

Antigen	Species	Tracer; separation technique	Specificity for β-LPH of: Leu-Enk	1–91	61–65	61–76	61–77	61–87	61–91	Sensitivity (pmol)	Ref.
Met-Enk/BSA	Guinea pig	[I^{125}] Met-Enk; Millipore	10	–	100	–	–	–	–	5–10	61
Leu-Enk/BSA	Guinea pig	[I^{125}] Leu-Enk; Millipore	100	–	10	–	–	–	–	5–10	61
Succinyl Met-Enk/ succinyl hemocyanin polylysine	Rabbit	[^3H] Met-Enk; dextran-charcoal	10	–	100	0	–	–	0	5	62
Leu-Enk/hemocyanin	Rabbit	[^3H] Leu-Enk; dextran-charcoal	100	–	10	0	–	–	0	1–2	62
Leu-Enk/BSA	Rabbit	[^3H] Leu-Enk; $(NH_4)_2SO_4$	100	–	20	–	–	–	–	0.1	63
Met-Enk/TBG	Rabbit	[^3H] Met-Enk; Millipore	0.3	–	100	0	–	–	0	0.2	64

Leu-Enk/TBG	Rabbit	[^{3}H] Leu-Enk; Millipore	100	–	<1	0	–	–	0	0.05	64
Leu-Enk/bis-diazotized benzidine/BSA	Rabbit	[I^{125}] Leu-Enk; double antibody	100	–	3.3	0	–	–	0	0.01	65
Met-Enk/BSA	Rabbit	[I^{125}] Leu-Enk; polyethylene glycol	<1	0	100	–	–	–	<1	0.01	66
Leu-Enk/BSA	Rabbit	[I^{125}] Leu-Enk; polyethylene gylcol	100	0	<1	–	–	–	<1	0.01	66
β-LPH$_{61\text{-}76}$/TBG	Rabbit	[I^{125}] β-LPH$_{61\text{-}76}$; double antibody	–	0.08[a]	0	100	–	0.1	0.05[a]	50 pg	67
β-LPH$_{61\text{-}91}$[a]/BSA	Rabbit	[I^{125}] β-LPH$_{61\text{-}91}$; double antibody	0	100[a]	0	0	–	100[a]	100[b]	50 pg	67
β-LPH$_{1\text{-}91}$[c]	Rabbit	[I^{125}] β-LPH$_{61\text{-}91}$; dextran-charcoal	0.1	71.4[d]	–	0.1	–	9.8[d]	100[d]	0.02	68

[a] Ovine.
[b] Ovine and porcine; 31,000-dalton precursor also cross-reacts.
[c] Human.
[d] Porcine.

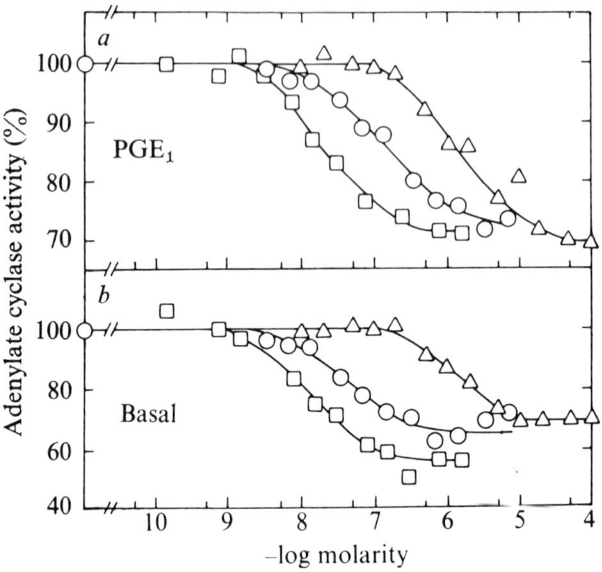

FIGURE 5 Basal and PGE_1-stimulated adenylate cyclase activity of neuroblastoma x glioma hybrid cell homogenates as a function of concentration of Met-enkephalin (□), Leu-enkephalin (○), and morphine (△). (From Ref. 79.)

VI. OPIATE RECEPTOR MULTIPLICITY

Receptor multiplicity is an established fact in many neurotransmitter systems. In the cholinergic system, nicotinic and muscarinic sites are readily distinguished. In the adrenergic system α_1-, α_2-, β_1-, and β_2-receptors can be recognized by specific anatgonists, and these discoveries have been exploited with the development of pharmacological agents such as the cardioselective β-blockers. Histamine receptors can similarly be separated into discrete populations, and recent work has lead to the development of specific H_2-antagonists as antiulcer agents (5).

The existence of pharmacologically differentiable populations of opiate receptors was first postulated by Martin (6) in 1967 based on biphasic dose-response curves obtained by Houde and Wallenstein with morphine-nalorphine mixtures in humans (83). Recently, Martin has extended this concept using the chronic spinal dog model and has postulated the existence of three distinct receptor populations producing different pharmacological syndromes (84). These receptors have been called μ, for which morphine is the prototype agonist; κ (ketocyclazocine); and σ (N-allylnormetazocine). Specific antagonists for these receptor populations do not exist, although apparent difference in in vivo pA_2 values for naloxone have been found for the μ and κ agents, morphine and pentazocine, respectively (85).

The relationship between these pharmacologically defined populations of receptors and the opioid peptide-opiate receptor system is not clear, but it is apparent that investigation of the probable heterogeneity of the opioid receptor population could lead to the development of drugs with more selective opioid action.

In the absence of specific antagonists for different receptor populations, evidence for heterogeneity of receptors can be obtained by simultaneous assay of agonists in several different assay systems (86). Variation in the rank order of potency of agonists in different bioassays suggests that receptor populations in the assay systems are not identical.

Initial studies with alkaloid-derived materials using the mouse vas deferens and guinea pig ileum preparations gave no indication of receptor heterogeneity in these systems (14). The first support for Martin's hypotheses at a receptor level was obtained during an assessment of the activities in vitro of a series of benzomorphans (87). These compounds had been shown not to substitute for morphine in the dependent monkey and included the prototype κ-agonist, ketocyclazocine. It was found that these agents were consistently less potent in the mouse vas deferens than in the guinea pig ileum when related to normorphine as a reference standard (Fig. 6). In addition, the pA_2 values for naloxone against the benzomorphans (7.9–8.05) were lower than those obtained for the more classical analgesic structures, such as morphine (8.5–8.7). These findings suggested that the guinea pig ileum contained a heterogeneous population of receptors and it was later proposed that the receptors recognized by morphine and ketocyclazocine in this tissue might be the μ and κ types suggested by Martin et al. (84).

The existence of two separate receptor systems, with closely related structural requirements, in the same tissue and performing the same function (i.e., inhibition of noradrenaline or acetylcholine release) is novel. In other cases where similar receptor systems have been found to exist (e.g., in the adrenergic system), these receptors perform opposing functions when found in the same tissue. As stated above, the evidence against a single receptor system in both mouse vas deferens and guinea pig ileum is largely based on the differing pA_2 values obtained for naloxone against the two groups of agonists. A recent report (88) has demonstrated a wide range of pA_2 values for naltrexone against a series of peptide agonists in the mouse vas deferens and, in the light of such findings, it is clear that relatively small differences in pA_2 values must be interpreted with some caution. Concrete evidence for κ-type receptors in the in vitro tissues will not be obtained until more specific antagonists at these putative sites are obtained.

The development of opiate receptor binding techniques and the availability of a range of different tritiated ligands of high specific activity has increased the number of bioassay systems available for the evaluation of opioid peptides, and these techniques have been applied in a parallel fashion, together with isolated tissue assays, to evaluate receptor heterogeneity with respect to the endorphins (7, 89).

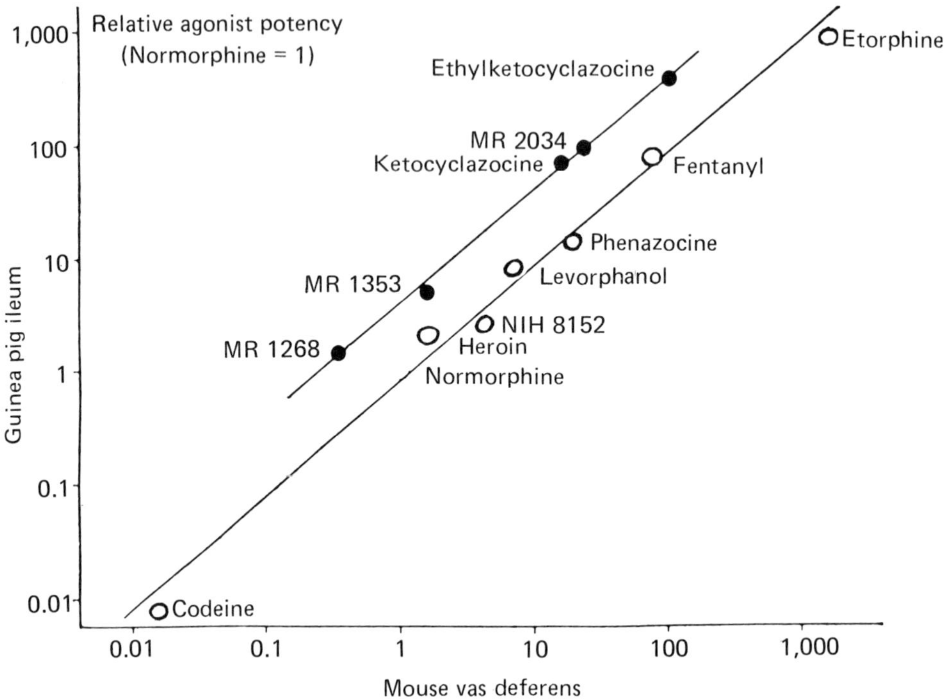

FIGURE 6 Relative agonist activities of various narcotic analgesic agonists in the mouse vas deferens and guinea pig ileum (normorphine = 1). The compounds fitting the regression line on the right substitute and those fitting the line of the left do not substitute for morphine in the morphine-dependent monkey. Mr 2034, (–)-α-(1R, 5R, 9R)-5, 9-dimethyl-2-(L-tetrahydrofurfuryl)-2′-hydroxy-6, 7-benzomorphan; Mr 1353, (±)-α-5, 9-dimethyl-2-(3-methylfurfuryl)-2′-hydroxy-6, 7-benzomorphan; Mr 1268, (±)-α-5, 9-dimethyl-2-(2-methylfuryl)-2′-hydroxy-6, 7-benzomorphan; NIH 8152, (±)-β-2, 9-dimethyl-5-n-propyl-2′-hydroxy-6, 7-benzomorphan. (From Ref. 7).

Results obtained in the guinea pig ileum and mouse vas deferens assays and in receptor binding studies using [^{3}H] Leu-enkephalin and [^{3}H] naloxone as ligands are summarized in Fig. 7. It can be seen that β-endorphin is equipotent on the two tissue preparations, whereas the shorter peptides, α-endorphin, Met- and Leu-enkephalin, are relatively more potent on the mouse vas deferens preparation. Morphine, by comparison, is more potent in the guinea pig ileum. The relationship between these results and the relative abilities of the peptides to compete for naloxone or Leu-enkephalin binding is striking. β-Endorphin is equipotent at displacing both ligands, and the shorter peptides are relatively more potent at displacing Leu-enkephalin; however, morphine is a very poor inhibitor of Leu-enkephalin binding. It is clear, therefore, that mouse vas deferens activity correlates well with Leu-enkephalin

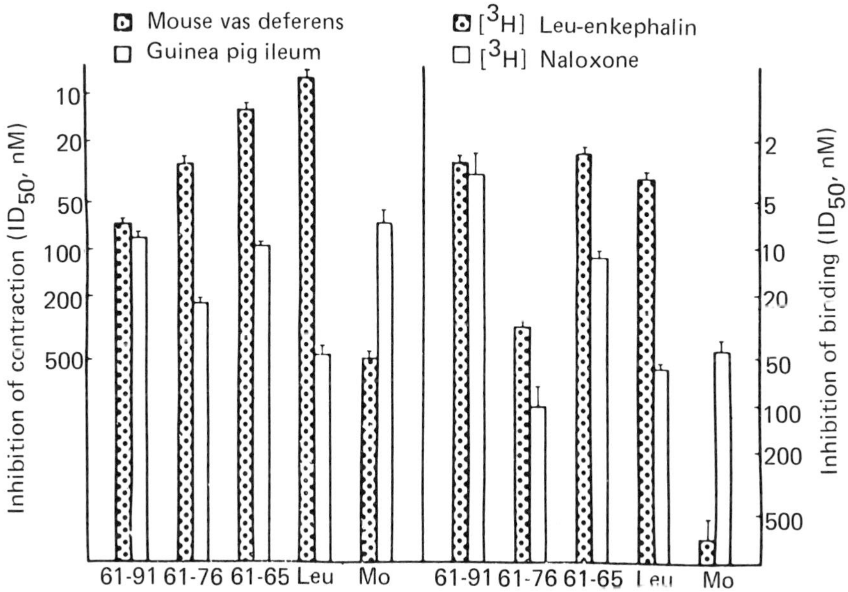

FIGURE 7 Agonist activities of various compounds in the mouse vas deferens and guinea pig ileum and their potencies to inhibit [^{3}H] Leu-enkephalin and [^{3}H] naloxone binding in homogenates of guinea pig brain (pH 7.4 at 0°C, no Na^+, 150 min). The numbers on the abscissa indicate the amino acid sequence of β-lipotropin; Leu, Leu-enkephalin; Mo, morphine. All peptides are synthetic (61–91, Ovine β-endorphin; 61–76, porcine α-endorphin; 61–65, Met-enkephalin and Leu-enkephalin (From Ref. 7.)

binding, whereas guinea pig ileum activity correlates better with naloxone binding in brain. Further evidence to support the theory that the peptides produce effects at a different set of receptors from the classical opiates in the mouse vas deferens is obtained by examining the effectiveness of naloxone in antagonizing the agonist effects of the compound on the mouse vas deferens and guinea pig ileum (Table 6). The K_e values for normorphine and the peptides tested differ by an order of magnitude in the vas deferens, a reflection of the relative lack of affinity which naloxone shows for the peptide receptors in this tissue. The same receptors, called δ-receptors by Lord et al. (32), are not responsible for the peptide actions in the guinea pig ileum, as the peptides are as readily antagonized in this tissue as is normorphine. This observation appears also to rule out any significant interaction of the peptides with putative κ-receptors in this tissue, as this type of interaction would also require more naloxone for reversal. It is interesting and perhaps significant to note that β-endorphin is a nonselective agent, in that it interacts with both μ- and δ-receptors with high affinity.

TABLE 6 Effectiveness of Naloxone in Antagonizing the Agonist Actions of Normorphine and Opioid Peptides in Isolated Tissues[a]

Agonist	Guinea pig ileum K_e (nM)	Mouse vas deferens K_e (nM)
Normorphine	1.89 ± 0.20 (4)	1.84 ± 0.20 (4)
Met-enkephalin	2.45 ± 0.26 (4)	22.6 ± 0.5 (4)
α-Endorphin	1.56 ± 0.15 (4)	22.5 ± 2.9 (4)
β-Endorphin	2.86 ± 0.42 (5)	21.7 ± 1.2 (3)
D-Ala^2-Met-enkephalin	2.55 ± 0.20 (4)	22.4 ± 2.7 (4)

[a]Results are means ± S.E.; the number of determinations is shown in parentheses.
Source: Data from Ref. 7.

The complexity of the opiate receptor system is further exemplified by the results obtained using the rabbit ear artery preparation (13; C. F. C. Smith, unpublished observations). In this tissue, structure-activity relationships differ significantly from those obtained on the ileum and vas deferens preparations (Table 7). Morphine, methadone, and pethidine have little affinity for the ear artery receptor, whereas other alkaloid-derived opiates (e.g., etorphine) and the enkephalins are potent inhibitors of the tissue response.

TABLE 7 Relative Inhibitory Potencies of Some Opiate Agonists in Guinea Pig Ileum, Mouse Vas Deferens, and Rabbit Ear Artery Preparations[a]

Compound	Relative potency (Met-enkephalin = 1) Guinea pig ileum[b]	Mouse vas deferens[c]	Rabbit ear artery
Met-enkephalin	1	1	1
Leu-enkephalin	0.3	1.8	0.8
D-Ala^2-Met-enkephalin	6.25	5.0	1.0
Morphine	1.5	0.1	<0.001
Normorphine	1.5	0.1	<0.001
Methadone	—	0.1	0.01
Pethidine (meperidine)	0.02	0.007	<0.001
Etorphine	400	100	1
Ethylketocyclazocine	280	1.7	0.3

[a]Methionine-enkephalin used as internal standard.
[b]Determined by cumulative-dose method.
[c]Determined by perfusion technique.

The potent activity of the endorphins in isolated tissue assays has stimulated much interest in the pharmacological profile of analogs, particularly of the shorter peptides, and many reports of structure-activity relationships are now available (90–94). It is interesting to analyze the results obtained in terms of the selectivity of these agonists for the receptor populations outlined above. Results obtained for selected compounds in parallel assay systems are reported in Table 8. It is apparent that relatively few analogs retain the ability of the natural pentapeptides to interact selectively with the δ-receptor. The simple analog D-Ala^2-Met-enkephalin shows a similar profile to the parent peptide, whereas, for example, the Tyr^1-N-methyl-Met-enkephalinamide is more morphinelike in its profile, showing relatively low potency in the vas deferens assay and in competition for Leu-enkephalin binding sites. The best example of a selective δ-receptor agonist appears to be the D-Ala^2-D-Leu^5 analog reported by Beddell and coworkers (91). In general, however, the smaller peptide analogs appear to show relatively higher affinity for the putative μ-receptor. Two compounds reported as producing potent analgesia in vivo, D-Met^2-Pro^5-enkephalinamide (93) and H-Tyr-D-Ala-Gly-Me-Phe-Met-(O)-ol (94), are illustrative of this point. Some agents have been reported which have considerably greater selectivity for μ-receptors than morphine does, and these are exemplified by the tripeptide derivative H-Tyr-D-Ala-Gly-NH$(CH_2)_2$-Ph (92).

It is clear, therefore, that a spectrum of activity exists, with the D-Ala^2-D-Leu^5 analog representing one extreme (i.e., selective mouse vas deferens activity) and the tripeptide, Tyr-D-Ala-Gly-NH$(CH_2)_2$-Ph, representing the alternative (i.e., selectivity for the guinea pig ileum receptors). The lack of specific antagonists makes it difficult to interpret the different structural requirements for activity in isolated tissue preparations, but it is certain that the receptor populations in these tissues differ in a significant manner. Do these differences have any real functional relevance in the whole animal? Results to date indicate that the differences can be mirrored in binding assays using brain synaptic membranes. It is not possible at present to relate specific pharmacological effects (e.g., analgesia) to specific receptor populations, as agents of sufficient selectivity have yet to be identified (92,94,95). Agents with selective action at different in vitro receptors might be expected, however, to produce different pharmacological syndromes in the whole animal. It is interesting to note, therefore, that the antinociceptive analog H-Tyr-D-Ala-Gly-Me-Phe-Met-(O)-ol possesses a range of non-morphine-like effects on gut and vascular smooth muscle in humans at low doses which were not reversed by nalorphine (96).

It can be postulated that these effects are the result of interactions with enkephalin receptors, for which morphine and nalorphine have little or no affinity and a parallel is seen in vitro in the rabbit ear artery preparation. These results and the demonstration in vitro of the poor affinity of naloxone for Leu-enkephalin binding sites in brain may be important in the interpretation of experiments designed to demonstrate a tonic involvement of endorphins in the control of pain transmission and mood (97). The lack of effect of naloxone in the absence of an exogenously

TABLE 8 Relative Inhibitory Potencies of Endorphin Analogs in Isolated Tissue and Binding Assays

	Isolated tissue		Binding assay[a]		
Compound	Guinea pig ileum[b]	Mouse vas deferens[c]	[^{3}H] Naloxone	[^{3}H] Naltrexone	[^{3}H] Leu-enkephalin
H-Tyr-Gly-Gly-Phe-Met-OH	1	1	1	1	1
H-Tyr-D-Ala-Gly-Phe-Met-OH	6.25	5.0	0.54 ± 0.13 (3)	–	1.67 ± 0.45 (3)
CH_3-Tyr-Gly-Gly-Phe-Met-NH_2	0.1	5.25	1.20 ± 0.1 (3)	–	0.08 ± 0.02 (3)
H-Tyr-D-Ala-Gly-Phe-D-Leu	32[d]	5.4[d]	–	0.26 (2)[e]	0.56 ± 0.10 (3)[e]
H-Tyr-D-Met-Gly-Phe-Pro-NH_2	0.29	14.0	–	–	–
H-Tyr-D-Ala-Gly-Me-Phe-Met-(O)-ol	0.69	26.5	–	–	–
H-Tyr-D-Ala-Gly-NH$(CH_2)_2$-Ph	0.02	4.36	–	0.433 ± 0.047 (3)[f]	0.009 ± 0.001 (3)[f]

[a]Results are means ± S.E.; the number of determinations is shown in parentheses.
[b]Determined by cumulative-dose method with Met-enkephalin as standard.
[c]Determined by perfusion technique with Met-enkephalin as standard.
[d]Data from Ref. 91.
[e]H. W. Kosterlitz et al., reported to the Committee on Problems of Drug Dependence, 1977.
[f]J. A. H. Lord, unpublished observations.

administered agonist may be interpreted as an indication of a lack of tonic action of the endorphins at receptors but may also be a reflection of the fact that naloxone may not antagonize the natural peptides effectively at a significant population of receptors. Development of new antagonists for these receptors is obviously of the greatest importance.

It remains to be seen whether the heterogeneity of the opiate receptor population, now clearly demonstrated, can be exploited therapeutically to produce agents of selective and useful pharmacological action.

ADDENDUM

The opioid peptide field is among the most rapidly moving areas of biological science and, as a result, it has been necessary to include a brief summary of some of the more important findings that have emerged between manuscript preparation and going to press.

Opiate Receptors in the Rat Vas Deferens

Lemaire et al. (98) demonstrated the presence of opiate receptors in the isolated rat vas deferens and claimed that these receptors differed from those in other isolated tissues in that they were peptide specific. Schulz et al. (99) have demonstrated the selectivity of this tissue for β-endorphin. In this study β-endorphin and β-$LPH_{61\text{-}78}$ showed an inhibitory potency similar to that demonstrated by these compounds in the mouse vas deferens and guinea pig ileum, whereas morphine was completely inactive. Met-enkephalin was virtually ineffective in this tissue and even the potent agonist etorphine was 100 times less effective than in the mouse vas deferens.

Nucleotide Regulation of Opiate Receptors

Like the opioid peptides, many other neurotransmitters also regulate adenylate cyclase activity. In some cases the receptors involved (e.g., β-adrenergic receptors) (100) are themselves regulated by nucleotides, and this has recently also been shown for opiate receptors in both brain membranes (101, 102) and in membranes prepared from neuroblastoma x glioma cells (103). Blume (101) showed that guanine nucleotides [guanosine triphosphate (GTP) and stable analogs] and sodium ions reduced the level of specific binding of dihydromorphine and other agonists and increased the rate of dissociation of the ligands from the receptors. Unlike the situation found with other systems showing nucleotide regulation, antagonist binding appeared also to be regulated by guanine nucleotides at the opiate receptor. Childers and Snyder (102) have confirmed the nucleotide effect on agonist binding but report that the binding of the antagonists naloxone and naltrexone is unaffected by GTP and stable analogs; and this point remains to be clarified.

Opiate Receptor Multiplicity

Recent studies reported by Chang and Cuatrecasas (104, 105) demonstrate conclusively the existence of opiate receptors in brain which show differential binding properties for morphine and its simple congeners and for enkephalins and their D-Ala[2] analogs. These data provide excellent support for the original observations made in 1977 by Lord et al. (7), who classified the receptors as μ and δ for the morphine and enkephalin receptors, respectively. An interesting parallel can be drawn between the situation found for opiate receptors and that observed for dopamine receptors. For dopamine, receptors have recently been classified into two subgroups; D-1 receptors, showing low (micromolar) affinity for the neurotransmitter, and D-2 receptors, showing high (nanomolar) affinity for dopamine (106). D-1-Dopamine receptors are coupled to adenylate cyclase, whereas D-2-receptors are not linked to this enzyme. Pert and Taylor (107), using nucleotide effects on receptor binding as diagnostic of coupling to cyclase, have recently hypothesized that opiate receptors showing low affinity for the enkephalins (μ-receptors) are coupled to adenylate cyclase, whereas receptors showing high affinity for the enkephalins (δ-receptors) are uncoupled, making the parallel with the dopaminergic system more extensive. Further work in this area will undoubtedly lead to some clarification of the nature and function of opiate receptors, and as mentioned in this chapter, such discoveries may have profound effects on the direction of the current search for novel pharmacological entities.

REFERENCES

1. J. H. Gaddum, *Pharmacology*, Oxford University Press, London, 1940.
2. J. Hughes, T. W. Smith, H. W. Kosterlitz, L. A. Fothergill, B. A. Morgan, and H. R. Morris, *Nature*, *258*: 577 (1975).
3. J. Hughes, *Brain Res.*, *88*: 295 (1975).
4. K. Starke, *Rev. Physiol. Biochem. Pharmacol.*, *77*: 1 (1977).
5. J. W. Black, W. A. M. Duncan, G. J. Durant, C. R. Ganellin, and M. E. Parsons, *Nature*, *236*: 385 (1972).
6. W. R. Martin, *Pharmacol. Rev.*, *19*: 493 (1967).
7. J. A. H. Lord, A. A. Waterfield, J. Hughes, and H. W. Kosterlitz, *Nature*, *267*: 495 (1977).
8. E. A. Gyang and H. W. Kosterlitz, *Br. J. Pharmacol. Chemother.*, *27*: 514 (1966).
9. G. Henderson, J. Hughes, and H. W. Kosterlitz, *Br. J. Pharmacol.*, *46*: 764 (1972).
10. W. D. M. Paton, *Br. J. Pharmacol. Chemother.*, *12*: 119 (1957).
11. J. W. Thompson, *J. Physiol.*, *141*: 46 (1958).
12. H. W. Kosterlitz and D. W. Taylor, *Br. J. Pharmacol. Chemother.*, *14*: 209 (1959).
13. J. Knoll, *Eur. J. Pharmacol.*, *39*: 403 (1976).
14. H. W. Kosterlitz and A. A. Waterfield, *Annu. Rev. Pharmacol.*, *15*: 29 (1975).
15. H. W. Kosterlitz and A. J. Watt, *Br. J. Pharmacol. Chemother.*, *33*: 266 (1968).
16. O. Arunlakshana and H. O. Schild, *Br. J. Pharmacol. Chemother.*, *14*: 48 (1959).

17. H. W. Kosterlitz, J. A. H. Lord, and A. J. Watt, in *Agonist and Antagonist Actions of Narcotic Analgesic Drugs* (H. W. Kosterlitz, H. O. J. Collier, and J. E. Villareal, eds.), Macmillan, London, 1972, p. 45.
18. A. A. Waterfield, J. A. H. Lord, J. Hughes, and H. W. Kosterlitz, *Eur. J. Pharmacol.*, *47*: 249 (1978).
19. J. Hughes, H. W. Kosterlitz, and F. M. Leslie, *Br. J. Pharmacol.*, *53*: 371 (1975).
20. C. B. Pert, D. L. Bowie, A. Pert, J. L. Morell, and E. Gross, *Nature*, *269*: 73 (1977).
21. A. Goldstein, L. I. Lowney, and B. K. Pal, *Proc. Natl. Acad Sci. U.S.A.*, *68*: 1742 (1971).
22. B. K. Pal, L. I. Lowney, and A. Goldstein, in *Agonist and Antagonist Actions of Narcotic Analgesic Drugs* (H. W. Kosterlitz, H. O. J. Collier, and J. E. Villareal, eds.), Macmillan, London, 1972, p. 62.
23. C. B. Pert and S. H. Snyder, *Science*, *179*: 1011 (1973).
24. C. B. Pert and S. H. Snyder, *Proc. Natl. Acad. Sci. U.S.A.*, *70*: 2243 (1973).
25. L. Terenius, *Acta Pharmacol. Toxicol.*, *32*: 317 (1973).
26. E. J. Simon, J. M. Hiller, and I. Edelman, *Proc. Natl. Acad. Sci. U.S.A.*, *70*: 1947 (1973).
27. C. B. Pert, G. W. Pasternak, and S. H. Snyder, *Science*, *182*: 1359 (1973).
28. E. J. Simon, J. M. Hiller, J. Groth, and I. Edelman, *J. Pharmacol. Exp. Ther.*, *192*: 531 (1973).
29. J. M. Hambrook and M. J. Rance, in *Opiates and Endogenous Opioid Peptides* (H. W. Kosterlitz, ed.) Elsevier/North-Holland, Amsterdam, 1976, p. 295.
30. T. T. Chau-Pham and W. L. Dewey, *Life Sci.*, *21*: 1337 (1977).
31. R. J. Hitzmann, B. A. Hitzmann, and H. H. Loh, *Life Sci.*, *14*: 2293 (1974).
32. J. A. H. Lord, A. A. Waterfield, J. Hughes, and H. W. Kosterlitz, in *Opiates and Endogenous Opioid Peptides* (H. W. Kosterlitz, ed.), Elsevier/North-Holland, Amsterdam, 1976, p. 275.
33. M. J. Kuhar, C. B. Pert, and S. H. Snyder, *Nature*, *245*: 447 (1973).
34. C. B. Pert, D. Aposhian, and S. H. Snyder, *Brain Res.*, *75*: 356 (1974).
35. I. Creese and S. H. Snyder, *J. Pharmacol. Exp. Ther.*, *194*: 205 (1975).
36. L. Terenius, *Proceedings of the Sixth Congress of Pharmacology*, Vol. 1., Pergamon Press, Oxford, 1976, p. 153.
37. W. A. Klee and M. Nirenberg, *Proc. Natl. Acad. Sci. U.S.A.*, *71*: 3474 (1974).
38. H. H. Loh, T. M. Cho., Y. C. Wu, and E. Leong Way, *Life Sci.*, *14*: 2231 (1974).
39. C. B. Pert and S. H. Snyder, *Mol. Pharmacol.*, *10*: 868 (1974).
40. I. Creese, G. Pasternak, and S. H. Snyder, *Life Sci.*, *16*: 1837 (1975).
41. L. Terenius and A. Wahlström, *Eur. J. Pharmacol.*, *40*: 241 (1976).
42. R. Simantov and S. H. Snyder, *Mol. Pharmacol.*, *12*: 987 (1976).
43. A. F. Bradbury, D. G. Smyth, C. R. Snell, N. J. M. Birdsall, and E. C. Hulme, *Nature*, *260*: 793 (1976).
44. G. W. Pasternak and S. H. Snyder, *Mol. Pharmacol.*, *10*: 183 (1974).
45. C. Y. Lee, T. Akera, and T. M. Brody, *J. Pharmacol. Exp. Ther.*, *202*: 166 (1977).
46. G. W. Pasternak, R. Simantov, and S. H. Snyder, *Mol. Pharmacol.*, *12*: 504 (1976).
47. R. Simantov, A. M. Snowman, and S. H. Snyder, *Brain Res.*, *107*: 650 (1976).
48. J. K. Chang, B. J. W. Fong, A. Pert, and C. B. Pert, *Life Sci.*, *18*: 1473 (1976).

49. J. M. Hambrook, B. A. Morgan, M. J. Rance, and C. F. C. Smith, *Nature*, *262*: 782 (1976).
50. R. Simantov and S. H. Snyder, *Eur. J. Pharmacol.*, *47*: 319 (1978).
51. A. M. Snowman and S. H. Snyder, *Mol. Pharmacol.*, *12*: 977 (1976).
52. H. W. Kosterlitz, personal communication.
53. R. Schulz, A. Herz, and M. Wuster, *Life Sci.*, *21*: 105 (1977).
54. B. M. Cox, A. Goldstein, and C. H. Li, *Brain Res.*, *115*: 285 (1976).
55. C. H. Li and D. Chung, *Nature*, *260*: 622 (1976).
56. C. Y. Lee, T. Akera, S. Stolman, and T. M. Brody, *J. Pharmacol. Exp. Ther.*, *194*: 583 (1975).
57. R. F. Squires and C. Braestrup, *J. Neurochem.*, *30*: 231 (1978).
58. R. S. Yalow and S. A. Berson, *Adv. Biol. Med. Phys.*, *6*: 349 (1958).
59. R. S. Yalow and S. A. Berson, *Clin. Chim. Acta*, *22*: 51 (1968).
60. S. Spector, A. *Rev. Pharmacol.*, *13*: 359 (1973).
61. R. Simantov and S. H. Snyder, in *Opiates and Endogenous Opioid Peptides* (H. W. Kosterlitz, ed.) Elsevier/North-Holland, Amsterdam, 1976, p. 41.
62. H. Y. Yang, J. S. Hong, and E. Costa, *Neuropharmacology*, *16*: 303 (1977).
63. B. A. Weissman, H. Gersham, and C. B. Pert, *FEBS Lett.*, *70*: 245 (1976).
64. D. Wesche, V. Höllt, and A. Herz, *Naunyn-Schmiedebergs Arch. Exp. Pathol. Pharmakol.*, *301*: 79 (1977).
65. J. Rossier, T. M. Vargo, S. Minick, N. Ling, F. Bloom, and R. Guilleman, *Proc. Natl. Acad. Sci. U.S.A.*, *74*: 4969 (1977).
66. R. J. Miller, J. K. Cheng, B. Cooper, and P. Cuatrecasas, *J. Biol. Chem.*, *253*: 531 (1978).
67. R. Guilleman, N. Ling, and T. Vargo, *Biochem. Biophys. Res. Commun.*, *77*: 361 (1977).
68. C. R. Snell, W. Jeffcoate, P. J. Lowrey, J. H. Rees, and D. G. Smyth, *FEBS Lett.*, *81*: 427 (1977).
69. G. J. Dockray, in *Hormones in Blood* (C. H. Gray and V. H. T. James, eds.) Academic Press, London, in press.
70. P. M. Barling, G. M. Hendy, and M. C. Evans, *J. Endocrinol.*, *66*: 307 (1975).
71. R. J. Miller, J. K. Chang, P. Cuatrecasas, S. Wilkinson, L. Lowe, C. Beddell, and R. Follenfant, in *Centrally Acting Peptides* (J. Hughes, ed.), Macmillan, London, 1978.
72. R. Mains, E. Eippler, and N. Ling, *Proc. Natl. Acad. Sci. U.S.A.*, *74*: 3014 (1977).
73. W. A. Klee and M. Nirenberg, *Proc. Natl. Acad. Sci. U.S.A.*, *71*: 3474 (1974).
74. S. K. Sharma, M. Nirenberg, and W. A. Klee, *Proc. Natl. Acad. Sci. U.S.A.*, *72*: 590 (1975).
75. J. Traber, K. Fischer, S. Katzen, and B. Hamprecht, *Nature*, *253*: 120 (1975).
76. M. Brant, R. Gullis, K. Fischer, C. Buchen, B. Hamprecht, L. Moroder, and E. Wünsch, *Nature*, *262*: 311 (1976).
77. W. A. Klee, A. Lampert, and M. Nirenberg, in *Opiates and Endogenous Opioid Peptides* (H.W. Kosterlitz, ed.), Elsevier/North-Holland, Amsterdam, 1976, p. 153.
78. A. Wahlström, M. Brant, L. Moroder, E. Wünsch, G. Lindeberg, W. Raynasson, L. Terenius, and B. Hamprecht, *FEBS Lett.*, *77*: 28 (1976).
79. W. A. Klee and M. Nirenberg, *Nature*, *263*: 609 (1976).

80. N. S. Agarwal, V. J. Hruby, R. Katz, W. A. Klee, and M. Nirenberg, *Biochem. Biophys. Res. Commun., 76*: 129 (1977).
81. M. Brant, C. Buchen, and B. Hamprecht, *FEBS Lett., 80*: 251 (1977).
82. M. Brant, K. Fischer, L. Moroder, E. Wünsch, and B. Hamprecht, *FEBS Lett., 68*: 38 (1976).
83. R. W. Houde and S. L. Wallenstein, *Fed. Proc., 15*: 441 (1956).
84. W. R. Martin, C. G. Eades, J. A. Thompson, R. E. Huppler, and P. E. Gilbert, *J. Pharmacol. Exp. Ther., 198*: 66 (1976).
85. A. E. Takemori, *Adv. Biochem. Pharmacol., 8*: 335 (1975).
86. C. H. Chang and J. H. Gaddum, *J. Physiol. (London), 79*: 255 (1933).
87. M. Hutchinson, H. W. Kosterlitz, F. M. Leslie, and A. A. Waterfield, *Br. J. Pharmacol., 55*: 541 (1975).
88. A. S. Ronai, I. Berzétei, and S. Bajusz, *Eur. J. Pharmacol., 45:* 393 (1977).
89. A. A. Waterfield, R. W. J. Smokum, J. Hughes, H. W. Kosterlitz, and G. Henderson, *Eur. J. Pharmacol., 43*: 107 (1977).
90. A. S. Dutta, J. J. Gormley, C. F. Hayward, J. S. Morley, J. S. Shaw, G. J. Stacey, and M. T. Turnbull, *Life Sci., 21*: 559 (1977).
91. C. R. Beddell, R. B. Clark, G. W. Hardy, L. A. Lowe, F. B. Ubatuba, J. R. Vane, S. Wilkinson, J. K. Chang, P. Cuatrecasas, and R. J. Miller, *Proc. R. Soc. Lond.* B, *198*: 249 (1977).
92. B. A. Morgan, J. D. Bower, K. P. Guest, B. K. Handa, G. Metcalf, and C. F. C. Smith, in *Peptides: Proceedings of the Fifth American Peptide Symposium* (M. Goodman and J. Meienhöfer, eds.), Wiley, 1977, p. 111.
93. S. Bajusz, A. S. Ronai, J. I. Szekely, L. Graf, Z. Dunai-Kovaks, and I. Berzetéi, *FEBS Lett., 76*: 91 (1977).
94. D. Romer, H. H. Büscher, R. C. Hill, J. Pless, W. Bauer, F. Cardinaux, A. Closse, D. Hauser, and R. Huguenin, *Nature, 268:* 547 (1977).
95. M. G. Baxter, R. L. Follenfant, A. A. Miller, and D. M. Sethna, *Br. J. Pharmacol., 59*: 523 (1977).
96. B. von Graffenried, E. del Pozo, J. Rowbicek, E. Krebs, W. Poldinger, P. Barmeister, and L. Kerp, *Nature, 272*: 729 (1978).
97. P. Grevert and A. Goldstein, *Science, 199*: 1093 (1978).
98. S. Lemaire, J. Magnan, and D. Regola, *Br. J. Pharmacol., 64*: 327 (1978).
99. R. Schulz, E. Faase, M. Wuster, and A. Herz, *Life Sci., 24*: 843 (1979).
100. M. E. Maguire, P. M. Van Arsdale, and A. G. Gilman, *Mol. Pharmacol., 12*: 335 (1976).
101. A. J. Blume, *Proc. Natl. Acad. Sci. U.S.A., 75*: 1713 (1978).
102. S. R. Childers and S. Snyder, *Life Sci., 23*: 759 (1978).
103. A. J. Blume, *Life Sci., 22*: 1843 (1978).
104. J. K. Chang and P. Cuatrecasas, *J. Biol. Chem., 254:* 2610 (1979).
105. J. K. Chang, B. R. Cooper, E. Hazum, and P. Cuatrecasas, *Mol. Pharmacol., 16*: 91 (1979).
106. J. W. Kebabian and D. B. Calue, *Nature, 277*: 93 (1979).
107. C. B. Pert and D. Taylor, in *Endogenous and Exongenous Opiate Agonists and Antagonists* (E. L. Way, ed.), Pergamon Press, Elmsford, N.Y. 1980.

chapter 5

Distribution of Opioid Peptides

Jean P. Rossier and Floyd E. Bloom*

The Salk Institute
San Diego, California

I. INTRODUCTION

Although the endorphins have only been known to neurobiologists for a short time, these endogenous morphinelike compounds have already become household words. Concepts of how these factors, largely peptides, may function, and how the effects of molecules so closely related to each other may differ, have undergone several rapid phases of revision. Definition of the roles and relationships between these substances has had to await the development of methods for optimal quantitation and cytological localization. In the case of peptides, the advent of immunological methods has allowed the entire pursuit to progress far more rapidly than for monoamines, amino acids, and other substances previously studied as neurotransmitters. This chapter reports on the present status of studies designed to determine the biological distribution of the endorphin peptides and is focused largely on a critical evaluation of reports attempting to locate and measure three molecules: β-lipotropin (β-LPH), β-endorphin, and the enkephalins Met-enkephalin and Leu-enkephalin.

II. PREPARATION OF ANTISERA

The explosion of the number of reports describing the distribution of the endorphins was made possible by the rapid acquisition of antisera prepared against the various opioid peptides. Usually, small peptides (haptens) are not sufficiently antigenic by themselves to act as haptens and induce an immune response and, therefore,

*Present affiliation: C.N.R.S. Laboratories, Gif-sur-Yvette, France

these small haptens must be coupled to a carrier molecule of higher molecular weight and greater antigenicity. Commercially available bovine serum albumin, ovalbumin, or thyroglobulin are often selected. In recent years, proteins from invertebrates (hemocyanin) or plants have also been used with great success (1).

All the antisera produced in various laboratories against β-endorphin, Leu-enkephalin, and Met-enkephalin were obtained after coupling these antigens to bovine serum albumin (2-6), ovalbumin (7), or hemocyanin (8, 9). The antisera prepared against β-LPH by C. H. Li did not require any coupling, because β-LPH is a large molecule (91 amino acids) with sufficient intrinsic immunogenicity (10, 11).

Numerous methods for coupling the peptides to the carrier proteins are in use. The carbodiimide and the glutaraldehyde methods are the most widely used. Because of its specificity in bonding the N-terminus of the hapten, we prefer to use bis-diazotized benzidine (2). For the opioid peptides β-endorphin, Leu-enkephalin, and Met-enkephalin, this NH-terminal amino acid is tyrosine in each case. Glutaraldehyde also achieves cross-linking between hapten and carrier but is less specific, and can give rise to more than one immunogen.

In general, the immunization procedure for endorphins was performed as follows: 0.5-2.0 mg of conjugates, emulsified in complete Freund's adjuvant, is injected into rabbits in numerous (around 40) intradermal sites in the back. Booster injections were performed at monthly intervals with half the dose of the antigen emulsified in incomplete Freund's adjuvant. Ten days after the last boost, animals were bled and the sera tested by radioimmunoassays.

Radioimmunoassays are particularly useful in testing the specificity of the sera obtained. A highly monospecific antisera will react only with its antigen and not with any other related molecule. In the case of β-endorphin, we have obtained a serum that does not cross-react with α-endorphin, Leu-enkephalin, and Met-enkephalin, but shows complete cross-reactivity with β-LPH. The absence of cross-reactivity with any of the enkephalins was the key factor in our demonstration that neurons containing β-endorphin in rat brain exist separately from those containing enkephalin (3, 12).

Until now, all the sera obtained in different laboratories against Met-enkephalin cross-react significantly (1-10% cross-reactivity) with Leu-enkephalin and vice versa. This cross-reactivity of the sera raised against the two enkephalins is particularly frustrating because without a monospecific serum, it is virtually impossible to know if the enkephalins Met-enkephalin and Leu-enkephalin are stored in different neurons, or if both are present in the same neurons.

III. DISTRIBUTION OF ENKEPHALINS

Using antisera developed independently in several laboratories against N-terminally conjugated enkephalins, a series of progressively refined reports have described the quantitative and cytological distribution (4, 6, 13-16) of these pentapeptides in the nervous system and other tissues.

A. Central Nervous System

Distributional studies on the content of enkephalins in brain were reported (17-20) before the availability of the specific radioimmunoassay. These data, obtained through the use of radioreceptor displacement assays on nonpurified extracts, provided numbers that can now be considered of doubtful significance. The original methods, in retrospect, gave poor recovery of endogenous peptides due both to incomplete inactivation of degrading peptidases or to suboptimal extraction procedures (see Ref. 21).

Simantov et al. (17) were the first to report the results of a regional assessment of rat brain with an enkephalin radioimmunoassay in which the antisera showed at least 10% cross-reactivity between Leu-enkephalin and Met-enkephalin immunogens. Unfortunately, the incomplete inactivation of degrading peptidases and suboptimal extraction procedures hampered this preliminary study in giving Met-enkephalin and Leu-enkephalin values tenfold less than those obtained shortly thereafter by Yang et al. (22). Yang et al. (22) presented more detailed results on rats killed with focused microwave irradiation, and antisera which also showed approximately 10% cross-reactivity between the two natural pentapeptides. Both studies indicated that the amounts of Met-enkephalin were some 5-10 times greater than Leu-enkephalin, that enkephalins were generally low in cortical regions and highest in diencephalic regions, and that enkephalins were highest of all in the corpus striatum. Similar results were also obtained by Gros et al. (7), Miller et al. (5), and Gillin et al. (23) but not by Simantov et al. (17, 18), who have reported that in cow brain the ratio of the levels of Met-enkephalin to Leu-enkephalin was 0.1. More recent studies have shown that the ratio of Met-enkephalin to Leu-enkephalin in cows was around 5-10 (24), as it is in other species (rat, rabbit, and guinea pig) (5, 7, 22, 25).

It is worthwhile to note that the values obtained by radioimmunoassay for Met-enkephalin and Leu-enkephalin were found to be in complete agreement with those obtained by chemical methods. In these chemical assays, Met-enkephalin and Leu-enkephlin are separated by various chromatographic methods and then each is separately assayed by radioimmunoassay (26, 27), by radioreceptor assay (24), or by biological assay(25). Alternatively, Met-enkephalin activity is destroyed by treatment with cyanogen bromide, which does not affect Leu-enkephalin. By differential assays before and after such treatment, values for both Met-enkephalin and Leu-enkephalin were obtained (24).

The distribution of immounoreactive (ir) Met-enkephalin and Leu-enkephalin in the rat obtained by radioimmunoassay is given in Table 1 (see also Refs. 28 and 29). The highest concentration in brain is seen in the globus pallidus, but the concentration in the pars nervosa of the pituitary is even higher. In these tissues the ratio of Met-enkephalin to Leu-enkephalin is 5 and 3, respectively. Other brain regions with high levels of (ir) enkephalins are whole striatum, hypothalamus, and thalamus. In these regions the ratio of Met-enkephalin to Leu-enkephalin is be-

TABLE 1 Distribution of Immunoreactive Met-enkephalin and Leu-enkephalin in Rat Brain and Pituitary

	ng/g tissue	
	(ir) Met-Enk	(ir) Leu-Enk
Striatum (whole)	600	100
Globulus pallidus	1750	350
Caudate and putamen	250	50
Hypothalamus	450	80
Thalamus	400	60
Pons	350	40
Hippocampus	200	20
Cerebral cortex	140	15
Cerebellum	100	7
Pituitary (whole)	700	60
Par nervosa	1900	600

Source: Values are from our laboratory (A. Bayon et al., in preparation).

tween 5 and 10. In the other regions where (ir) enkephalins are detectable, hippocampus and cerebral cortices, the ratio of Met-enkephalin to Leu-enkephalin is over 10. The brain region containing the lowest (ir) level is the cerebellum. Since no enkephalinergic fibers or enkephalinergic cell bodies have been reported by immunocytology in any layer of the cerebellum, one must question whether the presence of authentic enkephalin there has been established. However, nonpeptidic "morphine-like" material has been reported to exist in cerebellum (30, 31).

The estimates given in Table 1 are in general agreement with the recent quantitative regional and histological estimates of the distribution of the "opiate receptors" (32-34). Nevertheless, the distribution of the enkephalins and β-endorphin system is not always parallel with that of the opiate receptors. These differences are summarized later in this section.

Although recent studies of regional brain content of the enkephalin-containing regions have been more refined (35), the best guide to the distribution of enkephalin content in brain has derived from immunohistochemistry. All the studies that have described immunocytochemical distribution patterns are largely in agreement on the location of immunoreactive nerve terminals in untreated rats, and immunoreactive perikarya in rats pretreated with colchicine (4, 13). The following descriptions are based largely on the results of detailed studies by Uhl et al. (16, 23), Sar et al. (15), and by ourselves (unpublished results with antisera donated by R.J. Miller University of Chicago; see Fig. 1). This general agreement eliminates the necessity to postulate that slight differences in immunogens, in tissue fixation, antibody detection, or other covert causes of artifactual result have any significant bearing on the results. All the results are considered specific for enkephalins, although none per se is fully capable of absolute discrimination between Met-enkephalin and Leu-enkephalin. The reasons underlying the reproducible finding that colchicine pretreatment facilitates the localization of enkephalin-containing perikarya remain unclear, but the unproven assumption is that by disaggregating microtubules and depressing cellulofugal transport of stored peptide, immunoreactive materials accumulate with-

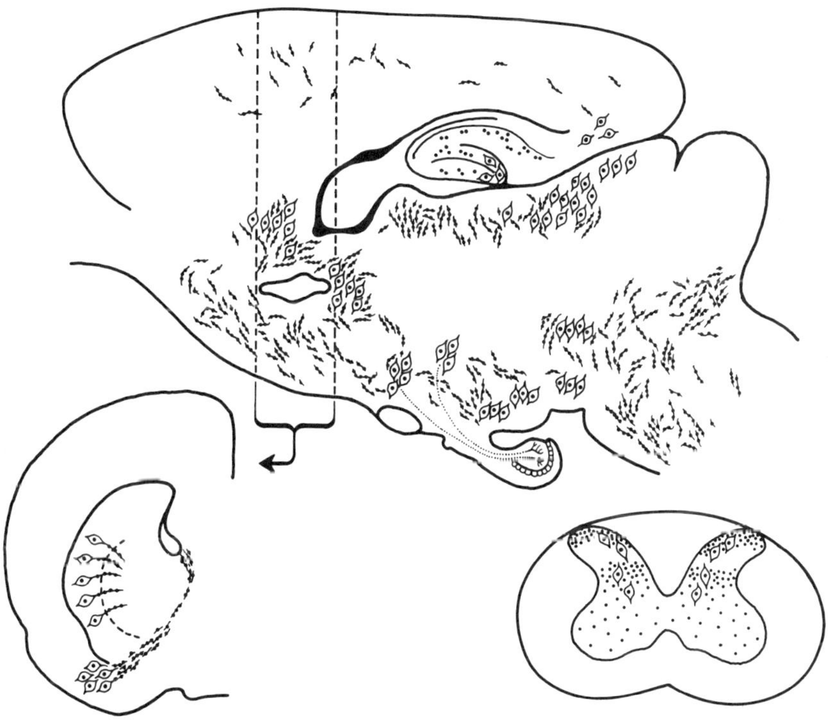

FIGURE 1 Schematic mapping of nerve cells and fibers exhibiting immunoreactivity for enkephalins in rat brain, compiled from various sources cited in the text. A sagittal section (above) indicates the major regions exhibiting staining of neurons and fibers. Dashed vertical lines indicate the plane of the section shown in the frontal view at the lower left to illustrate the presumptive circuits coursing between the caudate nucleus and the globus pallidus and between the central nucleus of the amygdala and the nucleus of the stria terminalis. At the lower right are mapped the cells and fibers typical of the spinal cord. Note that the pituitary lobes are totally unreactive except for fine nerve fibers entering the posterior lobe from the magnocellular nuclei of the hypothalamus.

in the perikayron. Recent work on the enkephalin-containing pathway between the magnocellular hypothalamic nuclei and the neurohypophysis (37) supports this general hypothesis (38).

If observations are restricted to colchicine-pretreated rats, enkephalin immunoreactive cells and fibers are detected throughout the central nervous system (see Fig. 1, based on Refs. 13-16, 36, 39, 40, and our own unpublished results). With four exceptions discussed separately below, no specific pathways have been described which relate specific immunoreactive perikarya with specific sets of nerve terminals, and there has been only one published report of electron microscopic localization of the immunoreactive elements (40).

In forebrain, enkephalin-reactive neurons are found in n. accumbens; the caudate nucleus and putamen, especially at the caudal pole; the interstitial nucleus of the stria terminalis; and the central nucleus of the amygdala. Nerve terminal-like patterns of immunoreactivity are densest in the globus pallidus and central nucleus of the amygdala, and show generally heavy innervation of the n. accumbens, the bed nucleus of the stria terminalis, and occasional patches of intense fiber staining around pyramidal cells in the posterior cingulate gyrus and in restricted patches within the hippocampus (Fig. 2). With high doses of colchicine, immunoreactive enkephalin neurons can also be observed in the molecular layer of the dentate gyrus and in the entorhinal area (F. Bloom et al., unpublished results).

In midbrain, immunoreactive neurons are found in both the supraoptic and paraventricular nuclei (37; Fig. 3) and in scattered smaller cells in the perifornical region and, more diffusely, in the lateral hypothalamus. Fibers have been seen in almost all hypothalamic nuclei, but are especially dense in the periventricular area, in the external layer of the median eminence, and the ventromedial nucleus. Thalamic nuclei exhibit mainly nerve fibers, which are less dense than in hypothalmic areas; in thalamus reactive fibers are present within the anterior intralaminar nuclei, but not in the paraventricular nucleus, according to Sar et al. (15).

Within the more ventral and caudal portions of the midbrain, positively reactive perikarya have so far been reported for interpeduncular nucleus, the dorsal cochlear nucleus, the medial vestibular nucleus, and the spinal portion of the vestibular nucleus, as well as in isolated small neurons throughout the pontine central gray and within the general confines of the reticular zone of the brain stem. Nerve fibers are found throughout the central gray as well, and specifically innervate those nuclei made popular by their monoamine content: the zona compacta of dopamine cells in the substantia nigra, the noradrenergic neurons of the locus coeruleus, and the serotonergic neurons of the midline raphe nuclei. Reactive fibers penetrate into the fourth, seventh, tenth, and twelfth cranial nerve motor nuclei as well as the n. tractus solitarius, and the spinal portion of the trigeminal nucleus and the substantia gelatinosa. In spinal levels, enkephalin reactive fibers are pronouced in the dorsal laminae I and II; some immunoreactive perikarya can also be seen within the dorsal horn.

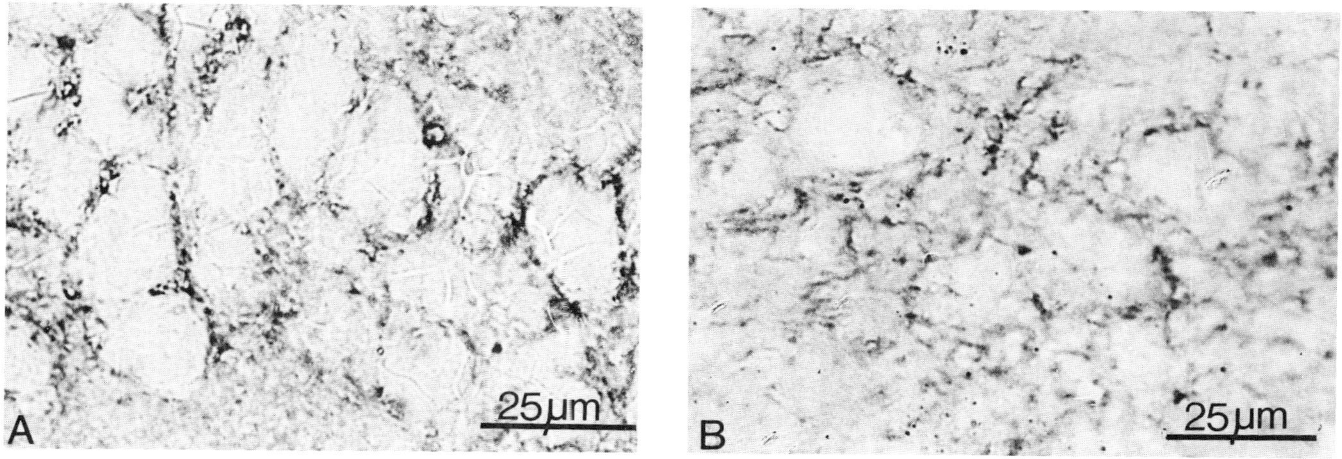

FIGURE 2 Two fields within the hippocampus exhibiting immunoperoxidase reactivity for antienkephalin sera. In (A), fiberlike staining is seen surrounding the pyramidal neurons at the junction between the CA3 field and the CA1 field. Clusters of punctate reactive boutons are seen but no typical extended fibers are present. In (B), more typical, fine fiberlike reactive elements are seen within the hilus of the dentate gyrus surrounding the large unreactive neurons seen in this region.

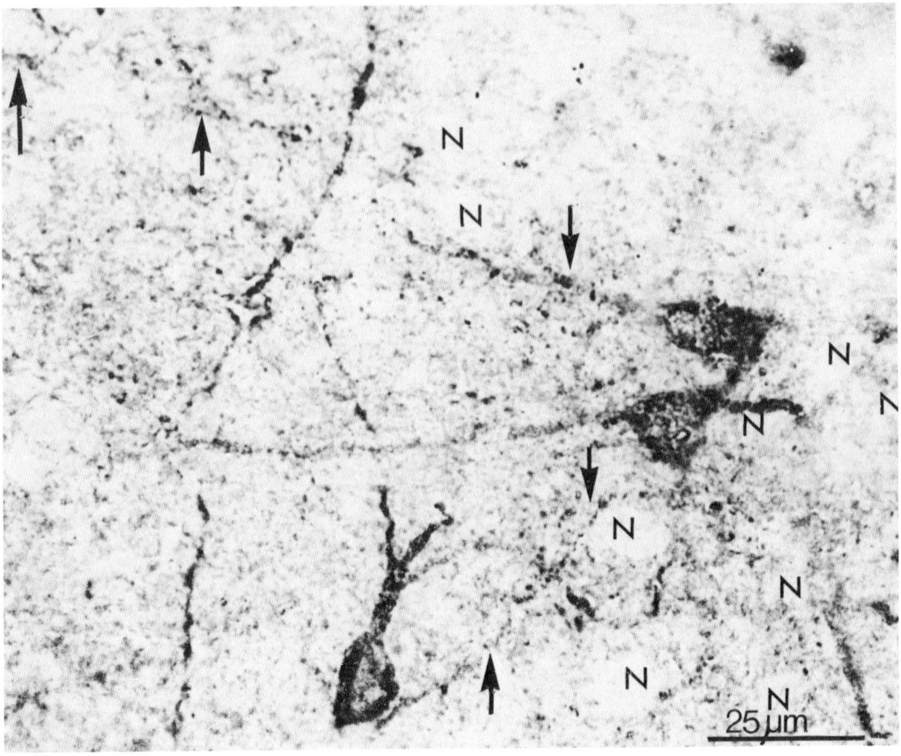

FIGURE 3 Immunoperoxidase reactivity to antienkephalin serum of neurons at the lateral edge of the paraventricular nucleus of the hypothalamus in an animal pretreated with intraventricular colchicine (25 μg, 24 hr). The entire neuronal structure is heavily immunoreactive except for the unreactive nucleus. The thickened dendritic extensions from the cell bodies extend across the field, while structures more indicative of nerve fibers (arrows) are seen in the neuropil surrounding unreactive nerve cells (N).

Although the technology for tracing connectivity patterns of neuronal circuits is currently undergoing a renaissance due to the advent of new orthograde and retrograde markers, only four possible enkephalin-containing circuits have so far been proposed (see Fig. 1), and these have been based either on the results of large transecting lesions or on direct tracing.

Hokfelt et al. (14) proposed on the basis of such lesions that the enkephalin-reactive neurons of the dorsal horn and of the spinal trigeminal nucleus are the source for the immunoreactive fibers of the spinal cord dorsal horn and superficial layers of the spinal trigeminal nucleus. Cuello and Paxinos (41) also used transections to propose that the enkephalinergic innervation of the bed nucleus of the stria terminalis arises from the central nucleus of the amygdala, based also on a pathway demonstrated earlier by De Olmos (43) without chemical designation. However, in other studies (44) after transections of the stria terminalis, no decreases of (ir) Met^5-enkephalin levels were observed in the bed nucleus of the stria terminalis. Direct retracing of pathways already known to exist also underlies the proposal by Rossier et al. (37) that the enkephalinergic neurons of the paraventricular and supraoptic nuclei provide the enkephalin-reactive fibers to the neural lobe. These fibers and neural lobe enkephalin content can also be shown to parallel functional or genetic changes in vasopressin content and are greatly decreased after lesions of the supraoptic and paraventricular nuclei. The hypothalamic pars nervosa enkephalinergic pathway may modulate neurohypophysial neurosecretion (37).

In brief, enkephalin-containing neurons are present throughout the entire rat central nervous system from cerebral cortex to spinal cord. Although limbic system, hypothalamus, central gray, and reticular formation are heavily innervated, neurons regarded both as sensory, motor, or vegetative in function all receive such innervation, making abstract presumptions of some definitive function extremely difficult to derive. In general, however, the enkephalin-containing cells are relatively short axon cells, and even the pathways proposed are only a few millimeters in length. Regions in which stimulation- and ablation-type studies (the unfortunate, but highly popular physiological testing strategy) might be most revealing are the central nucleus of the amygdala and the interpeduncular nucleus. As described below, both these regions are also devoid of β-endorphin reactive cells or fibers.

It would also seem worthwhile to compare these general immunocytochemical results with the distribution of the chemically detected or autoradiographically detected opiate binding properties. As acknowledged by Simantov et al. (45), there are at least five major discrepancies that remain unexplained: (1) receptors are very dense in caudate and putamen but not in globus pallidus, where the heaviest fibers are seen; (2) similarly, the caudate and putamen are perplexingly low in immunoreactivity for fibers, although some perikarya are seen here after colchicine treatments (14,15); (3) cerebral cortex, which has been shown to contain receptors by binding (see Ref. 29) and electrophysiologic studies (see Refs. 46 and 47), shows almost no immunoreactivity; (4) although nerve cells and fibers are exceedingly dense in the central nucleus of the amygdala, receptors are distributed more or less evenly throughout the entire amygdaloid complex; and (5) within the spinal cord the enkephalin-reactive fibers of the ventral gray regions are not represented by equivalent opiate receptor values. The colchicine injections required to demonstrate enkephalin-reactive perikarya have relatively little effect on the enkephalin content of most rat brain regions (38).

B. Pituitary

Recently, we detected significant amounts of immunoreactive (ir) Leu-enkephalin in extracts of the neurointermediate lobe of the rat pituitary (37) by radioimmunoassay. Negligible amounts of the pentapeptide were detected in the anterior lobe. In fact, in these assays, the concentration of Leu-enkephalin in the neurointermediate lobe was higher than in the globus pallidus, the brain region reported to contain the most dense enkephalinergic innervation (27; see Table 1). The high content of (ir) Leu-enkephalin in the neurointermediate lobe of the pituitary led us to pursue a more extensive investigation on its distribution and possible function (37).

The rat pituitary can easily be dissected into the anterior lobe (pars distalis) and the neurointermediate lobe. This latter is composed of the pars nervosa surrounded by the lobules of the pars intermedia. With a dissecting microscope, we isolated these three parts and assayed them by radioimmunoassay for β-endorphin and Leu-enkephalin. The major portion of (ir) Leu-enkephalin (76%) was found in the pars nervosa. The remaining (ir) Leu-enkephalin was equally distributed between the par intermedia and the pars distalis. Immunoreactive β-endorphin was present in both pars distalis and pars intermedia, as indicated in previous studies (3), but was almost absent from the pars nervosa (37).

These results suggested that the (ir) Leu-enkephalin in the pituitary was mainly concentrated in the pars nervosa. We have also found that (ir) Met-enkephalin was concentrated in the pars nervosa of the pituitary (see Table 1). Immunocytochemical studies revealed that fine varicose Leu-enkephalin nerve fibers were localized in pars nervosa. These fine fibers were more concentrated on the perimeter of the neural lobe than the center. These fibers were shown to arise from the hypothalamus, as they could be traced in favorable sections through the pars tuberalis and because lesions of the suprachiasmatic and paraventricular nuclei lead to loss of neurohypophysial enkephalin content (37; Fig. 4).

After pretreatment of the animals with colchicine, Leu-enkephalin immunoreactive cell bodies were also visualized in the paraventricular and supraoptic nuclei of the hypothalamus (Fig. 3).

The detection of a possible neuronal pathway between enkephalin immunoreactive neurons in the magnocellular hypothalamic nuclei and enkephalinergic terminals in the pars nervosa suggests two possible functional roles. As with other neurohypophysial hormones, enkephalin could be realeased as a neurohormone into the bloodstream together with vasopressin or oxytocin. This hypothesis seems unlikely since enkephalins have a very short half-life in the bloodstream (48). Alternatively, enkephalinergic fibers could somehow modulate the secretion of neurohypophysial hormones. Indeed, we found that severe dehydration decreases (ir) Leu-enkephalin in the neurointermediate lobe. We have also examined the distribution of enkephalin in the Brattleboro rat. In this strain the homozygous offspring are polyuric; these animals are completely unable to synthesize or secrete vasopressin (49). Compared to control littermates, the (ir) Leu-enkephalin levels in the neurointermediate lobe of Brattleboro rats are very low. Immuncytochemical studies of the enkephalin fibers in pars nervosa of the Brattleboro strain indicated that the number of enkephalin fibers here are decreased and their distribution and morphology somewhat dystrophic.

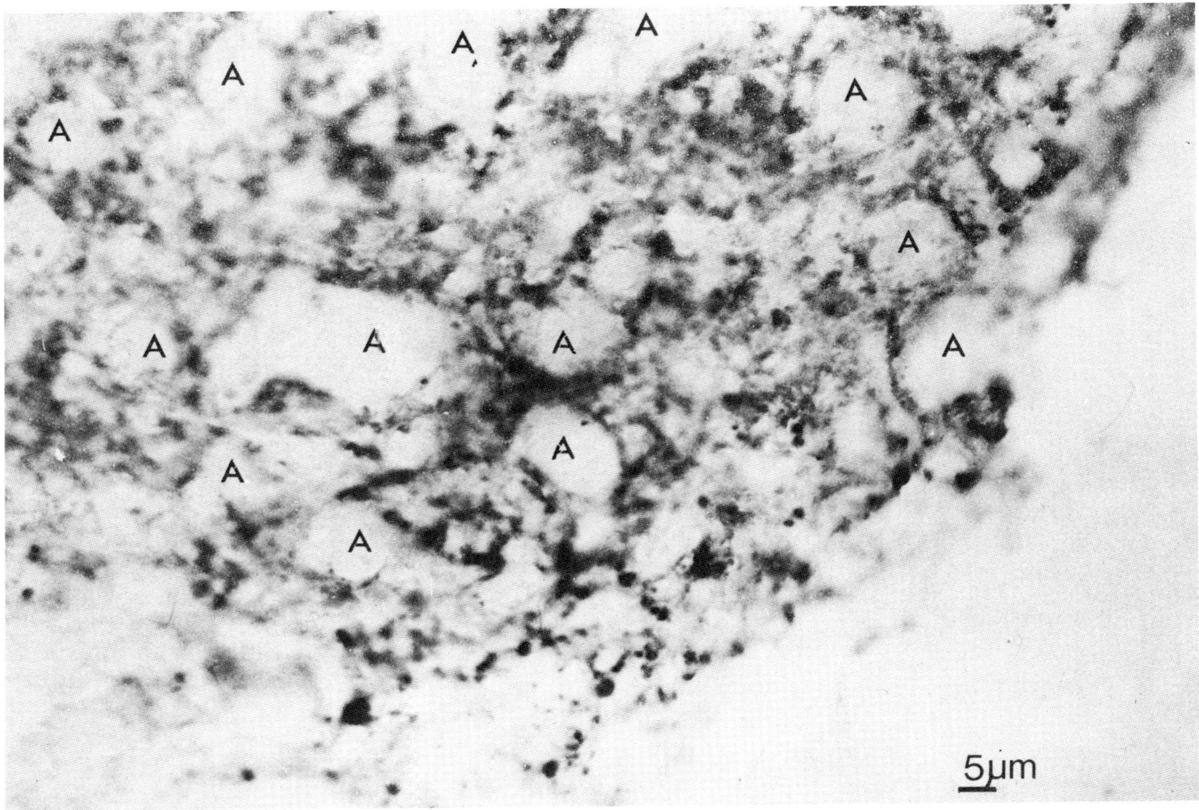

FIGURE 4 Immunoperoxidase reactivity to antienkephalin serum of nerve terminals within the posterior pituitary makes a dense plexus at the perimeter of the lobe around fascicles of unreactive axons (A9).

Morphine (50) or endorphin (51) injections are known to release vasopressin into the bloodstream and opiate receptors are also concentrated in the pars nervosa (52). We have, therefore, proposed that the enkephalinergic pathway and opiate receptors located on the neurohypophysial fibers may function to modulate vasopressin or their magnocellular hormonal secretion.

C. Gastrointestinal Tract

Although guinea pig intestinal muscle has been a primary bioassay target for detection and isolation for all the endorphins, determination of the presence of one or more of the endorphins in this tissue has received little attention (see Ref. 53) until quite recently. Puig et al. (54) suggested that an endogenous opiate could be undergoing release in vitro on the basis of a naloxone-induced reduction in the recovery from the decreased responsiveness to electrical stimulation which guinea pig ileum shows after high-frequency trains of stimuli. Subsequently, Elde et al. (6) made direct immunocytochemical recognition of enkephalinlike immunoreactivitiy in guinea pig myenteric plexus, and soon thereafter Polak et al. (55) reported that human pyloric antrum and duodenal mucosal cells showed immunoreactivity with antienkephalin sera.

Linnoila et al. (56) have recently reported a region-by-region analysis of the guinea pig and rat intestinal tract with both immunocytochemistry and radioimmunoassay of enkephalins. Immunopositive fibers, but no cell bodies, were most prevalent in stomach, duodenum, and rectum of the guinea pig; both the amounts and the number of fibers were more than 10 times less in the rat. Radioimmunoassay values roughly paralleled the enhanced fiber density seen in the stomach and rectum but with less marked variations. Interestingly, the fibers were considerably more reactive with anti-Met-enkephalin sera than with anti-Leu-enkephalin sera; by separate radioimmunoassay, the Met-enkephalin/Leu-enkephalin ratio was greater than 10. These differences were less marked in the duodenum and rectum. Within the small intestine, the fibers were seen to surround the ganglion cells of the Meissner's plexus, and were occassionally seen in the circular muscle; relatively few fibers were observed in the longitudinal muscle layer. Jejunum and ileum were even more sparsely innervated than duodenum. Fibers in the circular muscle layer of the colon were more reactive to anti-Leu-enkephalin sera than to anti-Met-enkephalin sera. A few immunopositive fibers were also observed in the walls of the common bile duct and gallbladder. On the basis of these observations it is difficult to predict why the isolated myenteric longitudinal muscle strip of the guinea pig has evolved into such a sensitive in vitro bioassay system. Nevertheless, the immunoreacitivty reported in intestinal nerve fibers in these studies would seem definitely to be intrinsic to the gut, as Schultzberg et al. (57) found that such intestinal fibers continued to exhibit immunoreactivity in fetal mouse intestines after 3 weeks of maintenance in organotypic cultures.

Recently, Schultzberg et al. (58) reported that rat, cat, and guinea pig adrenomedulla cells contained (ir) enkephalins. By immunofluorescence all the cells of the cat adrenomedulla were strongly visualized. Moreover, nerve terminals arising from the splanchnic nerves, as shown by transsection studies, also exhibitied (ir) materials. In this laboratory, we were able to confirm these findings in using immunocytological methods and radioimmunoassays on rat and hamster adrenals (unpublished).

IV. DISTRIBUTION OF β-ENDORPHIN

A. Radioimmunoassay of β-Endorphin

Table 2 shows the distribution of (ir) β-endorphin in rat brain and pituitary. The radioimmunoassay system used for measurement of β-endorphin is specific for the Leu^{14}-His^{27} segment of the molecule (2). Because β-endorphin is the COOH-terminal 31 amino acid fragment of β-LPH, this antiserum also binds on an equimolar ratio β-endorphin, β-LPH, and the 31,000-dalton prohormone (59-61). Attempts were

TABLE 2 Distribution of Immunoreactive Opioid Peptides in Rat Brain and Pituitary

	ng/g tissue	
	(ir) β-endorphin	(ir) Leu-Enk
Pituitary		
Whole	269.1	72
Adenohypophysis	128.1	4
Neurohypophysis and pars intermedia	1500.1	740
Brain		
Whole	108	25
Hypothalamus	490	120
Septum	234	85
Midbrain	207	32
Medulla and pons	179	30
Striatum	None	112
Globus pallidus	None	566
Hippocampus	None	13
Cortex	None	15
Cerebellum	None	5

Source: From Ref. 3.

made to separate the immunoreactive components by gel filtration. Extracts of whole rat brains were passed through a BioGel P60 column. Consistently, two peaks of immunoreactivity were resolved. One peak coincided precisely with the location of synthetic β-endorphin; the other peak was eluted in a broad zone of higher molecular weight (10,000-30,000) which did not coicide closely with the elution pattern of either β-LPH or the 31,000-dalton prohormone (3).

When similar gel filtration was performed with extracts of specific brain regions, striatum and cerebral, cerebellar, and hippocampal cortices were shown to contain only high molecular weight substances. As the serum used (RB 100) shows a slight cross-reactivity (0.001%) with myelin basic protein, we have proposed (3) that the reported presence of β-endorphin (62) in those specific regions—striatum, cerebral, cerebellar, and hippocampal cortices—was artifactual and presumably due to this slight cross-reactivity with myelin basic protein. Similar gel filtrations were performed with other brain regions. In the hypothalamus most of the (ir) β-endorphin was associated with authentic β-endorphin.

When the same regions (see Table 2 and Fig. 3) were assayed for β-endorphin and enkephalin, there was a clear-cut independent variation, from region to region, of the two classes of opioid peptides. Furthermore, globus pallidus and caudate nucleus, which contain large numbers of immunocytochemically detected enkephalin fibers, contained virtually no β-endorphin. Thus these data strongly suggested that β-endorphin and enkephalins are found in the brain within different neuronal systems. Such a view was also put forth later by other groups (39, 63, 64).

B. Pituitary

In the rat pituitary the total amount of (ir) β-endorphin determined by radioimmunoassay is equally distributed among the anterior and intermediate lobe (see Table 2). Since the volume of the intermediate lobe is much smaller than the anterior lobe, the much higher concentration of β-endorphin in the intermediate lobe becomes evident. When sizing experiments are performed, the elution pattern of (ir) β-endorphin in anterior and intermediate lobe differs considerably. The intermediate lobe contains mainly authentic β-endorphin. The anterior lobe (ir) β-endorphin is due mainly to β-LPH with equally smaller amount (around 5% of the total amount) of the 31,000-dalton prohormone and authentic β-endorphin (65-67; Rossier et al. in preparation).

We have reported that by immunocytology no (ir) β-endorphin was detected in the neurohypophysis, and this absence was confirmed by radiommunoassay (37). In rat pituitary as well as in mouse, kitten, pig, and frog pituitary, immunocytochemical studies indicate that (ir) β-endorphin is found in every cell of the intermediate lobe and in isolated cells—corresponding to those reactive to antisera against ACTH —in the adenohypophysis (68, 69; see Fig. 5).

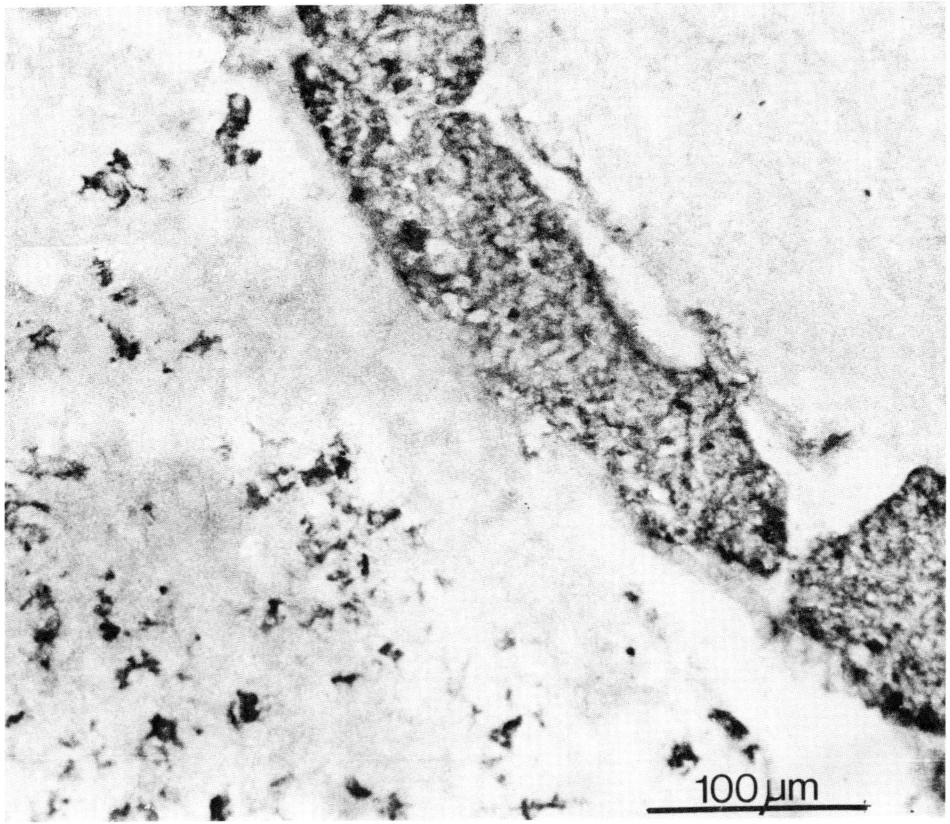

FIGURE 5 Immunoperoxidase reactivity to anti-β-endorphin serum of rat pituitary shows intense immunoreactivity of every cell of the intermediate lobe, and of corticotroph cells of the anterior lobe (lower left); there is no immunoreactivity within the posterior lobe (upper right).

C. Central Nervous System

Using the well-characterized anti-β-endorphin serum RB 100 of Guillemin et al. (2), we have examined in detail the distribution of β-endorphin immunoreactivity in the rat and mouse central nervous systems (68, 69). Even in untreated rats, immunoreactive neurons and neuronal processes exhibit immunoreactivity which is most pronounced within the diencephalin (see Fig. 6). The immunoreactive neurons exist exclusively within two adjacent clusters of the basal tuberal zone of the hypothalamus (Fig 7); these neurons are 1-20 μm in size, fusiform in shape, and extend from dorsolateral portions of the middle of the arcuate nucleus anterolaterally below the ventromedial nucleus, reaching almost to the lateral border of the hypothalamus. No other immunoreactive cells are observed, even after colchicine pretreatment sufficient to reveal enkephalin-immunoreactive neurons. Extensive nerve-fiber-like processes can be traced away from the β-endorphin immunoreactive neurons into the anterior hypothalamic area, where they turn dorsal into the stria medullaris to extend along the dorsal midline of the thalamus as far caudally as the dorsal raphe nucleus. From this level the fibers extend into the central gray, moving caudal and lateral toward the locus coeruleus. Caudal to the locus coeruleus, fibers become extremely difficult to detect. Specific nuclei in which there would appear to be extensive arborization of β-endorphin immunoreactive fibers are the supraoptic, periventricular, paraventricular, and suprachiasmatic nuclei of the hypothalamus, the dorsal and lat-

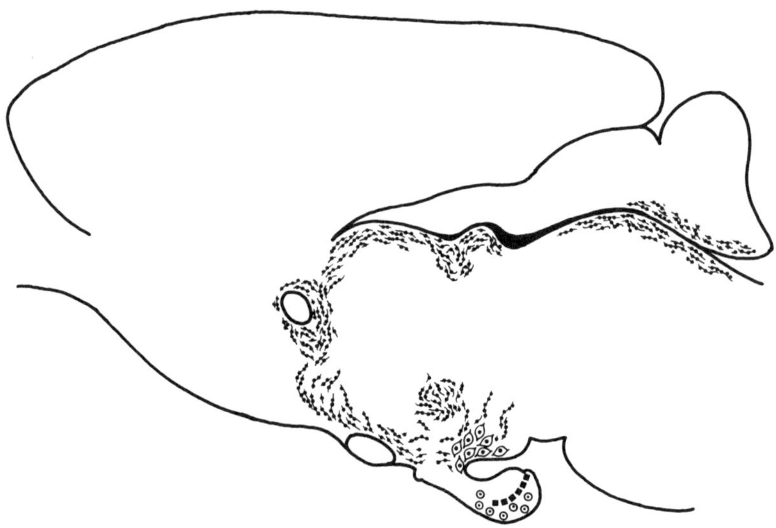

FIGURE 6 β-Endorphin distribution. Schematic mapping of immunoreactive nerve cells and fibers exhibiting reactivity with anti-β-endorphin serum. Also schematized are the reactive cells of the intermediate and anterior lobes of the pituitary. The contrasts in distribution with the enkephalin systems can be seen by comparison with Fig. 1.

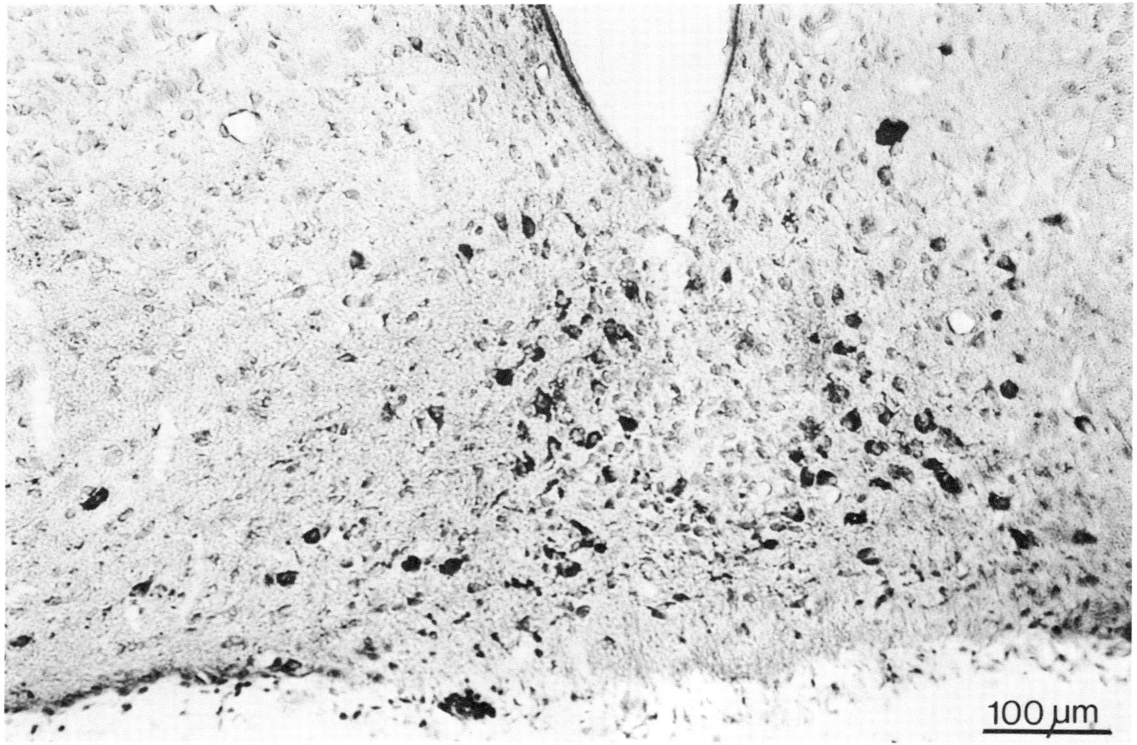

FIGURE 7 Immunoperoxidase reactivity to anti-β-endorphin serum of neurons in the basal midline hypothalamic zone, just posterior to the median eminence in the anterior premammilary region of the arcuate nucleus below the third ventricle. No colchicine pretreatment is required to demonstrate this specific immunoreactivity, and no additional reactive neurons can be seen in animals pretreated with colchicine in amounts sufficient to make the enkephalin-immunoreactive neurons demonstrable.

eral hypothalamic areas, and the median eminence. In the basal forebrain, neuropil staining is extensive in the nucleus accumbens, in the bed nucleus of the stria terminalis, and around the anterior commissure. Within the thalamus the main innervated target appears to be the paraventricular nucleus in both the anterior paired segment and the more posterior midline segment. Dorsal raphe and locus coeruleus are both innervated, but substantia nigra receives only a few fibers in the most lateral zone. Figure 6 summarizes the distribution of β-endorphin fibers and cell bodies in the rat brain and contrasts them with the several enkephalin-immunoreactive circuits, fibers, and cells (see above).

In comparison to the regional and cellular distributions of enkephalin-immunoreactive neurons and nerve fibers, it is of importance to note that those regions most dense in enkephalin fibers show no reactivity with these antiendorphin sera; globus pallidus, central nucleus of the amygdala, and interpeduncular nucleus are all negative for β-endorphin immunoreactivity, as is the whole of the substantia gelatinosa and dorsal horn. Direct comparisons of the β-endorphin reactive nerve fibers and those reacted in serial sections with anti-Leu-enkephalin sera (from R. J. Miller, University of Chicago) indicate that the β-endorphin fibers are larger and longer in a given region than Leu-enkephalin reactive fibers in the same region. Observations in serial sections of staining patterns with antisera to ACTH fragments (provided by D. Krieger, Mt. Sinai Medical School, and by R. DiAugustine, NIEHS, Research Triangle Park, NC) indicate that the regional distribution of this immunoreactivity is highly similar to β-endorphin as proposed by us for pituitary (68) and by Watson et al. (63) and us (68, 69) for brain.

These observations support the view first enunciated by us (3) that enkephalin and β-endorphin immunoreactivity exist within separate cellular systems in the brain of the rat. Similar observations have now been made in the mouse and pigeon brain (F. Bloom et al. and A. Bayon et al., in preparation). The distribution of β-endorphin immunoreactivity is superficially like that of luteinizing hormone releasing factor (LRF) immunoreactivity (70, 71): both systems arise from one or two groups of hypothalamic neurons, and both extend mainly to the diencephalin and dorsal midline thalamus. Nevertheless, a section-by-section comparison of the two patterns of immunoreactivity show substantial differences (F. Bloom et al., unpublised results), and are not in keeping with the suggestion that the same neurons may contain the same immunoreactive peptides (72). However, both the LRF-immunoreactive fibers and those reactive with antiserum to β-endorphin also innervate the circumventricular organs with regularity.

Finally, with regard to the suggestion (explored in more detail below) that immunoreactivity to β-endorphin is contained within the same structures exhibiting immunoreactivity to ACTH, and that ACTH and β-endorphin arise through a common precursor molecule (59, 60), it should be noted that the anti-β-endorphin serum RB 100 recognizes β-LPH as well as β-endorphin, and that uncharacterized antisera to human β-LPH (11) also give patterns of immunoreactivity similar—if not identical—

to those observed by us with RB 100 (69) and by Watson et al. (63, 64) with anti-ACTH serum. These data may be most conservatively explained, as we have proposed (69): namely, that β-LPH, β-endorphin, and ACTH may all coexist within the same neurons of the rat central nervous system (CNS) as they are known to do within the cells of the intermediate lobe and within the corticotrophic cells of the adenohypophysis (59, 60, 65, 67). The cells and fibers observed in the human hypothalamus with antisera to human β-LPH (73) are in keeping with this idea as well. Nevertheless, the question must be regarded as incomplete pending more detailed studies of the precise patterns and ultrastructural details of the neuronal elements stained with each of these antisera. Furthermore, unpublished observations by D. Smythe indicate on the basis of gel separation studies that rat brain, especially hypothalamus, contains no β-LPH-sized molecule, and mainly contains β-endorphin.

Critical weapons in these interpretations are the choice of the antisera and of the test tissues. In our hands, antisera to ovine or porcine β-LPH show no reactivity with rat pituitary or brain; if such lack of reactivity were to indicate that differences exist in the sequences or tertiary structure of rodent LPH, it is difficult to understand why rodent CNS and pituitary stain with the antiserum to human β-LPH prepared by Rao and Li (1977) because this latter serum is assumed to read the N-terminal region of β-LPH, where porcine, ovine, and human β-LPHs are identical. Furthermore, since Pelletier et al. (73) report that 20 μg/ml of β-LPH was needed to displace 100% of the [^{125}I]β-LPH trace, while 10 μg/ml of synthetic β-endorphin gave approximately 55% displacement of the β-LPH trace, it seems quite possible that the antihuman β-LPH (raised against unconjugated β-LPH) also reads β-endorphin. If that were the case, this uncharacterized β-LPH antiserum could not be used to prove or disprove the nature of the tissue constituent which exhibits immunoreactivity in rat brain. Our sizing experiments on the endorphin immunoreactivity of rat brain extracts (3) indicate that more than 67% of the β-endorphin immunoreactive material coelutes with synthetic β-endorphin, while the remainder was in some as yet uncharacterized higher molecular weight form.

Related to the controversy over the nature of the naturally stored β-endorphin, and its relationship to β-LPH, ACTH, and the 31,000-dalton common precursor (59, 60, 65-67, 74, 75) are the observations on sizing and bioassay of rat pituitary materials assayed by several groups of investigators. In these studies (65-67; 76), lesser amounts of β-endorphin were found with proportionately larger amounts of β-LPH in the anterior lobe of the pituitary, but only β-endorphin was found in the intermediate lobe.

Yet another controversial aspect of the distribution of endorphins is also associated with the relationship between pituitary endorphins and brain endorphin. Yalow and her colleague Moldow have suggested (77) that brain ACTH arises not from brain but from diffusion from the pituitary. This view stems from the correlation between ACTH tissue content and distance from the basal hypothalamus and infundibulum, and from their finding that certain commercially prepared hypophysectomized animals still exhibited ACTH immunoreactivity in plasma and in tissue scrapings from the sella turcica. This speculation on the nature of the brain ACTH source would therefore also be presumably leveled at the brain's β-endorphin content if it could be firmly established that β-endorphin and ACTH were made in (and released simultaneously from) the same cells. We have recently reinvestigated this problem to determine the validity of our earlier observations that brain and pituitary endorphin content were unrelated (3, 61). That conclusion was drawn on the basis of results obtained in rats which were maintained for several months after commercial hypophysectomy, and also on the basis of endocrine manipulations found to result in increases or depletions of adenohypophyseal endorphin and ACTH content. Devoting special attention to the issue of basal secretion in animals that showed no plasma β-endorphin or ACTH, and no detectable increase after ether stress, we also found no detectable ACTH or (ir) β-endorphin in scrapings of the sella turcica; yet these animals showed a distribution of β-endorphin and ACTH immunoreactivity indistinguishable from normal rats (R. Guillemin et al., in preparation).

V. CONCLUSIONS

Precise determinations of the distribution of the several endorphin peptides in central and peripheral nervous tissues have been accomplished by combinations of chemical separations, radioimmunoassays, and immunocytochemical localizations. The enkephalin-containing systems of the brain are distinct and independent from the three separate endorphin-reactive cell systems of the adenohypophysis, the intermediate lobe of the hypophysis, and the neuronal projection arising from the ventromedial regions of the basal hypothalamus. Enkephalin-immunoreactive fibers are also present in the sympathetic nervous system and in the adrenal medullary chromaffin cells of some species. These widely spread, overlapping, and independent systems of opioidlike peptides strongly favor the view that such substances perform many roles as communicative agents between nerve cells and their targets and suggests that pain suppression is but one aspect of their multifaceted physiology. Based on the distribution of these substances, physiological analysis is now urgently needed to make these determinations.

ACKNOWLEDGMENTS

This work was supported by USPHS Grants DA 01785, HD 09690, and AM 18811. We thank Nancy Callahan, Florence Rossier, and Elena Battenberg for assistance.

REFERENCES

1. D. Grouselle, A. Faivre-Bauman, and A. Tixier-Vidal, *Neurosci. Lett.*, *7*: 7 (1978).

2. R. Guillemin, N. Ling, and T. M. Vargo, *Biochem. Biophys. Res. Commun.*, *77*: 361 (1977).
3. J. Rossier, T. Vargo, S. Minick, N. Ling, F. Bloom, and R. Guillemin, *Proc. Natl. Acad. Sci. U.S.A.*, *74*: 4969 (1977).
4. S. J. Watson, H. Akil, S. Sullivan, and J. D. Barchas, *Life Sci.*, *21*: 733 (1977a).
5. R. J. Miller, K. J. Chang, B. Cooper, and P. Cuatrecasas, *Biol. Chem.*, *253:* 531 (1978).
6. R. Elde, T. Hokfelt, O. Johansson, and L. Terenius, *Neuroscience*, *1*: 349 (1976).
7. C. Gros, P. Pradelles, C. Rougeot, O. Bepoldin, F. Dray, M. C. Fournie-Zaluski, B. P. Roques, H. Pollard, C. Llorens-Cortes, and J. C. Schwartz, *J. Neurochem.*, in press (1978).
8. J. S. Hong, H. Y. Yang, W. Fratta, and E. Costa, *Brain Res.*, *134*: 383 (1977b).
9. S. Childers, R. Schwarcz, J. Coyle, and S. Snyder, in *Endorphins* (E. Costa and M. Trabucci, eds.), Raven Press, New York, 1978, pp. 161–174.
10. A. J. Rao and C. H. Li, *J. Peptide Protein Res.*, *10:* 167 (1977).
11. S. J. Watson, J. D. Barchas, and C. H. Li, *Proc. Natl. Acad. Sci. U.S.A.*, *74*: 5155 (1977b).
12. F. Bloom, E. Battenberg, J. Rossier, N. Ling, and R. Guillemin, *Proc. Natl. Acad. Sci. U.S.A.*, *75*: 1591 (1978).
13. T. Hokfelt, R. Elde, O. Johansson, L. Terenius, and L. Stein, *Neurosci. Lett.*, *5*: 25 (1977).
14. T. Hokfelt, A. Ljungdahl, L. Terenius, R. Elde, and G. Nilsson, *Proc. Natl. Acad. Sci. U.S.A.*, *74*: 3081 (1977).
15. M. Sar, W. E. Stumpf, R. J. Miller, K. J. Chang, and P. Cuatrecasas, *J. Comp. Neurol.*, *182*: 17 (1978).
16. G. Uhl, M. Kuhar, and S. Snyder, *Brain Res.*, *149*: 223 (1978b).
17. R. Simantov, A. M. Snowman, and S. H. Snyder, *Brain Res.*, *107*: 650 (1976).
18. R. Simantov, M. J. Kuhar, G. W. Pasternak, and S. H. Snyder, *Brain Res.*, *106*: 189 (1976).
19. G. W. Pasternak, R. Simantov, and S. H. Snyder, *Mol. Pharmacol.*, *12*: 504 (1976).
20. J. Hughes, *Brain Res.*, *88*: 295 (1975).
21. J. Rossier, A. Bayon, T. Vargo, N. Ling, R. Guillemin, and F. Bloom, *Life Sci.*, *21*: 847 (1977).
22. H. Y. Yang, J. S. Hong, and E. Costa, *Neuropharmacology*, *15*: 303 (1977).
23. J. C. Gillin, J. S. Hong, H. Y. T. Yang, and E. Costa, *Proc. Natl. Acad. Sci. U.S.A.*, *75*: 2991 (1978).
24. R. V. Lewis, S. Stein, L. D. Gerber, M. Rubinstein, and S. Udenfriend, *Proc. Natl. Acad. Sci. U.S.A.*, *75*: 4021 (1978).
25. J. Hughes, H. W. Kosterlitz, and T. W. Smith, *Br. J. Pharmacol.*, *61*: 639 (1977).
26. A. Bayon, J. Rossier, A. Mauss, F. E. Bloom, L. L. Iversen, N. Ling, and R. Guillemin, *Proc. Natl. Acad. Sci. U.S.A.*, *75*: 3503 (1978).
27. J. S. Hong, H. Y. T. Yang, W. Fratta, and E. Costa, *J. Pharmacol. Exp. Ther.*, *205*: 141 (1978).
28. R. J. Miller, J. K. Chang, B. Cooper, and P. Cuatrecasas, *J. Biol. Chem.*, *253:* 531 (1978).

29. S. H. Snyder and S. R. Childers, *Annu. Rev. Neurosci., 2:* 35 (1979).
30. A. R. Gintzler, M. D. Gershon, and S. Spector, *Science, 199*: 447 (1978).
31. S. Spector, J. Shorr, J. Finberg, and K. Foley, in *Endorphins in Mental Health Research* (E. Usdin, W. Bunney, Jr., and N. Kline, eds.), Oxford University Press, New York, 1979, pp. 569–575.
32. S. Atweh and M. Kuhar, *Brain Res., 124*: 53 (1977).
33. S. Atweh and M. Kuhar, *Brain Res., 129*: 1 (1977).
34. S. Atweh and M. Kuhar, *Brain Res., 134*: 393 (1977).
35. R. M. Kobayashi, M. Palkovits, R. J. Miller, K. J. Chang, and P. Cuatrecasas, *Life Sci., 22*: 527 (1978).
36. G. Uhl, M. Kuhar, and S. Snyder, *Brain Res., 149:* 223 (1978b).
37. J. Rossier, E. French, C. Rivier, N. Ling, R. Guillemin, and F. Bloom, *Nature, 270*: 618 (1977b).
38. A. Bayon, W. J. Shoemaker, and F. E. Bloom, *Proc. Natl. Acad. Sci. U.S.A., 75*: 3503 (1978).
39. J. D. Barchas, H. Akil, G. R. Elliott, R. B. Holman, and S. J. Watson, *Science, 200*: 964 (1978).
40. V. M. Pickel, T. H. Joh, D. J. Reis, S. E. Leeman, and R. J. Miller, *Brain Res., 160*: 387 (1979).
41. A. C. Cuello and G. Paxinos, *Nature, 271*: 178 (1978).
42. J. S. Hong, H. Y. T. Yang, and E. Costa, *Neuropharmacology, 16:* 451 (1977a).
43. J. De Olmos, in *The Neurobiology of Amygdala* (B. Eleftheriou, ed.), Plenum Press, New York, 1972.
44. C. Gros, P. Pradelles, F. Dray, G. Le Gal La Salle, and Y. Ben-Ari, *Neurosci. Lett., 10*: 193 (1978).
45. R. Simantov, M. J. Kuhar, G. W. Pasternak, and S. H. Snyder, *Brain Res., 106*: 189 (1977).
46. W. Zieglgansberger, E. French, G. R. Siggins, and F. E. Bloom, in *Effects of Opioids on Single Unit Activity,* Elsevier/North-Holland, Amsterdam, 1978.
47. R. A. Nicoll, G. R. Siggins, N. Ling, F. E. Bloom, and R. Guillemin, *Proc. Natl. Acad. Sci. U.S.A., 74*: 2584 (1977).
48. J. M. Hambrook, B. A. Morgan, M. J. Rance, and C. F. C. Smith, *Nature, 262*: 782 (1976).
49. H. Valtin, H. W. Sokol, and D. Sunde, *Recent Prog. Horm. Res., 31*: 447 (1975).
50. R. C. De Bodo, *J. Pharmacol. Exp. Ther., 82*: 74 (1944).
51. G. W. Bisset, H. S. Chowdrey, and W. Feldberg, *Br. J. Pharmacol., 62*: 370 (1978).
52. R. Simantov and S. Snyder, *Brain Res., 124*: 178 (1977).
53. T. W. Smith, J. Hughes, H. W. Kosterlitz, and R. P. Sosa, in *Opiate and Endogenous Opioid Peptides* (H. W. Kosterlitz, ed.), Elsevier/North-Holland, Amsterdam, 1976, pp. 57–62.
54. M. H. Puig, P. Gascon, G. L. Craviso, and J. M. Musacchio, *Science, 195*: 419 (1977).
55. J. M. Polak, S. R. Bloom, S. N. Sullivan, P. Facer, and A. G. E. Pearse, *Lancet, 1*: 972 (1977).

56. R. I. Linnoila, R. P. DiAugustine, R. J. Miller, K. J. Chang, and P. Cuatrecasas, *Neuroscience*, *3*: 1187 (1978).
57. M. Schultzberg, C. F. Dreyfus, M. D. Gershon, T. Hokfelt, P. Elde, G. Nilsson, S. Said, and M. Goldstein, *Brain Res.*, *155*: 239 (1978).
58. M. Schultzberg, J. M. Lundberg, T. Hokfelt, L. Terenius, J. Brandt, R. P. Elde, and M. Goldstein, *Neuroscience*, *3*: 1169 (1979).
59. R. E. Mains, B. A. Eipper, and N. Ling, *Proc. Natl. Acad. Sci. U.S.A.*, *74*: 3014 (1977).
60. J. L. Roberts and E. Herbert, *Proc. Natl. Acad. Sci. U.S.A.*, *74*: 5300 (1977).
61. J. Rossier, E. French, C. Rivier, N. Ling, R. Guillemin, and F. Bloom, *Nature*, *270*: 618 (1977).
62. D. T. Kreiger, A. Liotta, T. Suda, M. Palkovits, and M. J. Brownstein, *Biochem. Biophys. Res. Commun.*, *76*: 930 (1977).
63. S. J. Watson, H. Akil, S. Sullivan, and J. D. Barchas, *Life Sci.*, *21*: 733 (1977).
64. S. J. Watson, J. D. Barchas, and C. H. Li, *Proc. Natl. Acad. Sci. U.S.A.*, *74*: 5155 (1977).
65. A. S. Liotta, T. Suda, and D. T. Krieger, *Proc. Natl. Acad. Sci. U.S.A.*, *75*: 2950 (1978).
66. H. Yoshimi, S. Matsukura, S. Sueoka, M. Fukase, M. Yokota, Y. Hirata, and H. Imura, *Life Sci.*, *22*: 2189 (1978).
67. M. Rubinstein, S. Stein, and S. Udenfriend, *Proc. Natl. Acad. Sci. U.S.A.*, *74*: 4969 (1977).
68. F. Bloom, E. Battenberg, J. Rossier, N. Ling, J. Leppaluoto, T. M. Vargo, and R. Guillemin, *Life Sci.*, *20*: 43 (1977).
69. F. Bloom, E. Battenberg, J. Rossier, N. Ling, and R. Guillemin, *Proc. Natl. Acad. Sci. U.S.A.*, *75*: 1591 (1978).
70. G. E. Hoffman, K. M. Knigge, J. A. Moynihan, V. Melnyk, and A. Arimura, *Neuroscience*, *3*: 219 (1978).
71. L. A. Sternberg and G. E. Hoffman, *Neuroendocrinology*, *25*: 111 (1978).
72. G. Tramu, J. Leonardelli, and M. P. Dubois, *Neurosci. Lett.*, *6*: 305 (1978).
73. G. Pelletier, L. Desy, J. C. Lissitsky, F. Labrie, and C. H. Li, *Life Sci.*, *22*: 1799 (1978).
74. S. Nakanishi, A. Inoue, T. Kita, S. Numa, A. C. Y. Chang, S. N. Cohen, J. Nunberg, and R. T. Schimke, *Proc. Natl. Acad. Sci. U.S.A.*, *75*: 6021 (1978).
75. S. Nakanishi, A. Inoue, T. Kita, M. Nakamura, A. C. Y. Chang, S. N. Cohen, and S. Numa, *Nature*, *278*: 423 (1979).
76. R. Przewlocki, V. Hollt, and A. Herz, *Eur. J. Pharmacol.*, *51*: 179 (1978).
77. R. Moldow and R. S. Yalow, *Proc. Natl. Acad. Sci. U.S.A.*, *75*: 994 (1978).

chapter 6

Physiological Functions of Endorphins

Brian M. Cox and Eugene R. Baizman†*

Addiction Research Foundation
Palo Alto, California

I. INTRODUCTION

In the few years since the initial isolation and characterization of the enkephalins, extensive experimental studies in many laboratories have generated a considerable body of knowledge concerning the distribution, characteristics, and properties of the various endorphins. Nevertheless, it is somewhat premature, if not presumptuous, to attempt to assign specific physiological functions to endorphins at this time. It should be noted that the central nervous and endocrine systems contain several pharmacologically active peptides whose existence has been known for several years but for which there is as yet no clear understanding of specific physiological function. In this chapter we draw together experimental results which seem at present to offer significant pointers to possible or probable functions for endorphins, in the hope that this will facilitate the design of further experiments providing critical assessment of these potential roles.

We use the term *endorphin* as a generic descriptor to include all naturally occurring peptides that can activate opiate receptors. Met-enkephalin (Met^5-enkephalin), Leu- enkephalin (Leu^5- enkephalin) (1), and β-endorphin (2) are particular endorphins. The term *β-endorphin* will be used when activity has been unambiguously attributed to that peptide (e.g., by radioimmunoassay coupled with molecular size estimation). Where bioassay of tissue extracts has been employed without prior isolation of specific peptides, the more general term *endorphin* will be used.

Present affiliation:
*Uniformed Services University of Health Sciences, Bethesda, Maryland
†Sterling-Winthrop Research Institute, Rensselaer, New York

The location of endorphins in the central nervous system suggests a role in the regulation of nervous activity. Their concentration in pituitary gland suggests a possible hormonal function. In recent years, the distinction between neurotransmitters, neuromodulators, and hormones has become blurred. All communicate information from one cell to another. It is now widely accepted, following the pioneer studies of neurosecretion from the hypothalamohypophysial tract, that many neurons can secrete peptides to affect the functions of adjacent or distant cells. In this chapter we use the term *neurotransmitter* to refer to substances conveying information from one neuron to an adjacent cell in synaptic contact with it. The action of released neurotransmitter is short, thus allowing rapid response to a changing environment.

Neuromodulators are considered here as substances released from any type of cell to alter the excitability of neurons, and thus modulate the release or actions of neurotransmitters. Many substances that can be released into extracellular fluid could behave as neuromodulators, but proof that particular substances exert this function in specific physiological situations is generally not available. The term has value, however, in describing substances that do not share all the characteristics of neurotransmitters. In Sec. II and III we consider the evidence relating to a possible neurotransmitter or neuromodulator role for enkephalins and β-endorphin.

In the classical description by Starling, a hormone is defined as a substance released from a unique class of producing cells into the bloodstream to be transported to single or multiple distant target organs, where it regulates the function of those organs. The extent to which β-endorphin can satisfy that definition is discussed in Sec. IV. The possibility is also considered that endorphins may be transported from pituitary to serve a neuromodulator function in brain.

In Sec. V the use of indirect procedures in the study of endorphin function is discussed. Comparisons of the pharmacological effects of endorphins and opiate drugs with physiologically mediated phenomena, and examination of the effects of opiate antagonist drugs, have been utilized in predictions of physiological functions of endorphins. Finally, Sec. VI considers the role of endorphins in opiate addiction and dependence.

II. ENKEPHALINS AS NEUROTRANSMITTERS OR NEUROMODULATORS

A. Introduction

The purpose of the two sections following will be to evaluate critically current evidence for consideration of the enkephalins and endorphins as separate classes of novel peptide neurotransmitters or neuromodulators. We list the seven rather specific criteria developed for classifying a particular substance as a central neurotransmitter candidate (3-7) and concentrate on evidence relevant to a current understanding of the mechanism of action of the endogenous opioid peptides. The concept of opioid peptides as neurotransmitter candidates has received intensive recent attention (8–12); thus, these portions of the chapter will place special emphasis on new literature which has appeared in the last few years.

As described by Werman (3,4), a principal criterion characterizing a suspected neurotransmitter is one of "identity of action," which states that the substance should act similarly to the physiological transmitter at the synaptic level, mimicking the actions of presynaptic nerver stimulation. The subcriterion of "pharmacological identity" demands that agents modifying the action of the transmitter at the receptor should similarly affect the action of the exogenously applied substance. The presence of the transmitter itself in the nerve terminal is often interrelated with three auxiliary criteria; the presence (at or in the nerve terminal) of synthesizing enzymes; a mechanism(s) (either closely associated with or remote from the nerve terminal) for inactivating the transmitter (including diffusion, reuptake, and enzymatic breakdown); and the presence of biosynthetic precursors. Specific receptors interacting with the suspected substance are usually present in close proximity to presynaptic structures. *Collectability* of the transmitter after release refers to its detection, provided that inactivation is blocked, in extracellular fluid from the region of the activated synapse. According to Werman (4), only "collectability" and "identity of action" constitute the fundamental sine qua non for the demonstration of a neurotransmitter.

The following discussion describes the degree to which each of the two classes of opioid peptides fulfills these stringent requirements.

B. Location in the Nervous System

To begin assignment of a potential neurotransmitter/neuromodulator role for the pentapeptide enkephalins, we must clearly demonstrate their presence in central and peripheral neuronal elements associated with opiate receptor-mediated physiological processes. Unquestionably, the most significant recent advance in this area has been the pivotal development of immunocytochemical technqiues permitting visualization and mapping of enkephalinergic pathways and neuronal perikarya in the brain and periphery. An elegant summary of recent work on the immunohistochemically defined distribution of enkephalins (and larger endorphin) in the nervous system is presented in Chap. 5.

It is fair to summarize briefly that a widespread innervation of enkephalin-containing neurons and processes occurs within the central nervous system (CNS), in regions not only modulating sensory input (e.g., substantia gelatinosa of the dorsal horn; midbrain central gray; reticular formation; limbic areas), but also motor (e.g., caudate-putamen; globus pallidus) and autonomic outflow (e.g., hypothalamus; n. of the solitary tract) (13–20). Although quantitative differences have been noted consistently with respect to the relative radioimmunoassayable amounts of Leu-enkephalin and Met-enkephalin found in most brain regions (Met-enkephalin > Leu-enkephalin; 21-27), identical immunofluorescent staining patterns are observed for both pentapeptides in single brain sections sequentially treated with highly specific antisera (19, 20). Thus most studies suggest the presence of both enkephalins within the same neuronal elements.

Distribution of the pentapeptides generally parallels that of opiate receptors in the brain (28-33), intestine (21, 34, 35), and in other peripheral tissues, including sympathetic ganglia (19, 36, 37) and adrenal medulla (38, 39). Physiological functions influenced by opiates (vomiting, gut motility, cough, pupillary changes, motor effects, analgesia) thus appear to have neuroanatomical correlates which are rich in opiate receptors as well as enkephalins.

Furthermore, enkephalins, like opiate receptors, seem to be localized to subcellular fractions of brain, principally synaptosomal fractions, which reflect their presence at or in nerve terminals (40–44), and confirm immunocytochemical visualization within boutonlike structures (13-20; Chap. 4). It is generally agreed that classical neurotransmitters are localized principally in synaptic vesicles (5-7), and results from a recent study indicate the presence of enkephalins primarily within such structures (45). Caution is indicated, however, since presence per se within nerve terminals indicates neither ability to be released nor biological neuroeffectiveness once release is intiated.

C. Metabolism

The action of typical neurotransmitters is terminated at the synapse either by reuptake of the transmitter into presynaptic nerve terminals or glia, through metabolic inactivation by degradative enzymes, or by a combination of these mechanisms (3-7). Specific uptake mechanisms are virtually unknown for mammalian peptides, however (46). Thus work has centered on specific mechanisms responsible for the enzymatic catabolism of enkephalins in tissues in which they are located.

Early studies of the analgesic actions of the pentapeptides invariably demonstrated only transient behavioral effects without marked analgesia following heroic intraventricular or intracerebral doses (47-52). These results contrasted sharply with the prolonged analgesia and cataleptic actions of typical opiate alkaloids (49, 52-57) and the larger opioid peptides (58-62), when these substances are directly applied to appropriate brain structures. The low potency of enkephalins as analgesics has been attributed, at least in part, to rapid degradation of the peptides when exposed to enzymes from brain tissue. Rapid inactivation of enkephalins has been observed during incubation with brain homogenate (34, 49, 50, 62-69), isolated guinea pig ileum and mouse vas deferens (32, 70), rat plasma, neuroblastoma (71), and endothelial cells (72), and following intravenous (69, 73) and intracerebral injections (49, 60, 61, 65, 68). Since the finding that substitution of D-Ala^2 for Gly^2 in the pentapeptide moiety stabilized Met-enkephalin in vitro (50, 64, 68, 74) and simultaneously resulted in analgesia equivalent to β-endorphin or morphine in vivo

(49, 50, 60), additional evidence has accumulated for a principal role of metabolism in the poor antinociceptive actions of the native pentapeptides. For example, synthesis of a number of metabolically stable enkephalin analogs showing enhanced in vivo and in vitro biological activity has reinforced the hypothesis of rapid enzymatic degradation of enkephalins. With several notable exceptions (75-77), a general correlation was found between in vitro resistance to enzymatic degradation, and apparent increased receptor affinity in vitro (49, 50, 60), or in vivo analgesic potency (64, 66, 78).

The Tyr^1-Gly^2 bond has been shown to be cleaved by aminopeptidases. Thus release of free Tyr occurs, leaving the inactive fragments Gly-Gly-Phe-Met or Gly-Gly-Phe-Leu (63, 67, 68, 79). The hydrolysis is time, temperature, and concentration dependent (63-68, 78), and can be inhibited in a variety of preparations by the antibiotic protease inhibitors bacitracin (64, 66, 78) and puromycin (71, 80, 81), as well as several other reagents (82-84). Barclay and Phillips (80) reported that, in comparison with bacitracin, which had an IC_{50} value of 20 μM for inhibition of enkephalin-degrading enzyme complex in brain homogenate, puromycin (which resembles a tyrosyl analog of the peptides) was more potent (IC_{50} 0.8 μM; K_i = 200 nM). Without addition of such protease inhibitors, preincubation of enkephalins with washed rat brain membranes (or membrane fractions) at 25-37°C results in a 50-100% loss of intact peptide within 10 min or less when subsequently assayed (49, 50, 64, 66, 69, 78).

Substitution of Gly^2 with the unnatural amino acid D-Ala^2 greatly enhanced analgesic (49, 50, 60) and in vitro opioid potency (50, 64, 68, 74), producing a peptide similar in action and potency to morphine. This enhancement is apparently largely due to its resistance to plasma (63, 69, 73) and brain (50, 64, 68) aminopeptideases, and further supports the notion that degradation occurs at the Tyr^1-Gly^2 bond.

Binding of enkephalin but not D-Ala^2-Met^5-enkephalinamide was enhanced at 0°C (64), clearly suggesting enzymatic inactivation of the former. The L-Ala^2 analog is readily metabolized, indicating that it is the D-Ala^2 substituent, rather than the terminal amide, that confers most of the enzymatic resistance (50, 64, 68).

[^{3}H]-Leu^5-enkephalin degraded by aminopeptidase action in intact neuroblastoma cells (71) and in a membrane fraction of rat brain (81) proceeds at the same rate even in the presence of receptor-saturating (10 μM) concentrations of opiate narcotics, narcotic antagonists, native enkephalins, or metabolically stable enkephalin analogs (10^{-5} M), suggesting a lack of correlation between degree of receptor occupancy and rate of enkephalin hydrolysis. (Similar enkephalin-degrading activity has also been observed in neuroblastoma cells which do not bear opiate receptors; 71). Thus opioid/enkephalin receptors are probably not functionally coupled to the action of the enzyme. In the brain membrane fractions, bradykinin, angiotensin II, substance P, luteinizing hormone releasing factor (LRF), and vasopressin

(81) were found to inhibit the aminopeptidase. As in earlier studies, bacitracin (K_i = 32 μM) and puromycin (K_i = 0.23 μM) were also very effective inhibitors in both preparations, without interacting directly with opiate receptors or serving as substrates for the enzyme (81).

In contrast to the in vitro studies cited above, high-pressure liquid chromatographic (HPLC) analysis of enkephalin metabolites formed in situ following intraventricular infusion of [^{3}H]Met^5-enkephalin has revealed that the most rapid initial enzymatic hydrolysis of the pentapeptide occurs at the Gly^2-Gly^3 or Gly^3-Phe^4 bond, rather than at the amino terminal Tyr (77). Rat cerebrospinal fluid (CSF) did not metabolize the opioid, but rather metabolites in the ventricular perfusion fluid apparently resulted from its equilibration with a metabolically active brain compartment. Similar metabolites have been detected following enkephalin incubation with cultured human endothelial cells (72). Thus in addition to amino peptidase activity, another enzyme cleaves Met- and Leu-enkephalin to Tyr-Gly-Gly and Phe-Met or Phe-Leu. A similar (but not identical) enzyme(s) is apparently responsible for activation of angiotensin I and inactivation of bradykinin (72). Since only peptides with a free C-terminal are cleaved by peptidyl dipeptidase activity (72), resistance to the action of this enzyme may underlie the enhanced in vivo and in vitro activity of Met-enkephalin amide analogs of enkephalins (48, 66, 84).

The type of proteolysis described in these reports could be effective in rapidly degrading intraventricularly injected and peripherally administered enkephalins, as well as neuronally released pentapeptides, thus ensuring their short duration of action, consistent with behavior for a neurotransmitter.

A substrate-specific, high-affinity enkephalin-degrading enzyme isolated from a membrane fraction of mouse striatum has been described by Malfroy and colleagues (83). [^{3}H]Leu^5-enkephalin was rapidly cleaved to [^{3}H]Tyr and [^{3}H]Tyr-Gly-Gly. The enzyme, like that described by Craves et al. (77), appeared to be a C-terminal dipeptidase, cleaving at the Gly^3-Phe^4 bond.

Sterically protected enkephalin analogs showed markedly reduced affinity for the enzyme, while bacitracin exhibited some inhibitory potency. The most striking finding in this study was that, while both a high- and a low-affinity peptidase activity was observed, only the high-affinity fraction displayed a 60% increase in activity following a 3-day chronic morphine regimen in mice and rats. This remarkable observation, although requiring confirmation, suggests a feedback role for the enzyme in the development of tolerance and dependence due to chronic opiate receptor occupation.

In comparison to other peptidyl dipeptidases, the high affinity enkephalinase appears to be unique, exhibiting different substrate and inhibitor specificities (83), and is differentially distributed in brain, corresponding to the distribution of opiate receptors (85). In addition, it is a metallo enzyme, being inhibited by metal chelators such as EDTA and o-phenanthroline, whereas activity is restored following addition of Zn^{2+} (86). A similar enzyme has been described by Sullivan and coworkers (87).

Thus specific enkephalin-degrading enzymes have been localized to synaptic membrane fractions, as would have been predicted if the peptidase functions to inactivate the enkephalins in vivo. Enzyme activity apperas to be specific for the pentapeptides, several other neuropeptides [substance P, bradykinin, LRF, and thyrotropin-releasing hormone (TRH) being unaffected, or only weakly degraded (α-endorphin, β-endorphin; 83). Significantly, the high-affinity enzyme seems to have a heterogeneous distribution in brain, coincident with opiate receptor distribution.

Additional questions remain unanswered concerning enkephalin breakdown. Although several end products of proteolytic cleavage have been characterized in vitro and in situ, are these the sole products formed in vivo? Is the nature and degree of enkephalin metabolism the same throughout the brain, or do differences exist among cell groups? Most important, is the degradation of enkephalin subject to pharmacological and biological manipulation, and if so, what are the consequences? The development of specific enkephalinase inhibitors is an obvious direction for future research.

Although rapid metabolism of the opioid peptides in vitro and in vivo has been clearly demonstrated, some current work supports the notion that proteolytic cleavage alone is not the only determinant of the weak antinociceptive activity of the native enkephalins seen after intracerebral (i.c.) or intravenous (i.v.) administration. In several studies, the pharmacological effects of enkephalins on behavior (52, 88), the cardiovascular system (89), respiration (90), and body temperature (91) persists up to 2 hr. Dependence on Met-enkephalin has been established following osmotic perfusion of the pentapeptide into the periaqueductal gray (PAG), a finding inconsistent with rapid metabolic breakdown (92). Kinetic analysis of the metabolism of [^{3}H]Met^5-enkephalin shows an apparent half-life of 3.9 min (77) following ventricular perfusion, again suggesting that enkephalin, following central administration, should provide sufficient detectable analgesia. Met-enkephalin (10 mg/kg, i.v.) and D-Ala^2-Met^5-enkephalin (0.5–5 mg/kg, i.v.) both attain similar brain concentrations (metabolic half-life = 0.7 min), yet only the D-Ala^2 analog produced detectable analgesia (75). Previous studies have demonstrated that both opioids show similar receptor affinities in vitro, provided that metabolic breakdown of Met-enkephalin is blocked (50). Thus the relationship between in vitro potency, enzymatic stability, and analgesic efficacy remains unclear, and no satisfactory explanations for these discrepancies has been forthcoming.

Direct experimental evidence is still awaited to support the hypothesis (93) that the primary biosynthetic route to Met-enkephalin in brain involves conversion of β-lipotropin (β-LPH) to β-endorphin and eventually to the pentapeptide. In fact, recent findings strongly argue against this scheme, and suggest that major differences may exist in putative precursors of opioid peptides in brain (94–97).

Unlike the well-documented occurrence of β-endorphin, together with β-LPH, "pro-opiocortin," and adrenocorticotropin (ACTH) in the same or similar neurons and pathways in the brain (15–17, 98–101; and Chap. 4) and within the same cells in pituitary (98, 100, 102, 103; and Chap. 4), β-endorphin has not been detected following high-pressure liquid chromatographic analysis of extracts of striatum where enkephalins are present (94), or visualized immunocytochemically in the same neurons or fiber tracts with enkephalins in several other brain regions (16, 17, 98).

These studies imply that brain enkephalin may be produced via a biosynthetic pathway that is separate and distinct from that suggested for the larger opioid peptides (94, 104-107). Circulating β-LPH or β-endorphin of pituitary origin is probably not the source of enkephalin in brain, since hypophysectomy does not alter enkephalin content of brain (22, 108-110).

Furthermore, the current literature describes several high molecular weight opioid peptides, isolated from the CNS, which have not been completely characterized (94-97). Additional evidence for different opioid peptide precursors has been derived from analysis of other tissues such as the adrenal medulla (111, 112). Studies of labeled amino acid incorporation into enkephalins (113-115) have not yet permitted a complete elucidation of the enkephalin biosynthetic pathway.

As yet, no Leu^5-β-endorphin has been characterized in brain. Leu-enkephalin in brain presumably therefore arises from a novel precursor. Kanagawa and Matsuo (95), described isolation from porcine hypothalamus of "α-neo-endorphin," a Leu-enkephalin-containing 15-amino acid peptide with Arg-Lys-Arg immediately following the pentapeptide sequence, implying enzymatic cleavage from a larger cryptic prohormone. Perhaps the higher molecular weight peptides waiting to be sequenced (94, 96, 97) will turn out to include this novel opioid in one of their structures.

Thus it appears possible that Met-enkephalin and Leu-enkephalin in brain, and perhaps in intestine and adrenal medulla, may arise through novel biosynthetic precursor proteins, distinct from the pro-opiocortin system.

D. Evidence for Release of Enkephalins from Neurons

Among the most important criteria that a suspected junctional transmitter must fulfill, although probably the one most difficult to satisfy, is the demonstration of its release from prejunctional nerve endings when the appropriate nerve fibers are selectively stimulated. The isolated guinea pig ileum-myenteric plexus preparation provides a simple starting point for consideration of experiments suggesting that in vitro release of endogenous enkephalin may occur under certain well-defined conditions.

Since enkephalin is present in the myenteric plexus (12, 21), where opiates act to inhibit electrically evoked release of acetylcholine (ACh) (116), the effects of naloxone on ACh release from the myenteric plexus provided the first clue to opioid peptide participation. Waterfield and Kosterlitz (117) observed a 35% increase in ACh following naloxone pretreatment during field stimulation of this preparation. The increase was stereospecific, and implied that endogenous enkephalin modulated evoked ACh output. In experiments of Puig et al. (118), very high frequency (5-20 Hz) field stimulation of the longitudinal muscle-myenteric plexus preparation unmasked a short-latency poststimulation inhibitory response to subsequent (more usual) 0.1-Hz-evoked contractions. This response was about 55-70% naloxone reversible (10^{-8}-10^{-7} M), stereospecific, and in opiate-tolerant strips, exhibited cross-tolerance to morphine (119). These results, including the reports of Van Neuten et al. (120) on naloxone reversal of fatigue-induced inhibition of gut peristalsis, and the observation of a dose-dependent, naloxone-induced contracture of isolated ileum from stressed guinea pigs (121), imply that release of endogenous opioid material may be responsible for the stimulus-evoked inhibitions of intestinal muscle contraction. Furthermore, this neuronally mediated inhibition can be mimicked by the addition of exogenous enkephalin (or other endorphin) to the bath fluid (117). Direct confirmation of the electrically stimulated release of enkephalinlike material from the whole ileum preparation was obtained by Schulz et al. (122) by radioimmunoassay of bath fluid.

In a further study with preparations of myenteric plexus-longitudinal muscle preparations, stimulated at 10 Hz, McKnight et al. (115) found that by blocking enkephalin synthesis with cycloheximide and measuring tissue enkephalin concentration following a 1-hr period of stimulation, bioassayable enkephalins were reduced by 46%. Stimulation at lower (1 Hz) frequencies or for shorter time periods resulted in only small (5-18%) reductions. Reductions in enkephalin content were blocked by tetrodotoxin (0.3 μM).

Thus, together with its demonstrated presence in the nerve-plexus of the gut (12, 21, 34), the release of enkephalin appears to be neurally evoked and correlated with well-defined physiological activity (inhibition of intestinal motility); its actions are mimicked by exogenous application of authentic enkephalin; and both exogenous effects and endogenously evoked inhibition of contraction can be reversed by naloxone. The presence and release of enkephalin in the gut may serve to modulate ongoing physiological activity.

In the central nervous system, a direct demonstration of the release of a suspected neurotransmitter presumes (1) that the proper nerve pathway or set of axons has been identified and can be selectively stimulated; (2) that production and release of the transmitter occurs in physiological excess and can be detected in amounts secreted following excitation of nerve endings; and (3) that inactivation (diffusion, reuptake, metabolism, etc.) of the transmitter must be blocked (3-7).

The primary difficulty with application of these criteria in the CNS has been the inability of currently available techniques to detect release of small (synaptic) amounts of the peptide from a defined endorphinergic pathway without destroying the functional and morphological integrity of the region being examined (5). Thus only the resultant activity of a large population of heterogeneous neurons is reflected in these studies.

The earliest in vitro evidence for the presence and release of enkephalins from nerve terminals was provided by studies of brain synaptosomal fractions (34, 40), which were subjected to high K^+ ion in the medium. The finding of enkephalin release during chemically induced depolarization is necessary, but not sufficient per se to assume transmitterlike behavior.

Combining morphological studies and regional analyses of enkephalin-rich areas in the CNS with such techniques as brain slices has led to some intriguing evidence for the potential central release of opiatelike peptides.

Henderson et al. (123) reported a K^+-evoked, Ca^{2+}-dependent release of enkephalins (assayed on the mouse vas deferens) from perfused slices of guinea pig striatum. Another depolarizing agent, veratridine, was also effective in provoking peptide release in this study. Tetrodotoxin, which blocks Na^+ channels, abolished the veratridine effects (123).

Confirmation of these findings by Richter and colleagues (124) and Osborn et al. (125) has provided one added feature. K^+-evoked (but not basal) release of Met- and Leu-enkephalin immunoreactivity from superfused striatal slices was partly Ca^{2+}-dependent, and blocked by high Mg^{2+} concentrations. Interestingly, neither morphine (10 μM) nor naloxone (10 μM) altered basal or stimulated release of either enkephalin. Thus no evidence was obtained for possible autoregulation of release from enkephalinergic neurons of the CNS.

The globus pallidus, containing very high levels of the peptide, represents a likely region for the study of enkephalin release. Using superfused slices of rat globus pallidus as a model neuronal release system, Iversen et al. (126, 127) found that slow basal release (in the presence of bacitracin) of enkephalinlike immunoreactivity could be elevated 10- to 20-fold by a 6-min pulse of high K^+ (50 mM). Such release represented only 10% of total tissue enkephalin content. A much reduced release evoked by a second 6-min K^+ pulse clearly suggested exhaustion of releasable stores of the peptide, even though tissue content was 90% of nonstimulated control slices. Both spontaneous and K^+-evoked release were completely Ca^{2+} dependent, a requirement typical of secretion of other neurotransmitters (5–7, 128). However, in contrast to the neuropeptide substance P (129), the tissue content of which remains stable under these conditions, Iversen and coworkers (126, 127) reported a 60–70% loss of total enkephalin in tissue during the course of their experiements, suggesting a more labile storage pool of peptide subjected to rapid degradation by brain enzymes. It is possible that preparation of the slices themselves may have accelerated depletion of tissue enkephalin stores by releasing or activating brain peptidases. Not surprisingly, protection from enzymatic degradation was critical to the reproducible demonstration of basal and evoked release of peptide. Tissue content of enkephalin was similar whether or not bacitracin was present at the start of their experiments, implying that the peptide was protected at some intracellular site from bacitracin-sensitive degradative enzymes.

One major barrier to the study of in vivo release of the enkephalins has been the apparent rapid metabolism and inactivation of enkephalin once release has occurred. Following its inactivation, the peptide then cannot be detected by any of the currently available assay methods.

Initial suggestions that enkephalin may be released as a typical neurotransmitter in humans came from the work of Terenius and coworkers (130), who reported isolation of very small amounts of enkephalinlike material in human lumbar CSF, together with other components having opioid activity. This material was claimed to be similar in chromatographic behavior to authentic Met-enkephalin, but its exact identity and functional or pathological significance remain unknown. The presence of endorphins in CSF, and their possible pathological relevance, is discussed in Chap. 8.

E. Actions of Enkephalins: Electrophysiological Studies

Among the most stringent primary requirements for consideration of enkephalins as potential neurotransmitter candidates are the identity of action criteria and the requirement for pharmacological identity. The receptor-mediated effects of the endogenously released substance must be identical in all respects with the pharmacological actions of the exogenously administered peptide at the same synaptic site. An essential attendant criterion requires that antagonists of enkephalins also antagonize the actions of both endogenously released and exogenously applied peptide, blocking a particular physiological event associated with the transmitter. In addition, the presumed neurotransmitter must bind to the same specific receptors as the endogenous substance, and induce similar alterations in ionic conductances, producing changes in membrane electrical properties which ultimately alter cellular excitability.

This section evaluates recent pharmacological studies on the actions of the pentapeptides in a variety of systems, and concurrently examines the question of where and how they exert their effects at the neuronal level (see also the review by North; Ref. 131).

In the CNS it has been difficult to demonstrate that exogenous administration of a putative neurotransmitter produces the same effect as nerve terminal depolarization and that drugs which block the action of the natural transmitter at the receptor also exhibit similar selectivity toward the putative transmitter.

Generally, microiontophoretic application of enkephalins depressed the firing of neurons which were also depressed by opiates (132–151). Naloxone antagonism of the depressant effects of enkephalin (and opiates) on spontaneous or driven neuronal activity was reported by many (134, 135, 137, 139–143, 147, 148) but not all observers (132, 133, 136, 138). Two areas that were consistently excited by both opiates and the enkephalins included Renshaw cells of the spinal cord (149, 150), and hippocampal pyramidal cells (147, 150, 151).

In the hippocampus, excitatory responses to the pentapeptides are thought to result from their depressant effects on γ-aminobutyric acid (GABA)-ergic inhibitory interneurons (151–153). The resulting disinhibition of the pyramidal cells is naloxone and bicuculline sensitive (bicuculline is a GABA antagonist). Thus the effects of iontophoretically applied peptides depends not only on the specific receptors involved, but also on the intrinsic neuronal circuitry in the brain region being examined (153).

Rapid onset and fast recovery from enkephalin effects without the desentization or tachyphylaxis characteristic of morphine (134, 135, 139, 141, 145, 147) were common hallmarks of most but not all studies, and may be attributable to rapid metabolism (135, 144, 145, 147). Not surprisingly, the enkephalin-induced inhibitory effect on spontaneous or glutamate-evoked firing of units in the rat cortex and striatum showed cross-tolerance in morphine-tolerant/dependent rats (150, 151). Furthermore, the depressant actions of the opiates on brainstem neurons has been reported to be stereospecific (154-156).

In most brain regions, units were sensitive to both enkephalins and opiates, particularly in areas with a high concentration of endogenous enkephalin and of opiate receptors (21-33) [e.g., brainstem reticular neurons, thalamus, periaqueductal gray, caudate nucleus accumbens, locus coeruleus (132–151)] . Cerebellum and posterior cerebral cortex, sites insensitive to application of the peptides (139, 147), have low enkephalin content and lowest receptor density (30, 33). However, rat cerebral cortex displayed relatively low opiate receptor levels (30,33), yet demonstrated both excitations and inhibitions of cell firing (136-140, 147, 157). Tissue receptor density, therefore, may not relate directly with intensity of effect on a single cell.

In some studies, differential enkephalin effects were found on spinal cord dorsal horn neurons responding to noxious and nonnoxious peripheral stimuli (145, 149). Fairly selective reductions of nociceptive firing of laminae IV and V units were noted only after ejection of Met-enkephalinamide, D-Ala^2-Leu^5-enkephalin, or morphine onto the dendrites of these cells in the substantia gelatinosa. In contrast, nonselective depression of both types of firing resulted if the peptide or morphine was ejected directly onto the cell somata in the deeper layers. Each effect was antagonized by iontophoresed or systemic naloxone, however, suggesting the presence of opiate receptors in both regions examined. A general hyperpolarization of the cell somata in lamina IV and V (as seen in neurons of the myenteric plexus following enkephalin or opiate treatment; 158-160) could explain these nonselective effects, since similar depressions (not naloxone sensitive) were evoked by glycine and GABA at this site. In any case, application of morphine or the pentapeptides directly into the substantia gelatinosa, an area of termination of primary afferents and rich in opiate receptors, appears to selectively reduce firing of neurons believed to modulate pain transmission to the CNS evoked by nociceptive stimuli (165-168).

Significantly, while naloxone antagonised opioid actions in the dorsal horn, neither intravenous nor locally ejected antagonist increased nociceptive firing of neurons, suggesting that continuous local release of enkephalins was unlikely (145, 149). However, when administered into the substantia gelatinosa after morphine, naloxone actually enhanced nociceptive responses above control (145). This anomaly remains unexplained. In the CNS, the n. caudalis trigeminalis, containing the brainstem equivalent of the substantia gelatinosa of the cord, responds to iontophoresed enkephalin with naloxone-sensitive reductions in extracellularly recorded firing (181). Selectivity for noxious over nonnoxious stimuli was exhibited, as found for neurons in the dorsal horn.

Iontophoretically applied Met- and Leu-enkephalin excited about half the neurons examined in the n. reticularis paragigantocellularis (162). Bradykinin, injected intravenously excited these same neurons, and since the enkephalin effects were antagonized by systemic naloxone, specific opiate receptor-mediated activation of these neurons was likely. This area as well as its neighbor, the n. reticularis gigantocellularis, respond similarly to iontophoretic morphine (162), are selectively excited by peripheral noxious stimulation (162), and are the most highly sensitive sites in the medial medullary reticular formation for the production of analgesia (163). Significantly, they are thought to project to laminae I–II and V–VII of the spinal dorsal horn (164). The implication is that excitation of these neurons by opiates and opioid peptides may activate the descending component of a pain inhibitory system (responsive to bradykinin by a positive feedback loop) and thus lead to inhibition of nociceptive transmission at the cord level (162, 165–168).

Thalamic neurons responding to peripheral nociceptive stimulation were completely suppressed by iontophoretic application of GABA, Met-enkephalin, and D-Ala^2-D-Leu^5-enkephalin (136, 170). Peptide depressions were blocked by naloxone, but non-nociceptive responses were not examined for selectivity of depression of firing. The actions of both native peptide and stable analog were similar in onset and offset, suggesting diffusion, rather than metabolism, may terminate iontophoresed enkephalin actions in the neuropil.

Palmer et al. (157) suggest the possibility of functional differences in enkephalinergic responses of frontal cortex (where Met-enkephalin strongly depressed acetylcholine or glutamate-evoked firing) versus parietal cortex (where the peptide was much weaker). Alternatively, the opioid could be interacting with a neurotransmitter system with a differential distribution in cortical areas.

Questions have arisen concerning the exact synaptic site of action of the opiates and opioid peptides. Some workers suggest that opiate receptors are located on presynaptic nerve terminals (31, 155, 169), which raises the possibility that neuronal responses observed from iontophoresis may result from a presynaptic action affecting the tonic synaptic input onto the neuron under investigation. The actions of opiates to depress release of ACh from the myenteric plexus (116, 171) and the release of NE from the vas deferens (116, 172) clearly support this contention.

A dual pre- and postsynaptic localization for opiate receptors in the substantia gelatinosa of the spinal cord has been considered (33), based on anatomical observations and autoradiographic studies of opiate binding. An arrangment of interneurons making axoaxonic and axodendritic contacts with C-fiber terminals and dendrites of spinal cord cells is consistent with morphological data, and supports the possibility that enkephalins may be released from substantia gelatinosa interneurons to modulate incoming sensory information. Opiate receptor binding sites in the spinal cord, visualized by autoradiography (30, 31), are strictly localized to the substantia gelatinosa, and were reduced by 50% following dorsal root section (169), implying that at least half of the opiate receptors in the cord are located presynaptically.

Duggan et al. found that enkephalin, but not the depressant amino acids glycine and GABA, reduced spontaneous firing when ejected into the dendritic regions of the substantia gelatinosa (145), also suggesting a presynaptic site of action.

The actual membrane mechanisms underlying the changes in neuronal firing induced by the opiates or pentapeptides have been examined in several recent studies, which lend support to both pre- and postsynaptic actions.

Single neurons of the isolated, superfused guinea pig myenteric plexus responded to enkephalins in the perfusion fluid with rapid, concentration-dependent, naloxone-reversible inhibition of firing (143, 160), which was observed even in Ca^{2+}-free solutions (160). The pentapeptide was found to hyperpolarize the cell membranes in the preparation, preventing their excitation by reducing neuronal membrane resistance (143, 159, 160, 173). However, when enkephalin was iontophoresed directly onto the cell soma, no hyperpolarizations were observed, suggesting that the site of action of the peptide in myenteric neurons was not the soma membrane. Thus enkephalins may activate opiate receptors localized on cell processes, which induce hyperpolarization of the soma by electrotonic spread of current. Such membrane effects, which ultimately block neuronal propagation of action potentials, may be responsible for the opioid-induced inhibition of acetylcholine release from presynaptic cholinergic nerve terminals (116, 171, 172).

In contrast, enkephalins depress spontaneous neuronal activity, as well as postsynaptic excitatory actions of glutamate and acetylcholine in rat cerebral cortex, both effects being antagonized by naloxone (139, 157). Opiate receptor agonists were presumed to block the Na^+ conductance increase elicited by excitatory transmitters, such as glutamate (156). Thus the pentapeptides would inhibit neuronal firing by blocking transmitter-induced depolarization of the postsynaptic cell membrane (111). However, one cannot ignore a possible presynaptic action of glutamate, provoking release of the transmitter from a cell adjacent to that being recorded.

Furthermore, Zeiglgänsberger and colleagues (174, 175), consistently found that dorsal horn neuronal firing in laminae IV–VI (either synaptically evoked, glutamate-induced, or spontaneous) was inhibited by both Met- and Leu-enkephalin iontophoresed onto the neuron (175). Although extracellular and intracellular recording showed that these inhibitions were antagonized by naloxone, and the peptides non-selectivity reduced both noxious and nonnoxious evoked responses, these findings are at variance with those of Duggan et al. (145) and Davies and Dray (149). In the latter two reports, none of the opioids markedly affected spontaneous activity of spinal cord dorsal horn neurons, or neurons responsive to noxious stimuli, following direct iontophoresis onto the cell somata.

Since naloxone also antagonized the membrane depolarizations induced by glutamate as well as the peptides, Zeiglgänsberger et al. (174, 175) maintain that enkephalins induce blockade of a chemically excitable (e.g., glutamate) Na^+ channel, without altering membrane resistance or resting potential. The resulting decrease observed in the rate of rise of excitatory postsynaptic potentials (similar to that observed in vitro by Barker's group; Refs. 176 and 177) may reflect either a presynaptic depression of transmitter release, or a direct postsynaptic action.

Electrophysiological effects of opiates on cultured dorsal root ganglion-spinal cord cells are consistent with a presynaptic site of action. These cells, containing opiate receptors on their neuritic outgrowths (178), provide presynaptic primary afferent input to the dorsal horn (178). They respond to D-Ala^2-Met^5-enkephalin and Met-enkephalin in the medium with a reduction in the duration of evoked action potentials, but without changes in resting membrane potential or conductance (179). Naloxone completely reverses these effects, which were thought to involve an action of the peptides on inward Ca^{2+} currents (179).

In two recent studies of cultured mouse dorsal root ganglion-spinal cord cells, Barker's group (176, 177) has explored the mechanism of interaction of glutamate and enkephalin. Iontophoretic application of Leu-enkephalin depressed glutamate depolarizaions in a naloxone-reversible fashion. However, they argued for a noncompetitive interaction between the two substances, and suggested that the pentapeptides block glutamate activation postsynaptically, perhaps on the sodium ionophore without activating ionic conductances as do typical neurotransmitters. Membrane events for neurotransmitters, generally involving rapid activation of receptor-coupled ionic conductances, result in momentary alterations of membrane excitability (5–7, 176). Continued presence of the transmitter rapidly leads to block at the synapse through "desensitization." By contrast, the pentapeptides were found to display a long-lasting regulation of both voltage-independent and voltage dependent conductances, consistent with a neurohumoral mode of cell-to-cell communication. In addition, enkephalins were found to evoke excitatory effects (rapid depolarizations with action potentials) and increases in membrane conductance (176). Reversible depressions in membrane excitability without alterations in resting potential were also seen, suggesting that enkephalins may alter thresholds for conductance increases. These effects were generally naloxone-sensitive, and implied that both excitatory and inhibitory transmission may be effected by the peptides at specific synapses.

In summary, enkephalins usually depress firing of neurons in a variety of receptor- and enkephalin-rich brain areas, by a naloxone-sensitive, opiate receptor-mediated mechanism. Although neurons in the hippocampus and Renshaw cells of the spinal cord exhibit naloxone-reversible excitatory responses, the primary cellular effect, at least for the hippocampus, is inhibitory (basket cell depression), as in other brain areas. According to recent reports, this excitation may be behaviorally significant (180, 181).

Although enkephalins are basically morphinelike in their actions on single units, they are distinguished by their brief duration of action and somewhat reduced selectivity for depression of noxious over nonnoxious stimuli. Although disagreements exist as to the precise cellular mechanisms responsible for opioid action, furthur work with several novel in vitro systems may aid in clarification of some discrepancies.

It is clear that enkephalins can affect the behavior of neurons in several areas of the CNS implicated in the transmission of nociceptive information. The relevance of these actions to the production of opiate analgesia remains to be elucidated. In the spinal cord dorsal horn and its rostral extension, the caudal trigeminal nucleus, the peptides appear to influence sensory transmission with some selectivity. Differences in the neuronal responses among various brain regions may indicate receptor heterogeneity, or simply that opiate receptors mediating excitation and inhibition are located on different areas of the same neuron (e.g., cell soma, dendrites, or nerve terminals).

F. Interactions with Other Neurotransmitters

Primarily because opiate receptors are present in a variety of CNS areas also associated with other, classical neurotransmitters, the opioid peptides have been suggested to regulate the release of one or more of them, either in pain pathways or in other, more widespread areas of the brain and periphery. A variety of preparations have been used to assess these putative interactions and to compare them with the effects of opiate alkaloids. Predictably, the preparations initially examined for enkephalin effects were the mouse vas deferens and guinea pig ileum.

In the mouse vas deferens, exposure to normorphine (1 μM) or Met-enkephalin (0.5 μM) produced naloxone-reversible depression of norepinephrine (NE) release evoked by nerve stimulation (116, 182), but did not alter the amplitude or frequency of basal excitatory junction potentials, which presumably reflect spontaneous quantal release of NE from presynaptic nerve terminals. Met- and Leu-enkephalin (0.1-10 μM) also reduced K^+-evoked [^{3}H] NE release from the vas (183). Enkephalins, as well as opiates, may thus affect some process proximal to the stimulus-secretion coupling mechanism for neurotransmitter release, since only stimulation evoked (but not spontaneous) transmitter efflux was suppressed. In support of this concept, Met-enkephalin (2-8 μM) has also been demonstrated to reduce ACh release evoked by electrical stimulation of the guinea pig ileum-myenteric plexus preparation, an effect that is concentration dependent, correlated with the reduction in twitch height, and is fully antagonized by naloxone (116).

Intraventricular injection of Met-enkephalin (5-50 μg) or Leu-enkephalin (10 μg), like morphine and other narcotics (184), produced a dose-related suppression of spontaneous *in situ* release of ACh from rat cerebral cortex (185). The peptide effect is blocked by naloxone, and the actions of the opiate alkaloids in this preparation were stereospecific. The time course of the ACh suppression by the pentapeptides is remarkable (onset, 10 min; duration, 50 min) in view of the evanescent analgesic effects of intraventricular injection of Met-enkephalin (47-52), and suggests that alterations in cortical ACh output may not be involved with behavioral analgesia.

D-Ala^2-Met^5-enkephalinamide, in analgesic doses (10 μg), evokes significant increases in ACh levels in hippocampus within 15-30 min (186), an effect antagonized by naloxone and possibly relevant to peptide-induced excitatory effects on hippocampal neurons (151-153). ACh in cortex and striatum were unaffected. This elevation in levels may reflect a suppression of ACh release, since no effect on choline levels was observed in this study.

Met-enkephalin (0.1-10 μM) diminished the K^+-stimulated and electrically evoked ^{3}H-overflow from slices of rat occipital cortex preloaded with [^{3}H] NE, an effect that was antagonized by naloxone (187). It is curious that these investigators chose rat posterior cerebral cortex, since cells in this region were not responsive to iontophoretically applied Met-enkephalin (140), nor does the area contain a high opiate receptor concentration (30-33). Interestingly, however, naloxone alone added to the medium increased K^+-evoked but not electrically stimulated [^{3}H] NE release, an increase interpreted as a blockade of presynaptic opiate receptors inhibitory to NE neurons. Thus naloxone effects in two preparations imply participation of endogenous opioid peptides in the regulation of NE (187) and ACh release (184) from the cortex. In contrast, naloxone failed to affect resting or ouabain-stimulated release of ACh from rat striatal slices (188), suggesting a differential control of neurotransmitter release from this brain region.

Serotinergic systems have also received their share of attention. Following intracerebral injection of D-Ala^2-Met^5-enkephalinamide in the relatively high dose of 25-50 μg, Algeri et al. (189) found analgesia, immobility, and increased levels of 5-hydroxyindoleacetic acid (5-HIAA, a metabolite of serotonin), as well as elevated dopamine (DA) turnover in limbic forebrain areas. These effects were antagonized by naloxone. D-Ala^2-Met^5-enkephalinamide has no effect on NE turnover (190). It should be noted that 10 μg of this peptide, which produces profound analgesia when administered intracerebrally, produced no effect on 5-HIAA or NE levels in this study.

K^+-evoked release of [^{3}H] DA (and [^{3}H] ACh) from superfused slices of rat corpus striatum was significantly suppressed by Met-enkephalin (1-10 μM) (191). Naloxone (10 μM) again reversed the actions of the pentapeptide, but had no effect by itself on evoked transmitter release. Release of GABA from the hippocampus and histamine and serotonin from the hypothalamus was unaffected by Met-enkephalin, suggesting that despite the high concentration of opiate receptors and enkephalin in each of these brain regions, the peptide apparently exerts a selective regional suppression of the release of specific neurotransmitters (191). Not unexpectedly, the concentrations of peptides utilized in the majority of these studies (to 100 μM) was rather high, perhaps reflecting the fact that bacitracin was not present in the superfusion medium to retard catabolism.

Since enkephalin cell bodies and nerve terminals overlap in many CNS areas with those of DA, it is reasonable to consider an interaction between the two. Pollard at al. (192) described a reduction in opiate receptor binding ([^{3}H] Leu^5-enkephalin and [^{3}H] naloxone) to striatal membranes following injection of 6-hydroxydopamine (6-OHDA), or electrolytic lesions of the substantia nigra, presumably because of loss of DA nerve terminals. [^{3}H] Enkephalinamide binding to opiate receptors in substantia nigra was not altered by 6-OHDA lesions of the nigrostriatal pathway, but was reduced after knife cuts between striatum and substantia nigra (192). Thus enkephalinergic and dopaminergic circuitry appear to be intimately associated in these two areas. It should be noted that, while some partial agonist analgesics show affinity for DA receptors, a recent paper has shown that Met- and Leu-enkephalin, as well as β-endorphin, have no affinity for [^{3}H] spiroperidol binding sites in rat striatal homogenates (193).

The presence of high concentrations of opiate receptors and enkephalinergic neurons in the caudate nucleus and substantia nigra suggests that the peptides may exert a regulatory role on the output of DA in striatum, perhaps resulting in modified behavior (e.g., opioid-induced catalepsy or hyperactivity). The similarities in the biochemical effects of opiates and opioid peptides on striatal DA metabolism have been proposed by several investigators to be a link in the biochemical correlate of the profound motor effects exerted by these agents *in vivo* (194-200). For example, following intraventricular and intracaudate injections of Met-enkephalin (100-200 μg) or D-Ala^2-Met^5-enkephalinamide (6-50 μg), only the metabolically protected analog (and morphine) elevated striatal homovanillic acid (HVA) levels after 45 min (201,202). This increase was temporally correlated with the onset of peak motor effects (catalepsy and rigidity), and was reversed by naloxone. It was inferred that stimulation of DA turnover resulted from presynaptic activation of opiate receptors on striatal DA nerve terminals, since kainic lesions of striatal cell bodies did not alter the peptide-induced biochemical effects.

One further observation of interest suggests that enkephalin metabolism and DA metabolism may be linked in the rat striatum. Chronic (but not acute) regimens of haloperidol, pimozide, or chlorpromazine, all potent neuroleptics and DA receptor antagonists, increased enkephalin synthesis in the striatum (197), and exerted profound cataleptic effects when injected into this tissue (197, 199). Clozapine, a neuroleptic with minimal Parkinsonian side effects, failed to evoke similar biochemical effects. Thus, chronic receptor blockade, which induces an apparent increase in DA synthesis, also increases enkephalin metabolism, further suggesting a regulatory role for the pentapeptides in the striatum.

It should be noted that despite these numerous indications of a function for enkephalins in the striatum, the critical neuroanatomical focus for the cataleptic actions of opioids is suggested by Pert and coworkers (198,199), and by Browne et al. (200), to reside in the PAG and not in the striatum. Direct intracaudate microinjections of either morphine or the pentapeptides did not alter motor activity. Thus the cataleptic actions of the opiates after intracerebral or systemic administration may not result from their observed effects on striatal DA turnover; or alternatively, the opiate action on striatal DA turnover is mediated through some other region of the brain.

There is evidence that enkephalins interact with DA neurons in other brain areas. Bilateral microinjections of D-Ala2-Met5-enkephalinamide (0.03-2 μg) into the A_{10} area of the ventral tegmentum (origin of the cell bodies of mesolimbic DA fibers supplying the forebrain) produces transient behavioral stimulant effects similar to those seen following stimulation of this pathway. The effects were blocked by naloxone (203).

Enkephalins have also been suggested to interact with acetylcholine (ACh) in the striatum (188). Inhibition of ouabain-evoked ACh release from slices of rat striatum was observed with morphine, D-Ala2-Met5-enkephalinamide, and DA itself, only if the slices were obtained from 6-OHDA-pretreated rats. Opposite effects on ACh release were observed in slices from intact animals. Both effects were antagonized by naloxone, however, suggesting a complex interaction (perhaps involving disinhibition of striatial cholinergic neurons) among the various neurotransmitters and peptides of the straitum.

More recently, intracaudate injections of morphine (30 nmol) or β-endorphin (2 nmol) were reported to reduce GABA turnover in the caudate nucleus, while increasing it in the globus pallidus. GABA turnover was unaltered in several other brain regions examined (204). Local naltrexone injections antagonized these reciprocal changes, as well as simular alterations produced by subcutaneous injections of morphine. It was suggested that enkephalins might regulate GABA-ergic neurons in the caudate, since muscimol, a GABA agonist, induces both catalepsy and elevated GABA turnover when injected into the globus pallidus (205). In this system, it is likely that the pentapeptides are interacting with opiate receptors within the striatopallidal pathway that has recently been identified (206, 207).

Opioid peptides also interact with other peptidergic systems in the CNS and periphery. Studies of enkephalin interactions with substance P (SP) are the best documented. This undecapeptide, claimed to be an excitory transmitter released from primary afferent fibers involved in central pain transmission (208-210), shares a unique CNS distribution with enkephalin in intimate association with pain pathways (211). A number of other similarities exist in the behavior of SP and enkephalin. Both appear to be localized in high concentration in association with small-diameter afferent fibers of sensory ganglia in the substantia gelatinosa of the dorsal horn of the spinal cord (212). Antobodies directed against enkephalin label nerve cell bodies of apparent interneurons in the substantia gelatinosa, while SP-positive immunoreactivity is localized in primary sensory afferent axons (14, 211, 212). Both types of peptidergic neurons appear in close association with catecholamine terminals in the CNS (45). SP nerve terminals, like a substantial proportion of opiate receptors (169), disappear following dorsal root section (212), and [^{3}H] SP binding is increased 2-3 weeks after transection of the roots (213). SP, like enkephalin, appears to require a Ca^{2+}-dependent mechanism for release (123, 126, 214), and SP applied iontophoretically primarily affects neurons within laminae IV and V of the dorsal horn (215) as well as those of the n. caudalis trigeminalis (161), which respond selectively to noxious stimuli.

Early in vivo studies reported that mice injected intracerebrally or intraperitoneally with SP not only showed long-lasting analgesia in the hot plate test, which surprisingly proved naloxone reversible, but these animals also exhibited cross-tolerance to SP when chronically morphinized (216). Malick and Goldstein also observed analgesia following SP microinjection into the rat PAG, although others report hyperalgesia (218).

Frederickson et al. (219) have confirmed that low doses of SP (1-5 ng) elicit analgesia in the mouse after central administration. Higher doses, however, lost their analgesic effect, becoming hyperalgesic when combined with naloxone. Combination of SP and baclofen (to block postsynaptic effects of SP) restored the analgesic effect. The authors suggested that a presynaptic action of SP to release endogenous opioid peptides may be responsible for induction of analgesia, whereas at higher doses a direct postsynaptic excitatory response predominated. Dual opposing roles were thus proposed for SP and enkephalins in regulating neuronal activity in CNS pain pathways.

Another study showing naloxone-reversible analgesia and hyporeactivity with SP injected intraperitoneally or subcutaneously (1-5 μg) concurrently reported increases in DA and reduction in 5-HT turnover (220). SP, however, did not block naloxone precipitated withdrawal jumping in tolerant mice, agreeing with biochemical studies showing its lack of opiate agonist activity (221).

Morphine as well as the opioid peptide analog D-Ala^2-Met^5-enkephalinamide, produced stereospecific, naloxone-reversible suppression of K^+-stimulated SP release from slices of the SP-rich rat trigeminal nucleus (210). Although bacitracin was present in the superfusion fluid to retard enkephalin catabolism, very high concentrations of opiates (10 μM) were required. However, the substantia nigra, another CNS region with high SP concentration, was not sensitive to opiates or peptide inhibition of K^+-evoked release (210), again substantiating a selective regional CNS interaction of the enkephalins with a neurotransmitter-like substance. It has been proposed that primary afferent terminals may form excitatory SP synapses in the substantia gelatinosa with dendrites of lamina IV and V neurons. Local enkephalin containing inhibitory interneurons might form inhibitory synaptic contacts with the primary afferent nerve terminals to modulate release of SP. This relatively simple model, as suggested by Jessel and Iversen (210), may represent the morphological substrate of the "gating process" in the spinal cord (222). Mudge et al. (179), extending the observations of SP-enkephalin interaction to cultures of dorsal root ganglion cells, have reported the D-Ala^2-Met^5-enkephalinamid (10 μM) inhibited K^+-evoked release of SP, possibly by modulating the Ca^{2+} component of the action potential evoked in the sensory neuron. The effects of the opioid were blocked by naloxone (50 μM).

In summary, the enkephalin pentapeptides, like the opiate alkaloids, appear to exert their effects on numerous transmitter-like substances in the periphery as well as in specific brain regions. In most cases, enkephalins are inhibitory to the stimulus-evoked release of the transmitter, while spontaneous release appears unaffected, implying an interaction of the peptide with the stimulus-secretion coupling mechanism.

Of the putative neurotransmitters examined, SP is probably of greatest relevance to the analgesic action of the enkephalins, principally because of its strategic CNS location. Complex interactions in the basal ganglia with a number of neurotransmitters point to an enkephalin involvement in this brain region, perhaps in the mediation of the cataleptic effects of opioids. However, it is difficult at this point in time to assign definitive functional roles to other specific enkephalin-neurotransmitter interactions.

G. Effects on Cyclic Nucleotides

Cyclic nucleotides, acting as second messengers in the cellular response to neurotransmitter-receptor interactions, have been strongly implicated in the process of synaptic transmission (223). Consideration of the cyclic nucleotides as intracellular mediators of the biochemical response to opiate receptor stimulation has naturally led to examination of the influence of the enkephalin pentapeptides on their metabolism. The principal model system utilized for these studies has been the cultured neuroblastoma x glioma hybrid cell line containing a high density of opiate binding sites and displaying many of the properties of neurons (224-227).

Opiates exert a stereospecific, naloxone-reversible inhibition of basal (228) and PGE_1-stimulated adenylate cyclase activity (224-226), and block the PGE_1-induced rise in cAMP in these cells (229). This inhibitory activity of opiate agonists roughly paralleled their in vitro binding (226, 230). Similar, though short-lasting effects, blocked by naloxone, were observed independently by two groups (231-234), when Leu- or Met-enkephalin were added to the incubation medium. Thus the response to both peptide and opiate appears to be receptor mediated, and to involve similar populations of receptors in this preparation. In contrast, neither the peptides nor morphine inhibited adenylate cyclase activity in homogenates of receptor-free parent glioma cells (226-232).

Incubation of cells for 12-97 hr with continuously saturating concentrations (10 μM) of enkephalin produced a delayed increase in adenylate cyclase activity and returned both cAMP and cyclase to normal levels. Thus these cells exhibited a form of tolerance and dependence in response to prolonged incubation with the peptides (157,158), and adapted to the enkephalins (as to the opiates) with an increase in adenylate cyclase activity.

Dopamine-stimulated (but not basal secretion of) adenylate cyclase of monkey amygdaloid nucleus homogenates was completely inhibited by morphine and the enkephalins in a naloxone-reversible manner (235). Only the peptides (Met-enkephalin, D-Ala^2-Met^5-enkephalinamide) exhibited a bell-shaped dose-response curve, with maximum inhibition at 0.1 μM but no effect at 10 μM. Thus opioid receptors were proposed to interact with the catalytic unit of the DA-stimulated cyclase.

Alterations of neostriatal cyclic GMP metabolism have been observed following *in vivo* administration of the opioid peptides. Intrastriatal D-Ala^2-Met^5-enkephalinamide (12-50 μg), like morphine, reduces cyclic GMP levels in cerebellum (236). The biochemical effect was blocked by naltrexone, suggesting that opiate receptors in the caudate may influence cyclic nucleotides in other brain areas.

Blume's studies have provided evidence that opiate receptors may be regulated by an interaction with guanine nucleotides (237). GMP-p (NH) p, a stable analog of guanine monophosphate, as well as several other guanine nucleotides tested, reduced stereospecific binding of both [^{3}H] opioid agonists and antagonists and increased their dissociation rate from the receptor. [^{3}H] Leu- and Met-enkephalin were similarly affected. Childers and Snyder, in a similar study (238), were able to demonstate selectivity of the guanine nucleotides for inhibition of binding of agonists (including opioid peptides) but not for antagonists, a phenomenon well known to occur with Na^+ ion. Similar findings were later confirmed by Blume (239). Since guanine nucleotides are thought to affect receptor sensitivity by coupling the receptor to adenylate cyclase, these findings at the receptor level may be relevant to the postsynaptic actions of opioids and opioid peptides. To date it is not known if the receptor-mediated actions of opioids on neuronal activity result from a functional integration of cyclic nucleotide systems with membrane events, such as ion fluxes or membrane fluidity. There is some evidence that manipulations which increase and maintain intracellular cAMP levels do not alter normorphine-induced inhibition of neuronal firing of neurons in the isolated, perfused guinea pig ileum myenteric plexus (240).

Despite the findings that opiates and endogenous opioid peptides alter metabolism of cyclic nucleotides in vitro and in vivo, and selectively reduce binding of opioid agonists, there is no evidence to suggest that the acute actions of opioids on these systems is relevant for the production of analgesia. However, adenylate cyclase does appear to be implicated in the development of adaptive changes in tolerance, following prolonged exposure of cell cultures to opiate and opioid peptides.

H. Heterogeneity in Opiate Receptor Properties

Since the original work of Martin et al. (241, 242), contrasting the neurophysiological and behavioral effects in the spinal dog following administration of several opiate alkaloid congeners, evidence has been accumulating to support the concept of heterogeneous opiate receptors in the CNS and periphery. The concept that multiple opiate receptor subpopulations may be involved in the actions of opiates or opioid peptides is intriguing, especially in view of the multiplicity of potential endogenous ligands, and is indirectly supported by the demonstration of multiple receptor subclasses for several other putative neurotransmitters.

Lord and coworkers have suggested the existence not only of subpopulations of brain opiate receptors, but have also shown that guinea pig ileum and mouse vas deferens displayed differential relative sensitivities to morphine and the opioid peptides (243, 244). Morphine was found to be more potent in the guinea pig ileum than in the mouse vas deferens, whereas enkephalin had the reverse potency relationship. In the mouse vas deferens, enkephalins required more naloxone for antagonism than did the alkaloid (243, 244); β-endorphin, on the other hand, was equipotent in both assay systems.

On this basis, Martin's concept of a μ (morphine)-receptor was applied to the guinea pig ileum, and a mixed population of μ and δ (peptide)-receptors in the mouse vas deferens was proposed. Enkephalins have a higher affinity for δ-receptors than for

μ-receptors, the difference being greater for Leu-enkephalin than for Met-enkephalin. In contrast, morphine and related alkaloids have a higher affinity for μ-receptors than for δ-receptors, while β-endorphin has approximately equal affinity for both receptor subtypes (244). Recently, strain differences were reported in the sensitivity of the vas deferens to opioid peptides or to opiate alkaloids have suggested that in this tissue, the two receptor subclasses are under differential genetic control (245, 246).

In in vivo studies, Martin's work in the dog has been extended, using the intact, unrestrained dog, to delineate the disparate behavioral, EEG, and sleep effects of μ-, κ- and δ-agonists, and their differential sensitivity to naloxone antagonism (247). However, a more rigorous pharmacological analysis for receptor heterogeneity that can be used in vivo is determination of antagonist pA_2 values, Yaksh and coworkers (248) found the naloxone gave similar pA_2 values against both morphine and D-Ala^2-Met^5-enkephalinamide in measurements of analgesia after intrathecal administration directly to the spinal cord in rats. In another similar study, intraventricular injections of D-Met^2-Pro^5-enkephalinamide, β-endorphin, and morphine, in intact mice, produced similar pA_2 values with naloxone for hot plate analgesia, again suggesting that these compounds interacted with the same type of receptor to mediate this effect (249). In the rat tail flick assay, however, the pA_2 values for the opioid peptides were higher than that for morphine, raising the possibility of receptor heterogeneity in this assay system (249).

Further evidence for heterogeneity in opiate receptors comes from ligand binding studies. Recent work with high specific activity iodinated analogs of enkephalins, and with ^{3}H-labeled narcotics, has indicated that the binding site for enkephalins is similar but not identical to that for [^{3}H]naloxone (250, 251).

Scatchard analysis revealed the presence of two high-affinity binding sites, one which selectively binds the peptides, and another which has a higher affinity for the narcotics (252). Binding of both is pH and temperature dependent, and is selectively reduced by physiological concentration of Na^+ and increased by Mn^{2+} (252). The binding of labeled opiates and labeled opioid peptides are displaced by various agonists, partial agonists, and peptides with different rank orders of potency in the two systems (252-257). In general, narcotics are less able to displace bound [^{3}H]-peptide than to displace [^{3}H]-naloxone. Enkephalins, by contrast, more readily displace bound peptides than bound [^{3}H] naloxone. Thus different receptors, as proposed by Martin (241, 242), Lord et al. (243, 244), and Chang and Cuatrecasas (252), or alternative modes of interaction with the same receptor (257), might explain these findings.

Recent work has suggested that the brain regional distributions of the two receptor subtypes may be different. Support for such a finding comes from in vivo studies of Frenk et al. (258), who report that the analgesia obtained after Met-enkephalin injections into the ventrocaudal PAG and the electroencephalogram (EEG) seizure activity observed when the peptide (or morphine) is administered into the dorsomedial thalamus, may be mediated through μ- and δ-receptors, respectively, since higher doses of naloxone were required to antagonize the enkephalin-induced seizure activity. However, although other explanations, such as a differential distribution of degradative enzymes for the peptides in brain, could explain these findings, it is significant that Chang et al. recently reported that homogenates of a number of brain areas do demonstrat a differential distribution of opiate receptor subtypes in binding studies (254).

At this point in time, it has not been possible to relate a specific subclass of opiate receptors in the CNS to a neuronal system or pathway utilizing a particular endorphin, although the findings or differential distribution in brain of opiate receptor subclasses make such a possibility very appealing.

III. β-ENDORPHIN AS A NEUROTRANSMITTER OR NEUROMODULATOR

A. Introduction

At the initial discovery of opioid peptides in extracts of fresh bovine pituitary (259), in commercial preparations of ACTH (260, 261), and in MSH-containing extracts (261, 262), it was clear that these endogenous substances were much larger than the previously isolated enkephalins.

These initial findings assumed particular significance when the pentapeptide sequence of Met-enkephalin was recognized as identical to residues 61-65 of the pituitary peptide β-lipotropin (β-LPH) (263). Thus in the search for other related opioid peptides in the gland, an untrikonapeptide was isolated from camel (2) and porcine pituitary (264), found to consist of residues 61-91 of β-LPH, and unlike β-LPH itself, displayed typical opioid activity *in vivo* and *in vitro* (2, 58-62, 264-266). This substance, now termed β-endorphin, has generally been characterized as the opioid peptide present in highest concentration in the pituitary of all mammalian species examined, including the human (267), and contains as its amino terminal residues, the pentapeptide sequence of Met-enkephalin. Of the endogenous opioid peptides thus far characterized, three fail to bear this common pentapeptide sequence: Leu-enkephalin, Leu^5-β-endorphin (see Sec. IV.C), and α-neo-endorphin (95). The finding of opioidlike material in pituitary gland has proved a major impetus toward examination and elucidation of a potential neurohormonal role for β-endorphin.

In a search for larger endorphins in brain, early radioimmunoassay and gel filtration studies succeeded in demonstrating the presence of β-endorphin (17, 23, 24, 268) as well as β-LPH in the CNS (15, 101, 268-270). The hypothesis of a role for β-LPH as a prohormone for β-endorphin arose (93, 2), reinforced by immunocytochemical studies showing similar distribution patterns for the two peptides in CNS and pituitary (Chap. 5; 15-17, 98-103) (see also the review by Krieger and Liotta, Ref. 271). ACTH and β-endorphin probably coexist in the same group of hypothalamic neurons (16).

The presence of higher molecular weight opioid-containing material in brain (21, 23, 94-97, 101) and pituitary (98-100, 102, 271, 272) has been confirmed by several techniques, including immunocytochemistry (see Chap. 5) and HPLC analysis of brain extracts. Although the majority remain cryptic, at least one of these species, a 31,000-dalton protein thought to represent the precursor to both ACTH and β-LPH in pituitary (104-107, 272) and possibly in brain (15, 16, 98), has been identified and sequenced following complementary DNA cloning techniques (106).

A similar high molecular weight precursor has not yet been characterized to explain the presence of Leu-enkephalin in brain, although the isolation and structure of α-neo-endorphin (95) suggests that such a precursor should exist. It is likely that the several recent reports describing opioid material in brain, different from that of the known series (94, 96, 97), will resolve this question when the materials are sequenced.

At this juncture it appears very likely that regional differences between the more restricted CNS locations of β-endorphin and the diffuse enkephalin innervations constitute presumptive evidence for separate and distinct enkephalinergic and endorphinergic cell bodies and pathways in brain (Chap. 4, 13-15).

The distribution of β-endorphin in pituitary and brain is covered thoroughly in Chap. 5. The remainder of this section considers β-endorphin as a potential endogenous neurotransmitter/neuromodulator substance, and compares its properties, metabolism, and actions in the CNS with those of the enkephalins.

B. Metabolism

The following subsection concentrates on those aspects of β-endorphin inactivation relevant to its possible neuroregulator role in brain or pituitary.

In marked contrast to the enkephalins, β-endorphin is relatively stable to degradation by enzymes present in a variety of in vitro preparations (67, 68, 79, 273-275). The profound analgesic and behavioral effects after CNS microinjections of the peptide also clearly support a long half-life (51, 52, 58-60, 62, 84).

Metabolism of β-endorphin in several in vitro preparations involves a series of sequential catabolic cleavages by enzymes with widely differing specificities, derived from both the soluble and membrane fractions of brain (67, 68, 79, 275-280). Enzymatic breakdown apparently proceeds initially via endopeptidase cleavage at the 77-81 region, while directly sparing the enkephalin sequence at the N-terminal. γ-Endorphin and α-endorphin appear to be the primary metabolic products at neutral or acid pH, respectively, with formation of only small amounts of Met-enkephalin providing some supportive evidence for a precursor-product relationship (68, 273, 279). The shorter sequences are much more susceptible to both carboxy- and aminopeptidases, since bacitracin significantly prolongs their half-life without altering that of the parent untrikonapeptide (273, 274). Slow release of Tyr^{61} from β-endorphin, as reported by several investigators (67, 68, 274, 277), also indicates the action of an aminopeptidases, although it is uncertain whether the amino acid is subsequently released from the shorter metabolic fragments via exopeptidase activity, following initial endopeptidase attack.

Preferred conformational characterisitcs appear to play a crucial role in slowing the hydrolysis and inactivation of β-endorphin, thus probably bestowing its typically longer duration of action (275, 278, 279). A recent finding that β-endorphin may adopt a partial helical conformation in lipid solutions supports this possibility (281). The conformation of β-endorphin may favor hydrolysis at the 16–20 region while retarding direct enzymatic attack of sequences closer to the N-terminal of the peptide, thus slowing enkephalin production. Even in the presence of bacitracin, only small quantities of the pentapeptide were detectable after stepwise degradation of β-endorphin by brain homogenate, suggesting that the Met^5-Thr bond is not cleaved directly, but may proceed through hydrolysis at adjacent sites, followed by sequential activity of a carboxypeptidase at the cleavage point (68, 273, 274, 277).

Endopeptidase activity was found associated with lysed as well as intact synaptosomal membranes, did not copurify with those membrane components bearing opiate receptors, and was found distributed uniformly throughout the sucrose density gradient (273, 275). These findings suggested that the enzyme was not exclusively associated with the opiate receptor complex.

Palmour et al. (282) reported that free [^{125}I]Tyr was the principal product when [^{125}I]β-endorphin or [^{125}I]Leu^5-β-endorphin were incubated with a soluble fraction from brain, liver, or kidney homogenates, but other longer peptides, including [^{125}I]Tyr-Gly-Gly-Phe and [^{125}I]Tyr-Gly-Gly-Phe-Met (or Leu), were also generated in small amount. A half-life of 9–12 min was reported for β-endorphin in the absence of bacitracin. In washed brain membrane preparations, however, the half-life was extended to 2 hr for both endorphins. Thus the β-endorphin-degrading activity appeared to be principally in the soluble fraction and not associated with membrane-bound opiate receptors.

The half-life of β-endorphin following its intravenous administration in rats was estimated by radioimmunoassay to be about 10 min (283). β-LPH had an even shorter half-life than β-endorphin.

Storage of β-endorphin in inactive form within secretory cells of the pituitary may involve formation intracellularly of α-N-acyl derivatives (284). Such modified peptides possessed neither potent analgesic activity nor significant opiate receptor affinity, but were cross-reactive with antisera used for radioimmunoassay of β-endorphin. The possibility that such acylation occurs in vivo as a further means of inactivation (or even conservation) of the peptide might be considered.

In summary, little is known of the distribution, properties, cofactor requirements, or substrate specificities of the series of catabolic enzymes responsible for β-endorphin degradation. Furthermore, pituitary enzymes which specifically metabolize β-endorphin have not yet been identified. A comparison of the mode of degradation of the peptide in both pituitary and brain may prove of considerable interest.

As with the enkephalins, labeled peptides were not accumulated in brain slice preparations, suggesting lack of high-affinity uptake system (273, 274). Degradation thus appears to occur extracelluarly, although in this study it is probable that some of the observed breakdown occurred through intracellular enzymes liberated from the surface of the slice.

The significance of these enzymatic processes in the regulation of the turnover and availability of β-endorphin at its site of action in the pituitary or brain is unknown. Possibly, discrete mapping studies localizing specific enzymes involved in its breakdown may offer a clue to function. Since enzymes releasing β-endorphin from β-LPH have been localized to the adenohypophysis and pars intermedia of the pituitary (285), a neuroendocrine role for the larger opioid peptide seems strengthened, as does the putative precursor-product relationship between β-LPH and β-endorphin. Their common biochemical ancestry and unique tissue localization within the pars intermedia and pars distalis suggested that cleavage of pituitary ACTH to α-MSH or β-LPH to β-MSH and β-endorphin may occur at discrete anatomical sites to subserve a specilized neurohormonal function. Brain and pituitary probably contain several endopeptidases, each with differing specificities, which may be involved in the conversion of the prohormones to their active fragments. High-affinity, substrate-specific degrading enzymes, such as those found for the enkephalins, have yet to be characterized in either location for the larger opioid peptide.

C. Evidence for Release of β-Endorphin from General Tissue

Studies on the release of β-endorphin have primarily focused on the pituitary gland, and are discussed below (Sec. IV. B). However, some measurements of release of β-endorphin from brain slices in vitro are now being reported. When slices of rat hypothalamus were depolarized by K^+, a three- to fourfold elevation over basal levels of β-endorphin-like immunoreactivity (β-EI) was detected (286), resembling similar experiments with enkephalins (Sec. II.D). The release was Ca^{2+} dependent and produced significant depletion of tissue-releaseable stores of peptide, since a second K^+ pulse released only half as much peptide. However, only about 2% of the total tissue content of peptide was released. The gel filtration profile of the released material suggested the presence of larger species (including β-LPH).

There are indications that release of β-endorphin from neurons can occur in vivo. Two groups (98, 287, 288) have studied the effects of direct electrical stimulation of defined brain regions in humans on the levels of β-endorphin in CSF. In patients with intractable pain, electrical stimulation of the periventricular thalamus (98) or PAG region (288), both areas containing enkephalin and β-endorphin fibers, has evoked analgesia accompanied by progressively elevated levels of β-EI in sequential samples of third ventricular CSF. Increases as large as 13- to 20-fold over prestimulation levels have been reported (287). Coupled with earlier reports of naloxone reversibility of stimulation produced analgesia in rat (289) and humans (290), these results suggest that released β-endorphin or other opioid peptide might be implicated in the mechanism of stimulation-produced analgesia.

D. Actions of β-Endorphin; Electrophysiological Studies

The electrophysiological actions of the larger opioid peptide have been examined in a number of studies, and generally appear to be qualitatively similar to those of morphine and the enkephalins, although the latter produce more evanescent effects and are generally more rapid in onset. Methodological problems associated with reliable ejection of the peptide from micropipets, as reported earlier (147), have been overcome.

Extracellular recordings of neurons in the isolated, perfused myenteric plexus responded to β-endorphin (and the enkephalins; Sec. II. E) with a concentration-dependent, naloxone-reversible inhibition of cell firing, suggesting mediation by specific opiate receptors (173). These effects, from low β-endorphin doses (1-300 nM), may be due to hyperpolarization of the cell soma in this preparation (158-160). Furthermore, since these inhibitory actions were also observed in Ca^{2+}-free solutions, they were deemed not to be mediated by induced alterations of ongoing inhibitory transmitter release, or changes in transmembrane Ca^{2+} fluxes.

A systematic survey of peptide actions on a number of sensitive brain areas was described by Nicoll and coworkers (147) in a study comparing the neuronal actions of α- and β-endorphin with those of Met-enkephalin. The larger endorphins exhibited several interesting properties. Their inhibitory effect on spontaneous or glutamate-evoked firing was generally similar in onset to the enkephalins, but surprisingly, the responses in brainstem were only of marginally longer duration. The caudate nucleus and thalamus exhibited the highest proportion of cells inhibited by both peptides. A higher percentage of cells in cerebral cortex and brainstem were excited by β-endorphin compared to the pentapeptide, suggesting some divergence in their pharmacologic effect and raising the possibility of different subpopulations of opiate receptors differentially responsive to either the larger or smaller peptides. β-Endorphin, like the enkephalins, uniformly excited hippocampal pyramidal cells. Excitatory as well as inhibitory actions of the peptides were blocked by naloxone in all brain regions (147).

Simultaneous recordings from adjacent hippocampal cells have provided evidence that this apparent excitatory effect of β-endorphin may result from an inhibition of hippocampal interneurons, thus exciting the adjacent pyramidal cell (153). The inhibitory neurotransmitter GABA was implicated in these experiments, since the opioid-mediated excitation could be antagonized by the GABA antagonist bicuculline, as well as by naloxone. The excitation of hippocampal neurons evoked by opioid peptides may be manifested behaviorally by nonconvulsive, EEG-defined limbic seizures, which are commonly observed following intraventricular injections of β-endorphin (180).

Recently, recordings from a novel superfused preparation of hippocampal cells transplanted in oculo (291) have confirmed the naloxone-sensitive actions of β-endorphin in eliciting epileptiform spiking. The relevance of this excitatory effect in the hippocampus to seizure generation as well as to other behavioral expressions of opioid peptide actions merit further investigation.

In summary, the actions of β-endorphin on electrical activity of neurons do not markedly differ qualitatively from those of Met-enkephalin, although a longer duration of action for the larger peptide was expected due to its slower hydrolysis.

The electrophysiological results are thus somewhat at variance with the prolonged behavioral actions of centrally administered β-endorphin reported in a number of studies. This seems to indicate that, at the single cell level, resistance to enzymatic metabolism is not critical for prolonging the actions of β-endorphin, but other factors, such as diffusion of the peptide away from the synaptic cleft, may participate in a relatively rapid termination of its action at the receptor.

Confirmatory work is needed before it can be assumed, without reservation, that microiontophoretically applied β-endorphin produces effects at the single cell level entirely similar to Met-enkephalin. Indeed, Nicoll et al. (147) have suggested that the effects of the larger and smaller peptides may be different depending on the particular brain region examined.

E. Interactions of β-Endorphin with Other Neurotransmitters

As was true for the enkephalins, the effects of β-endorphin have been examined on the release and actions of several neurotransmitters in a variety of preparations in order to clarify its potential role as a modulator of neurotransmission in the CNS. Predictably, such studies have resulted in numerous claims that the primary effect of β-endorphin at the synapse is due principally to its interactions with one or another of the more well established neurohumoral transmitters.

Arbilla and Langer (292) were unable to confirm the first report of Loh and coworkers (293), which showed that β-endorphin (or morphine) inhibited K^+-stimulated striatal dopamine release from brain slices. Possibly, differences in K^+-ion concentration or exposure time in the brain slices contributed to this major discrepancy. However, β-endorphin (0.6-2.0 μM) and morphine (10 μM) did suppress K^+-evoked release of NE from occipital cortex (292). These actions were reversed by naloxone (3 μM) and were supportive of an opiate receptor-mediated presynaptic neuromodulator effect of the opiate and the peptide in the regulation of NE release.

It should be recalled that rat occipital cortex contains few opiate receptors compared to rat striatal tissue (30, 33), and exhibits rather low concentrations of β-endorphin (23) and enkephalin (21-27). Striatal tissue, on the other hand, also contains little or no β-endorphin in this species, as measured by radioimmunoassay (23), but appears to be moderately high in both enkephalin and opiate receptors (20-21, 30, 33). Thus assignment of any physiological role for endogenous β-endorphin in the regulation of neurotransmitter release in these brain regions would be premature.

Recently reported interactions of opiates with intrinsic GABA-ergic neurons of striatum suggest that morphine may activate enkephalin receptors located on these neurons, thus lowering GABA turnover in caudate, while raising it in globus pallidus (294, 295). Thus dopaminergic and GABA-ergic mechanisms have been implicated in studies of the behavioral and biochemical effects of β-endorphin, in attempts to relate some of the observed behavioral effects of the peptide, such as akinesia, to modifications of neurotransmitter metabolism in striatum. Low intraventricular doses of β-endorphin (1 μg), but not Met-enkephalin (100 μg), induced behavioral hyperexcitability, while higher doses of the peptide (5 μg) evoked behavioral depression and catalepsy (195). Dose-dependent elevations of striatal homovanillic acid (HVA) levels were temporally correlated with the development of catalepsy, and both behavioral and biochemical effects were antagonized by naloxone. On a molar basis, morphine was 14 times as potent as the peptide in producing HVA increases, but only 0.6 times as effective in producing catalepsy. Although β-endorphin may activate DA metabolism via an opiate receptor mediated pathway, clear differences exist in its potency relative to morphine.

In a contrasting in vivo study, Izumi and colleagues (196) found that intraventricular β-endorphin administration slightly reduced striatal and midbrain dopamine turnover without altering steady-state levels of DA or NE in a number of brain regions. Serotonin levels in midbrain were reduced, although the significance of this reduction is obscure. Interestingly, apomorphine (224) as well as L-dopa (296) also antagonized β-endorphin-induced akinesia. However, naloxone was not administered to confirm that the reported biochemical alterations resulted from opiate receptor interactions.

GABA turnover is reduced in the caudate nucleus, but elevated in globus pallidus and substantia nigra following intraventricular or intrastriatal injection of β-endorphin (1–10 μg). These effects, similar to those observed with morphine and the enkephalins (294), suggested that the actions of GABA in the globus pallidus may be relevant to the production of catalepsy. Muscimol, a GABA agonist, induces similar effects when injected into the globus pallidus, but not into substantia nigra (294, 295). The biochemical and behavioral effects of β-endorphin were blocked by naltrexone. Although the effects of β-endorphin in this system are clearly opiate receptor mediated, the complex neuronal circuitry of the striatum precludes any definitive statement of its putative functional or pathological role.

It is important to recall that β-endorphin and a number of other opioid peptides have no affinity for neuroleptic binding sites, at least in striatum (193). Thus the profound motor effect resulting from central administration of the opioid peptide are unlikely to result from direct interaction with DA receptors. In the nigrostriatal pathway there is also evidence for dopaminergic inhibitory control of ACh release within the caudate (188). The presence of opiate receptors here and in other limbic regions (e.g., n. accumbens) has led to examination of opiate and peptide effects on release and turnover of ACh in these areas. The implication in these studies has been that opiate receptors modulate ACh metabolism indirectly by presynaptic regulation of dopamine receptors impinging on ACh neurons. β-Endorphin, like morphine, when administered intraventricularly, reduced ACh turnover in four of five brain regions (cortex, hippocampus, globus pallidus, and n. accumbens) (296, 297). ACh turnover in the caudate nucleus, however, was unaffected by either opiate or peptide, suggesting a fairly site-specific action of these agents. Steady-state levels of

ACh in all brain regions examined were unchanged. In the hippocampus, the reduction in ACh turnover as well as the production of analgesia and catalepsy by intraventricular β-endorphin (ID_{50} = 1.8 nmol/brain) were dose related and temporally correlated. Both biochemical and behavioral effects of the peptide were blocked by naltrexone. The results suggested that endogenous β-endorphin acting in several selected brain regions on specific opiate receptors of cholinergic neurons (or excitatory afferents to these neurons) may serve to reduce ACh metabolism and thus decrease firing of these neurons.

A further study by the same group (298) showed that intraseptal microinjections of both β-endorphin and morphine selectively decreased ACh turnover rate only in hippocampus, without the production of analgesia or catalepsy. β-Endorphin proved to be approximately 100 times as potent as morphine in depressing hippocampal ACh turnover, and the actions of both agents were antagonized by naltrexone administered either intraseptally or systemically. The authors suggested that this highly localized reduction in ACh turnover may reflect an inhibition by the peptide of cholinergic neurons with cell bodies located in the opiate receptor-rich medial septum and fibers projecting to the hippocampus. Clearly, the dissociation of the behavioral effects of β-endorphin from the biochemical changes associated with ACh turnover suggests that opiate receptors in CNS areas outside the established analgesic pathways (165-168) may selectively modify neuronal (or behavioral) activity not directly related to analgesia. Possibly, other effects of the opiates can be correlated with reduced ACh turnover in these restricted brain regions.

In support of this contention, β-endorphin (10 μg, i.v.t.) elevated hippocampal ACh levels, but produced no changes in the ACh content of cortex or striatum (186). The biochemical effects paralleled the development of analgesia (30 min), and both effects were antagonized with naloxone. Since choline content was unaffected in any brain region examined, it was suggested that the peptide may suppress ACh release from cholinergic neurons, rather than increase its synthesis. Obviously, more work is required to directly relate the biochemical changes observed in these studies to altered behavior. It is tempting to speculate that the differential potency of morphine and β-endorphin in altering the activity of brain cholinergic neurons indicates the existence of different classes of opiate receptors in these brain regions, located either presynaptically or postsynaptically. With regard to the limbic seizure activity generated by intraventricular β-endorphin (180), such a suggestion is compatible with the observation that equimolar doses of morphine failed to elicit similar epileptiform activity (180).

Substance P release from superfused, K^+-treated slices of rat trigeminal nucleus also appears to be modulated by β-endorphin (IC_{50}, 0.5 μM) as it is by Met-enkephalin analogs (210). However, in slices of rat substantia nigra, which contains very high concentrations of SP, as does the trigeminal nucleus, no significant inhibition of SP release by β-endorphin (or 10 μM morphine) was observed. Presumably, not all SP-containing neurons carry opiate receptors that regulate peptide release.

F. Effects of β-Endorphin on Cyclic Nucleotides

The actions of β-endorphin on the adenylate cyclase-cAMP system in neuroblastoma x glioma hybrid cells has also been studied to compare its effects with those of morphine and the enkephalins.

The initial report that the pituitary contained opioid material behaving similarly to morphine in the neuroblastoma x glioma cell system was made by Goldstein and coworkers (299). A partially purified endorphin preparation of approximately 3000 daltons prepared from porcine MSH concentrate produced naloxone-reversible inhibition of basal and PGE_1-stimulated cAMP levels. This material was assumed to be principally β-endorphin, although related opioid peptides may have contributed to the total activity.

In the same system, β-endorphin was found to be less potent by an order of magnitude than the inhibitory effects of Met-enkephalin on PGE_1-stimulated cAMP (234). Wahlstrom et al. also showed that β-LPH_{61-69} and β-LPH_{61-75} were effective in concentrations of 10 and 60 nM, respectively, while Met-enkephalin reduced cAMP levels at 3 nM concentration (300). Brandt et al., in another study, confirmed that the endorphins suppressed PGE_1 elevations of cAMP at IC_{50} values of 5, 10, and 40 nM (for β-endorphin, α-endorphin, and γ-endorphin), while the IC_{50} of Met^5-enkephalin was about 1 nM. Naloxone reversed the actions of the opioid peptides and morphine (234).

In the Wahlstrom et al. study, the order of potency for the peptides appeared similar in both the receptor binding assay and in the cAMP system of the neuroblastoma x glioma hybrid cell system, suggesting that binding to similar receptors in both preparations was likely. Interestingly, the cultured cell system was found to be much less sensitive to the opiate alkaloids than to the opioid peptides, whereas the larger peptides were found to be approximately equipotent in both assays. This difference in relative potency suggests a possible parallel with the potency differences found for the peptides and opiate alkaloids in guinea pig ileum and mouse vas deferens (243, 244), and implies that the opiate receptors in neuroblastoma x glioma hybrid cells selectively bind δ-receptor agonists.

IV. ENDORPHINS AS HORMONES

A. Introduction

Much of the opioid activity in pituitary gland is attributable to β-endorphin, although there is evidence that other opioid peptides are present (301-303). Possible physiological roles for these other peptides have not yet been explored. The discussion in this section is therefore mainly concerned with β-endorphin.

The high concentration of β-endorphin in pituitary gland (see Chap. 5) naturally suggested that this peptide might function as a hormone, released from the gland by appropriate stimuli to be carried by the circulation to distant target organs. The synthesis of β-endorphin as a coproduct in the synthesis of ACTH, β-MSH, β-LPH, and α-MSH (see Chap. 2), and its storage in the form of the precursor, β-LPH, in intracellular granules that also contain ACTH (102) imply that β-endorphin might be mobilized by factors that promote release of these peptides, to play a role complementary to that of ACTH or MSH. An alternative hypothesis, that β-endorphin in pituitary is simply a by-product of ACTH synthesis now rendered redundant by evolution, cannot be rejected at present. However, the apparent conservation over a range of mammalian species from rodents to humans of the amino acid sequences of the peptide that confer high potency as an opiate receptor agonist or protect against rapid degradation by exopeptidases, whereas other regions with no known function near the amino terminus of β-LPH show considerable species variation, suggests that β-endorphin offers advantage to species survival as an opiate receptor ligand.

In establishing a hormonal role for β-endorphin it will be necessary to show (1) its release form the pituitary gland by specific stimuli, (2) its transport in blood, and (3) its action on some distant target organ that is adequately sensitive to the concentrations of free peptide in blood which result from the application of releasing stimuli.

B. Release of Endorphin from Pituitary

Very sensitive and specific assays are required for the demonstrtation of the release of β-endorphin into blood. However, the concentration of endorphin activity in the pituitary gland is such that the content of the separated lobes of a single rat pituitary can be estimated by measuring the displacement by a gland extract of radioactive opiate receptor ligand from receptors in brain tissue (304). Radioimmunoassays for β-endorphin have also been developed (305, 306). These assays can be used to measure gland content, and are also sensitive enough to allow the measurement of circulating β-endorphin in animals.

An indirect approach to the demonstration of release of endorphin is to measure changes in pituitary gland content following the application of possible releasing stimuli. The synthetic relation of β-endorphin and ACTH and MSH naturally suggests that procedures that provoke the release of these peptides might also release endorphins. The high concentration of β-endorphin in the pars intermedia (103, 302), where MSH is also stored, made this an interesting tissue to consider initially. A number of stimuli have been shown to induce changes in pituitary MSH content associated with increased release into the circulation. However, different groups have frequently obtained conflicting results in experiments utilizing similar procedures. Thus Howe and Thody (307) have reported that bilateral lesions of the paraventricular nucleus of rat hypothalamus increased neurointermediate lobe MSH content, and increased circulating levels of β-MSH (308). In contrast, Taleisnik and coworkers (309) observed a fall in pituitary MSH levels. In each case the gland levels were estimated by bioassay. Another stimulus acting on the hypothalamohypophysial system, dehydration through hypertonic saline loading, has given similar divergent results, both in respect to changes in neurointermediate lobe vasopressin (310) and MSH (311-313) stores. It seems likely that measurements of gland content are complicated by multiple effects of the applied stimulus; both release of peptide and synthesis of new peptide are promoted. Thus dehydration has been shown to cause both the release and synthesis of vasopressin (314). The relative balance of these two actions, a balance that may be influenced by many factors, will determine whether gland content increases, decreases, or remains unchanged.

In studies of pituitary endorphin content, bilateral lesions of the paraventricular nucleus (PVN) were found not to change gland levels. However, a controlled suckling stimulus in lactating rats (a stimulus acting through the PVN to induce oxytocin release from the neurophypophysis) increased neurointermediate lobe endorphin without affecting the levels of endorphin in the anterior lobe (315). A longer term stimulus to neurohypophysial hormone release, dehydration induced by administration of hypertonic saline, reduced neurointermediate lobe endorphin levels substantially, while having a lesser effect on anterior lobe endorphin (315, 316). This treatment is known to produce histological changes in the pars intermedia (317). Rats of the Brattleboro strain, with diabetes insipidus of genetic origin, had lower neurointermediate lobe endorphin content (and concentration, expressed per milligram of protein) than Sprague-Dawley rats of equivalent weight (316).

The changes in neurointermediate lobe endorphin content resulting from suckling or dehydration are presumed to result from increased synthesis of endorphin and increased release into the circulation. So far, however, no measurements of circulating levels of β-endorphin following application of these stimuli have been reported. Thus the available evidence suggests that, while pituitary endorphin stores do not depend on the integrity of the paraventricular nucleus, stimuli provoking transport, synthesis, and release of neurhypophysial hormones affect the storage and release of neurointermediate lobe endorphin. Direct stimulation of endorphin release by vasopressin, and subsequent regulation of vasopressin release by endorphin, has been proposed (316).

Recently, it has been shown that immunoreactive Leu-enkephalin and Met-enkephalin are present in varicose nerve fibers localized in the pars nervosa of rat pituitary, at a total enkephalin concentration of about 4 pmol per lobe (318). This level was reduced by about 60% by dehydration induced by replacement of drinking water by 2% NaCl solution over a period of 5 days, a stimulus which also substantially depletes vasopressin stores. Neural lobe enkephalin levels were also lower in polyuric homozygous Brattleboro rats than in heterozygote littermate control with normal urine production. The possible functions of endorphins in control of neurohypophysial hormone release are discussed in Sec. IV. D.

ACTH release is provoked by procedures lowering the circulating levels of corticosteroids such as adrenalectomy, and by stress. Guillemin and his colleagues have shown that pituitary β-endorphin content is increased following adrenalectomy. (319). This increase presumably occurred in the anterior lobe, since Mata et al. (316), using a bioassay, did not find changes in neurointermediate lobe endorphin following adrenalectomy. The elevation of gland content was accompanied by an increase in the circulating level of β-endorphin (319). Severe stress has also been shown to affect anterior lobe endorphin content, and to increase circulating levels of plasma β-endorphin. Thus the application of inescapable electric shocks to rats through the floor of the cage resulted in a decline in anterior lobe endorphin of greater magnitude with increasing duration of stimulation. Rats treated in this way had elevated plasma levels of β-endorphin, measured by radioimmunoassay (32). The severe acute stress of limb fracture increases plasma β-endorphin levels by 50% (314). These studies by Guillemin and his colleagues (319, 320) have shown a close parallelism between the release of β-endorphin and ACTH.

Both foot shock and limb fracture are inherently painful procedures. Since endophins are potent analgesics when they gain access to appropriate structures in the central nervous system (see Chap. 7), it is possible that the release of β-endorphin from the pituitary provoked by these stimuli occurs as a consequence of the painful nature of the stimulus. Rats can also be stressed by immobilization in various ways, an insult that increases plasma corticosterone (321), presumably as a result of ACTH release. This stress is not painful to the animals. Nevertheless, rats immobilized for 3 hr had lower anterior lobe endorphin levels than control rats kept in the home cage (315). It appears that release of endorphin from the anterior lobe is not dependent on the presence of a nociceptive component of the applied stress.

β-Endorphin release has also been studied in in vitro pituitary preparations. A K^+-evoked, Ca^{2+}-dependent release of β-endorphin immunoreactivity (β-EI) occurs from isolated whole rat pituitary (322), anterior lobe (323), primary pituitary cell cultures (324, 325), and pituitary tumor cells (326). Incubation of the isolated pituitary gland (323) and dispersed anterior pituitary cells (320–322) with purified hypothalamic corticotropin releasing factor (CRF) promoted a dexamethasone-sensitive release of β-EI, as well as ACTH and β-LPH secretion. Thus CRF or glucocorticoids may function physiologically as regulators of pituitary secretion of these hormones. Several other substances (ACTH itself, SP, opioid peptides, naloxone) were ineffective in evoking β-EI release from anterior lobe, up to a concentration of 10 μM. In addition to control by dexamethasone, release of β-EI from whole pituitary is inhibitied by DA (327). Secretion for isolated cells is stimulated by α-adrenergic agents (epinephrine, NE, phenylephrine), which also release ACTH (324, 325), thus implicating catecholaminergic mechanisms in secretions of the peptides. ACTH, in low concentrations (10^{-7} M) is effective in suppressing release of β-endorphin from anterior pituitary lobes, when secretion is evoked by CRF (322, 323).

Less specific hormonal releasing agents (dibutyryl-cAMP, theophylline, 3-isobutylmethylxanthine) evoke similar actions on basal β-endorphin secretion (324, 325). Preincubation of cultured pituitary cells with dexamethasone nonselectively suppresses spontaneous release of β-EI and ACTH from this preparation, as well as that evoked by a number of secretagogs (324, 325).

β-Endorphin stores in discrete areas of rat pituitary may be under differential control. Herz's group found that although basal efflux of β-EI from isolated anterior lobes was lower than that for intermediate lobes, a 50 mM K^+ pulse only evoked β-endorphin secretion from adenohypophysis (322). They suggest the possibility that isolation of pituitary may result in disinhibition and maximum activity in the intermediate lobe cells, rendering them insensitive to further stimulation. The finding generally supports previous studies in which secrtagogs are usually ineffective in altering hormonal release from pars intermedia (e.g., ACTH; Ref. 328).

Evidence does suggest that intermediate lobe may be under tonic inhibitory neural control (317, 329), and that precursor processing to β-LPH and hence to β-endorphin in this lobe may occur more readily than in anterior lobe (330). For example, Herz and coworkers find that β-EI and β-LPH were released in parallel from isolated anterior lobe, but only basal secretion of β-EI was detected for intermediate lobe (323). The implication is clearly that release, regulation, and metabolic processing of peptides in anterior and neurointermediate lobes may differ markedly. Whereas adenohypophyseal secretion is controlled by specific releasing factors, the intermediate lobe may be under tonic inhibitory control by the CNS.

Although further studies of factors regulating endorphin release from the pituitary gland are needed, some consistent findings are beginning to emerge. Release of ACTH from the anterior pituitary is accompanied by the release of β-endorphin and/or β-LPH in comparable amounts (319). Measurement of the endorphin content of the separated lobes of the pituitary suggest that the endorphin released in stress derives principally from the adenohypophysis (315).

The release of β-endorphin from the pars intermedia into the circulation is less well established. Indirect evidence suggests that factors resulting in the secretion of neurohypophysial hormones also release endorphin from the pars intermedia. Thus it becomes necessary to assume that the stores in the two lobes of the pituitary are controlled by separate mechanisms. There is increasing evidence that the processing and release of ACTH- and MSH-containing peptides in pars intermedia and pars distalis are also differentially regulated (331, 332).

C. Endorphins in Blood

Initial attempts to demonstrate the presence of endorphin in blood utilized bioassay procedures. These assays have the advantage that material isolated from a body fluid such as blood with activity in a bioassay must be presumed to have some functional relevance. However, bioassays suffer from the disadvantages (1) that they are insensitive relative to radioimmunoassay; (2) that where several active substances of unknown structure but similar pharmacological properties coexist, it is difficult to determine the relative contribution of the various active substances; and (3) that the assay may readily be invalidated by other nonopioid substances present in crude extracts.

Several reports of the presence in blood of substances active in opiate bioassays have appeared. In each case the active principal(s) have not yet been identified, but the reported properties of the crude extracts suggest that the active materials are not identical. Pert et al. (333) measured displacement (by extracts of human and rat plasma) of [^{3}H]naloxone binding to opiate receptors in homogenized brain membranes. They described a low molecular weight lipophilic substance, which they termed "anodynin," that differed from previously isolated opioid peptides in its physical properties and sensitivity to enzymatic degradation. Injection of the partially purified extract into the PAG region of the brain of conscious rats resulted in a mild analgesia that could be antagonized by naloxone. In plasma from hypophysectomized rats, the level of anodynin was less than 5% of control levels, suggesting that the pituitary gland was implicated in the maintenance of the circulating levels of this substance. However, no further information on the chemical nature of anodynin, or its relation to pituitary endorphins derived from β-LPH, has been forthcoming. Opioid materials in blood and other body fluids have been described by Schulz et al. (334) and by Cox et al. (335). There was high variability in the levels of these substances. The absence of information on their chemical structure, or of their relationship to the pituitary gland, precludes further discussion of their relationship to a possible hormonal role of β-endorphin.

Radioimmunoassays utilizing antisera specific for sequences of the β-endorphin molecule can detect much lower concentrations of this peptide than bioassay, with some certainty that only the peptides containing the appropriate amino acid sequence will be measured. However, there can also be some ambiguity in the interpretation of radioimmunoassays. Both prohormones (336, 104) and some biologically inactive metabolites will contain the amino acid sequence recognized by the antibody, and will therefore contribute to some extent to the observed immunoreactivity if they are present.

Employing an antiserum raised to β-endorphin that specifically recognizes the amino acid sequence in the 20–27 position of β-endorphin, Guillemin and his colleagues (319) have identified a β-endorphin-like material in rat plasma. Estimates of the apparent molecular weight of the active material by gel filtration chromatography suggest that the activity is almost entirely attributable to β-endorphin rather than to the precursor β-LPH. In normal rats, the reported plasma concentration was about 1.5 ng/ml (0.4 nM), dropping to undetectable levels following hypophysectomy or treatment with dexamethasone. In contrast, adrenalectomy increased the circulating level about sixfold. These experiments suggest a striking parallelism in the changes in plasma concentration of β-endorphin and ACTH. Coincident release of β-endorphin and ACTH was also obtained following the severe stress of limb fracture (319). Another severe stress that has been shown to elevate plasma β-endorphin levels is the application of inescapable footshock over periods of up to 1 hr (320). The elevation of plasma β-endorphin following stress has been confirmed by others (337). Currently available data on the resting levels of β-endorphin in rat plasma and changes produced by experimental manipulation are summarized in Table 1. The values for β-endorphin in rat represent total β-endorphin-like immunoreactivity,

TABLE 1 Plasma Concentrations of β-Endorphin, β-LPH, and ACTH[a]

	Plasma Concentration [fmol/ml (pM)]		
	β-Endorphin immuno-reactivity (reference)	β-LPH immuno-reactivity (references)	ACTH immuno-reactivity (reference)
1. Rat			
Resting levels	440 (319)	–	180 (319)
	86 (338)	–	4 (342)
	125 (337)	–	–
After adrenalectomy	2560 (319)	–	2010 (319)
	–	–	80 (342)
After limb fracture	1030 (319)	–	420 (319)
After footshock (60 min)	1320 (320)	–	650 (320)
Handling stress	970 (337)	–	–
2. Humans			
Resting levels	–	5 (339-341)	21 (339)
	<0.5 (344)	5 (344)	–
	1.7 (345)	11 (345)	–
	6.2 (346)	12 (346)	–
	2.4 (347)	9 (347)	–
	7.1 (348)	13 (348)	–
After insulin hypoglycemia	–	25 (339)	95 (339)
	–	61 (341)	50 (341)
Hypopituitarism	–	<3 (340)	<3 (340)
Cushing's disease	–	2-10[b] (340)	25-180 (343)
	–	24-270[b] (341)	–
	–	10 ± 13[c] (339)	37 ± 4 (339)
Addison's disease	26 (349)	–	–
Nelson's syndrome	–	100-798[b] (340)	Up to 2000 (343)
	–	440-5600[b] (341)	–
	–	77 ± 39[c] (339)	180 ± 80 (339)
	197 (349)	–	–

[a] Note that values for plasma β-LPH for Ref. 341 have been computed from the published values for β-MSH immunoreactivity. It has been shown that material in human plasma that reacts with β-MSH antibodies is exclusively of the 10,000-dalton molecular weight range, and probably is intact β-LPH (350). β-LPH cross-reacts 100% with the β-MSH antisera B7 used by Gilkes et al. (341).
[b] Range.
[c] Mean ± S.E.

which is predominantly attributable to β-endorphin and not to β-LPH in the rat, according to Guillemin et al. (319).

The concentration of β-endorphin in human plasma is substantially lower than in the rat. Gel filtration analysis of the β-endorphin-like immunoreactivity in human plasma is mainly attributable to β-LPH (344-350), the molar ratio of β-LPH to β-endorphin varying from 1.8 to greater than 10 in different studies (Table 1). Data on changes in circulating β-endorphin levels in humans in response to experimental procedure or in pathological conditions are only now being accumulated. However, the levels of β-LPH, together with those of ACTH, are elevated by experimental procedures such as the induction of hypoglycemia by administration of insulin, and in Cushing's disease and Nelson's syndrome. In contrast, the level of both peptides is lower in hypopituitarism (Table 1). These results support the contention that β-endorphin, or its precursor β-LPH, is released from the pituitary at the same time as ACTH. No data are presently available concerning the possible release of β-endorphin or β-LPH in humans by stimuli releasing neurohypophyseal hormones.

Recently, the presence in hemodialysates from psychotic patients of Leu^5-β-endorphin has been reported (351) (see Chap. 8). This finding seemed to be of considerable significance since this peptide, a putative precursor of Leu-enkephalin, had been sought in brain and pituitary of experimental animals without success. The peptide reported to be isolated from the hemodialysates was identified as the Leu^5 analog of β-endorphin by standard peptide sequencing procedures. This structure is supported by measurements of its activity relative to that of several variants of β-endorphin, including Met-$(O)^5$-β-endorphin in five assay systems (guinea pig ileum, mouse vas deferens, displacement of [^{3}H]etorphine from opiate receptors in brain membranes, and radioimmunoassays utilizing two antisera with differing cross-reactivities; 352). The presence of a peptide related to β-LPH in hemodialysates is not in itself surprising since it has been shown that material cross-reacting with β-MSH antisera (presumably β-LPH; 350) is elevated during renal dialysis, although plasma ACTH levels were in the normal range (353). It was noted that the levels of β-MSH-like immunoreactivity in the plasma appeared to increase with the number of years in which the patient had been subjected to dialysis. However, in the studies on psychotic patients, the amount of Leu^5-β-endorphin recovered from the dialysates declined with repeated treatment in parallel with the reduction in psychotic symptomatology (351).

In an attempt to confirm the presence of elevated levels of the Leu^5 variant of β-endorphin in psychotic patients, Ross et al. (354) have assayed total β-endorphin-like immunoreactivity in plasma samples taken from 98 schizophrenic subjects, using an antisera with equal affinity for Met^5- and Leu^5-β_h-endorphin. The levels of immunoreactivity did not differ greatly from the values observed in 42 normal subjects. There was no difference in levels associated with diagnostic category or medication. Furthermore, no immunoreactivity was detectable in dialysates from nine schizophrenic and eight nonpsychotic renal patients. Thus the presence of high concentrations of a variant of β-endorphin in schizophrenic subjects has not been confirmed. At present, both the natural occurrence of Leu[5]-β-endorphin and its association with psychopathological states remain uncertain.

D. Target Organs for Circulating Endorphins

Opiate receptors are present in several peripheral tissues. The utilization of in vitro preparations of receptor-bearing tissues such as the guinea pig ileum and mouse vas deferens was fundamental to the discovery of endorphins (259, 260, 355). The opiate receptors found in these tissues have properties similar to those of receptors in the central nervous system with respect to stereospecificity, antagonism by naloxone, and the relative potencies of a series of alkaloid and synthetic opiates (171, 357-359). Opiate effects can also be demonstrated in a number of other tissues that have not received such extensive study (Table 2). Table 3 lists peripheral tissues in which stereospecific opiate binding sites have been detected.

Table 2 shows that opiate receptors are located in a number of disparate autonomically innervated smooth muscles. The receptors are located in structures with both cholinergic and adrenergic innervation, although not all tissues with autonomic innervation are sensitive to opiates. In experimental preparations, the demonstration of the presence of opiate receptors in a particular tissue has generally been achieved in one or two species only. Thus the guinea pig ileum-myenteric plexus preparation is the best known in vitro model for opiate action, but opiate effects are much less readily observed in ileum preparations from other laboratory animals under the same conditions. However, enkephalins are present in both rat (360) and rabbit (361) ileum, and stereospecific binding of opiates can be detected in homogenates of rabbit and rat ileum (371). These observations suggest that opiate receptors may be present in similar structures in several species, but that activation of these receptors produces rather subtle effects that are not always demonstrable under the particular conditions prevailing in isolated tissue preparations.

Opiate receptors in peripheral tissues appear to be located for the most part on the cell bodies and processes of neurons innervating smooth muscle. Activation of these receptors results in a reduction in the output of neurotransmitter from the receptor-bearing neuron, except in the dog intestine, where serotonin is released (Table 2). This type of presynaptic modulation of transmitter release appears to be charactertistic of opiate action both in the central and peripheral nervous system (see Sec. II. F).

A number of difficulties arise in considering these peripheral opiate receptor-bearing neurons as target structures for β-endorphin released from pituitary gland. Some peripheral tissues, such as the myenteric plexus, contain intrinsic neurons in which enkephalins are found (360, 361); other endorphins may also be present. Release of enkephalin or other endorphin from the guinea pig myenteric plexus in response to high-frequency electrical stimulation has been demonstrated (118, 372).

TABLE 2 Opiate-Sensitive Peripheral Tissues[a]

Tissue	Species	Effect of opiates	References
Myenteric plexus	Guinea pig	Inhibition of acetylcholine release from cholinergic neuron	357, 362
Myenteric plexus	Guinea pig	Inhibition of the depressant effects of sympathetic nerve stimulation	363
Intestine	Dog	Stimulation of release of 5-hydroxytryptamine	364
Heart	Rat, rabbit	Inhibition of acetylcholine release from vagus nerve	365
Nictitating membrane	Cat	Inhibition of noradrenaline release from sympathetic neuron	366, 367
Vas deferens	Mouse	Inhibition of noradrenaline release from sympathatic neuron	172, 359
Vas deferens	Rat	Inhibition of electrically stimulated contraction by β-endorphin	368, 369
Vascular smooth muscle	Rat	Contraction of aortic strip; dilation of mesenteric arterioles	370

[a] The criteria for determining that an effect is exerted through opiate receptors are (1) stereospecificity and (2) antagonism by a specific opiate antagonist. For most of these tissues, stereospecificity has not been examined. However, in most tissues antagonism by naloxone or nalorphine has been demonstrated.

TABLE 3 Peripheral Tissues with High-Affinity Stereospecific Binding Sites for Opiate Drugs[a]

Tissue	Species	References
Myenteric plexus	Guinea pig	35
Myenteric plexus	Rabbit, rat	371
Vas deferens	Mouse	371
Posterior pituitary	Bovine	388
Kidney	Guinea pig, rabbit	373
Liver	Guinea pig	373
Adrenal medulla	Bovine	371, 374

[a]Stereospecific binding sites for opiates in myenteric plexus, vas deferens and posterior pituitary have properties resembling those of opiate binding sites in brain. The stereospecific opiate binding sites in kidney and liver have anomalous properties, and do not bind opioid peptides to a significant extent.

Thus, in the myenteric plexus, local stores of endorphin might be an important source of activating ligands for the opiate receptors. However, no endorphin of any kind has as yet been found in other receptor-bearing tissues, such as the mouse vas deferens. The presence of an endorphin circulating in blood might explain the existence of these otherwise apparently redundant receptors. Furthermore, receptors may be activated both by locally released neurotransmitter, and by hormone carried in blood. This situation would be analogous to the activation of adrenoceptors by noradrenaline released from sympathetic neurons, and by adrenaline released from the adrenal medulla and transported in blood to the receptors.

A major difficulty in accepting the hypothesis that β-endorphin is released from the pituitary to function as an agonist at these peripheral opiate receptors is the discrepancy between the concentration of β-endorphin in plasma and the apparant affinity of the receptors for β-endorphin. The concentration of β-endorphin in rat plasma following the very severe stress of limb fracture or repeated inescapable footshock does not rise above 1.5 nM (Table 1). The most potent stimulus for elevation of plasma β-endorphin so far discovered, adrenalectomy, does not increase plasma levels above 3 nM. The concentration of β-endorphin required to give 50% of maximal effect in the isolated guinea pig ileum preparation is in the range 20–80 nM (116, 352). This value corresponds to the concentration giving 50% receptor occupancy (35, 375). Thus when β-endorphin release is stimulated maximally, opiate receptor occupany is only 5–10% (Table 4). (The unphysiological nature of adrenalectomy should be emphasized. In most stress situations, receptor occupancy would be substantially lower than this.) In the mouse vas deferens (116, 352) and rat vas deferens

TABLE 4 Fractional Receptor Occupancies for Observed Plasma Levels of β-Endorphin

Condition	Plasma level[a]	Fractional receptor occupancy[b] (f)
1. β_c-endorphin/rat		
Resting	0.1–0.5 nM	0.003–0.016
After adrenalectomy	2.6 nM	0.08
2. β_h-endorphin/humans		
Resting	<0.001–0.007 nM	$0–1.2 \times 10^{-4}$
Nelson's syndrome	0.197 nM	0.003

[a] Plasma levels taken from Table 1.
[b] Calculated from relation: f = endorphin concentration/(endorphin K_D + endorphin concentration); β_c-endorphin K_D assumed to be 30 nM; β_h-endorphin K_D assumed to be 60 nM (352).

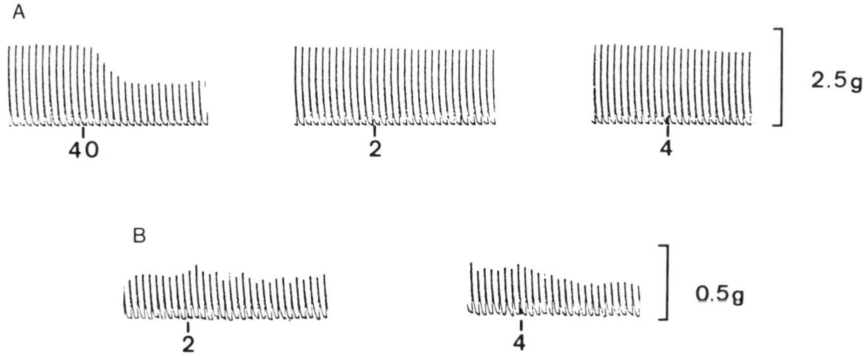

FIGURE 1 Threshold effects of β-endorphin on guinea pig ileum. With electrical stimulation of the isolated myenteric plexus-longitudinal muscle preparation at 80 V, 250 μs, 0.1 Hz, giving maximal responses, β-endorphin at a bath concentration of 40 nM gave 50% inhibition. At 2 nM and 4 nM, the effects of β-endorphin were barely detectable. When the duration of the electrical stimulus was reduced to 10 μs, giving submaximal responses, these low concentrations of β-endorphin produced a greater inhibition of the stimulated response. The concentration of β-endorphin in the plasma of rats after adrenalectomy was between 2 and 3 nM (320). It is possible that the function of the myenteric plexus might be modified by this concentration of β-endorphin in vivo. Figures under the trace indicate the concentrations of ovine β-endorphin applied to the tissue at the points indicated. The tissue was washed several times between each segment of trace. (A) Responses to maximal stimulation; (B) responses to submaximal stimulation. Vertical deflections of the pen represent contractions induced by the electrical stimulus. A resting tension of 1 g was maintained throughout. The calibration bars indicate the additional tension induced by the stimulus.

(which is selectively sensitive to β-endorphin; 368, 369), the potency of β-endorphin is no higher. In such isolated preparations, β-endorphin at a concentration of 4 nM or less has only marginal effects on release of transmitter in response to maximal electrical stimulation (Fig. 1). However, somewhat greater inhibition can be obtained when submaximal stimulation is employed. Thus it is not impossible that low fractional receptor occupancy is compatible with significant physiological effect. Detailed experiments on the behavior of peripheral opiate sensitive tissues in vivo after administration of β-endorphin in doses giving an appropriate plasma concentration will be required to determine if the occupation of such a small fraction of receptors is functionally relevent.

In humans the situation is even more problematic since the circulating concentration of β-endorphin in the absence of known releasing stimuli is at least tenfold lower than in rats. Levels that might be attained following application of releasing stimuli have not been determined. Furthermore, opiate receptors (from lower mammals) have a somewhat lower apparent affinity for the human variant of β-endorphin than for the ovine form (352). The affinity of human opiate receptors for human β-endorphin has not been reported.

Similar difficulties arise in consideration of opiate receptors in the central nervous system as targets for pituitary β-endorphin if it is assumed that access to the receptor is from the general circulation. Thus in the presence of sodium at concentrations equivalent to those present in extracellular fluid (i.e., CSF), central opiate receptors are no more sensitive to endorphins than peripheral opiate receptors (376, 377). Furthermore, the blood-brain barrier interposes a significant obstacle to the penetration into the central nervous system of blood-borne endorphins. While β-endorphin is very active as an analgesic after direct application to the brain, it is uncertain whether even massive intravenous doses of the peptide produce any analgesia (378, 379). The low concentrations of β-endorphin in peripheral plasma that are achieved following release from the pituitary are entirely insufficient to produce detectable effects by direct action on opiate receptors in the CNS.

These arguments lead to the examination of other possible functions for β-endorphin in blood and pituitary. It is possible that β-endorphin plays a purely intrapituitary role. Morphine has been shown to stimulate the release of vasopressin in vivo (380). Intraventricular injections of β-endorphin or enkephalins have been shown to stimulate the release of immunoreactive Arg-vasopressin into the circulation of rabbits (381), and the release of material with vasopressinlike biological activity in water-loaded rats (382). However, in a recent report, intraventricular administration of β-endorphin to rats without prior water loading has been reported to lower plasma Arg-vasopressin immunoreactivity (383). An antidiuretic effect of intraventicular enkephalin (384) or β-endorphin (385, 386) has been clearly demonstrated in water-loaded rats. In this case, it is not certain that the antidiuresis can be attributed to vasopressin release, since the effects of β-endorphin and vasopressin administration on the urine content of Na^+ and K^+ were reported to be different (386). The substantial reduction in urine Na^+ and K^+ concentration induced by the intraventricular injection of 1 μg of β-endorphin was partially antagonized by naloxone (1 mg/kg, i.p.).

Indirect evidence suggests that opiates might inhibit the release of oxytocin in mice. Morphine (10 mg/kg, s.c.) substantially reduced the milk yield from lactating mice, the effect being completely antagonized by an equal dose of naloxone (387). Milk ejection induced by oxytocin injection was not affected by morphine; a centrally mediate inhibition of oxytocin release by morphine was therefore proposed.

It is probable that endorphins and opiate drugs can modulate neurohypophysial hormone release at several sites. Stereospecific opioid binding sites are present in posterior lobe of bovine pituitary (388), and enkephalin-containing never fibers have been demonstrated in rat pars nervosa (318). β-Endorphin from anterior lobe or pars intermedia might also gain access to hormone release sites in pars nervosa (see below and Fig. 2). However, β-endorphin and morphine are reported not to influence spontaneous vasopressin release when incubated with rat pars nervosa in vitro (381, 382). Evidence for a hypothalamic site of action is clearer. Vasopressin release can be provoked by the localized administration of morphine into the supraoptic nucleus of hypothalamus (380).

The reported discrepancies in the effects of β-endorphin or enkephalins on vasopressin release in rats (383, 384) might be related to actions on different types of opioid receptors, or to the presence or absence of prior water loading. The prior treatment of the animals may also be important in determining the absence or presence of opioid effects on hormone release in in vitro studies. Presently available evidence raises the possibility that endogenous opioids might both modulate the osmotic or other regulatory mechanisms in hypothalamus and the hormone release mechanisms in pars nervosa. Further studies are needed to clarfiy these actions. Other effects of endorphins in the maintenance of water balance must also be considered, since opiate anatagonists depress fluid comsumption in thirsty rats (389).

Morphine has also been shown to stimulate or inhibit the release of anterior pituitary hormones such as ACTH, luteinizing hormone (LH), thyroid-stimulating hormone (TSH), growth hormone (GH), and prolactin (PRL) (390). However, there is no evidence to suggest that these effects result from an action of morphine within the pituitary. Thus neither morphine nor β-endorphin release GH or PRL from anterior pituitary cells in culture (391). Opiate receptors have not been detected by radioligand binding studies in the anterior lobe of pituitary (388). It is probable that morphine influences, and endorphins participate in, the regulation of anterior pituitary function through opiate receptors located in the hypothalamus or other brain structures (see Sec. V. B).

Recent evidence has suggested a mechainism by which pituitary peptides might gain direct access to the hypothalamus. The direction of blood flow in the vasculature of the hypothalamohypophysial tract has been disputed for many years (392-394). In anesthetized rats the concentration of many pituitary hormones in blood passing to the anterior lobe of the pituitary in the long portal vessels has been shown to be several orders of magnitude higher than in peripheral venous blood (395). The simplest explanation of this apparent anomaly is that substances can pass from both lobes of the pituitary to the median eminence, and return to the pituitary via the long portal vessels. Anatomical structures that would permit this retrograde flow of hormone have been described by Page et al. (396, 397). They have shown that a common capillary network connects the posterior lobe of the pituitary with the median eminence. These vessels receive an arterial input at each end; the direction of blood flow through these vessels will depend in part on the relative pressures of each arterial input. It is also probable that flow in these vessels is controlled by the local release of vasoconstrictor or vasodilator substances. The external plexus of the median eminence provides a switching station in which blood from the neuro-

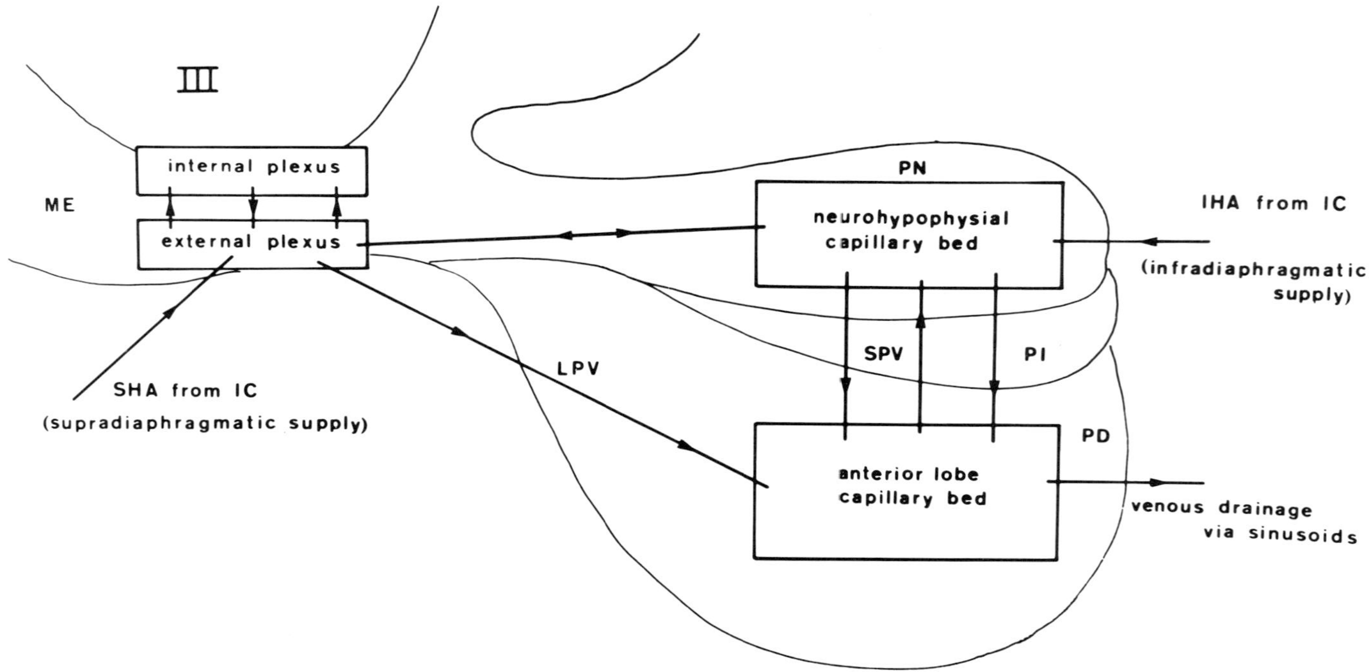

FIGURE 2 Schematic diagram of the vascular connections of the rabbit (from ref. 396). The direction of flow in the vessels between pituitary and median eminence will be determined by the relative pressures in the supradiaphragmatic and infradiaphragmatic arterial supplies. Such differences might occur despite their common origin from the internal carotid artery since the superior hypophysial arteries above the diaphragmatic sella are bathed in cerebrospinal fluid, while the anterior and inferior hypophysial artieries are bathed by venous blood in the cavernous sinus. Regulation by local release of vasoconstrictor and vasodilator substances is also possible. Flow from the anterior lobe capillary bed to the neurohypophysis via SPV is suggested by the observations of Oliver et al. (395). IHA, Inferior hypophysial artery; SHA, superior hypophysial; IC, internal carotid artery; SPV, short portal vessels, LPV, long portal vessels; PN, pars nervosa (infundibular process); PI, pars intermeida; PD, pars distalis; ME, medain eminence, III, third ventricle.

hypophysis can be routed to the interior plexus lying in close proximity with the third ventricle, or directly into the long portal vessels supplying the anterior pituitary (Fig. 2). This complex vascular system allowing retrograde flow in the pituitary stalk would make possible the transport of β-endorphin, after diffusion from the pars intermedia into the neuronal lobe capillary network, to the hypothalamus. Here it could act on local opiate receptors, pass into the fluid of the third ventricle to act at other sites in the brain, or return via the long portal vessels to the anterior pituitary.

Oliver et al. (395) found that under their experimental conditions the ratio of peptide concentrations in portal blood returning to the anterior pituitary to those in systemic arterial blood was 68 for TSH, 116 for LH, 196 for prolactin, 448 for ACTH, 407 for β-MSH, and 141 for vasopressin. It should be noted that the surgical procedures necessarily employed in collecting portal blood will have altered the pressure relationships in the pituitary vasculature, and thus may have artifactually changed hormonal flow patterns. Bergland et al. (398) have partially overcome this problem by sampling blood from the internal carotid artery above the pituitary, or from the superior saggital sinus, in anesthetized sheep. The plasma concentrations of prolactin and growth hormone from these vessels were substantially higher than those found in the cervical carotid artery below the pituitary in the majority of animals. If the concentration ratios found by Oliver et al. (395) are applicable to β-endorphin, it seems probable that the concentration of this peptide reaching the hypothalamus under conditions of retrograde flow in the hypothalamohypophysial tract would be well into the range required to give substantial occupancy of opiate receptors located either in the hypothalamus or elsewhere in the brain in reasonable proximity with the third ventricle.* The low concentration of β-endorphin in the peripheral circulation may simply reflect the dilution of blood from the hypothalamo-hypophysial circulation in the large volume of peripheral blood.

The hypothesis that β-endorphin is transported from pituitary to hypothalamus is supported by the recent observation that hypophysectomy results in a 50–80% decline in the β-endorphin content of the hypothalamus, while the levels in other brain regions were unaffected or increased (399). However, when severe stress that elevates peripheral plasma β-endorphin levels was applied to rats, hypothalamic content of β-endorphin was found to decrease slightly (319), and not increase, as appears to be predicted by the retrograde-flow hypothesis. Further studies are needed to determine the circumstances in which a significant transport of β-endorphin from pituitary to brain might occur.

One further possible function for β-endorphin needs to be considered. It is conceivable that the peptide exerts a function entirely unrelated to its ability to activate opiate receptors. For this purpose it would be necessary for β-endorphin receptors (probably with higher affinity than opiate receptors) to exist on some peri-

* A recent abstract has reported that β-endorphin-like immunoreactivity is indeed present at a relatively high level in portal blood in the rat (507).

pheral or central structure. β-Endorphin action at such sites would not be affected by opiate receptor ligands and their existence could be detected only by a search for very high affinity binding sites for radiolabeled β-endorphin, although their existence might be inferred by the demonstration of a particular deficiency state arising from the removal of β-endorphin by hypophysectomy that could only be corrected by readministration of β-endorphin. Until it can be shown convincingly that β-endorphin in pituitary does not act on opiate receptors, it is not likely to be worthwhile to pursue this speculation further.

V. FUNCTIONAL STUDIES INDICATING A PHYSIOLOGICAL ROLE FOR ENDORPHINS

A. General Considerations

The physiological functions of endorphin might be predicted on the basis of the pharmacological actions of opiate drugs, assuming that these drugs act on opiate receptors that are normally concerned in physiological regulation when activated by endogenous opiates. Thus, since opiate drugs are analgesic, it could be inferred that endorphins normally regulate the perception of, and the response to painful stimuli. This argument ignores the possibility that extrajunctional receptors for endorphins might exist, where exogenous drugs could exert significant but unphysiological effects on neuronal activity. Furthermore, the consequences of long-term receptor occupation following the administration of an opiate drug might be different for overall animal behavior from the consequences of the brief receptor occupation resulting from the release of the enkephalin from a nerve terminal. Nevertheless, assuming that endorphins exert some functions through opiate receptors, it is likely that some of the actions of opiate drugs will mimic the normal effects of physiologically released endorphin.

The possible role of endorphins in such a system can be further evaluated by the use of specific opiate receptor antagonists, such as naloxone or naltrexone. The effects produced by these drugs at moderate doses seem to be specifically associated with their ability to block opiate receptors (400), although actions at other sites are implicated when high doses of drug are given (401). Thus it is reasonable to conclude that pharmacological effects produced by moderate doses of naloxone or naltrexone result from the antagonism of physiologically (or pathologically) released endorphin. This experimental approach can thus provide a priori evidence that the function of the system affected by the opiate antagonist is in some way regulated by endorphins. This conclusion requires support from additonal independent evidence, since it will not be entirely surprising if actions of naloxone are subsequently discovered that are not mediated by endorphin receptor blockade. The converse conclusion can be drawn with some certainty. If the normal functioning of a system is not affected by the administration of an adequate dose of an opiate antagonist, it is very unlikely that endogenous opioids acting through opiate receptors are concerned in the normal regulation of that system. However, the demonstration that endorphins can induce tolerance (see Sec. VII) suggests that endorphin (opiate) receptors are not continuously occupied by endorphins. Prolonged receptor occupation would result in the reduced effectiveness of released endorphin and thus be self-defeating. It seems likely that endorphins are released for short periods in response to specific stimuli. It is therefore necessary to examine the effects of an opiate antagonist under conditions in which the provoked release of endorphins seems likely.

Determination of an adequate dose or concentration of naloxone or naltrexone, and the appropriate duration of exposure to the drug, require some consideration. Evidence is accumulating that the actions of endorphins on opiate receptors in tissues such as the mouse vas deferens are less readily antagonized by naloxone or naltrexone than are the actions of alkaloid opiates such as morphine (244, 402). This discrimination does not occur in all tissues; endorphins and morphine are equally antagonized in the guinea pig ileum. In the mouse vas deferens, the apparent affinity of naloxone, when estimated by its ability to antagonize enkephalin, is about tenfold lower than when estimated from its ability to antagonize normorphine (244). Quantitative studies of the comparative potency of naloxone in antagonizing behavioral effects of endorphin and morphine have not been reported, but estimates of the relative affinities of different peptide and alkaloid ligands for opiate receptors in homogenized brain membranes suggest that at least some of the receptors in brain resemble the receptors in mouse vas deferens more than they resemble the receptors in guinea pig ileum (244). Thus it is possible that a dose of naloxone that reduced the effectiveness of morphine by a factor of 2 might fail to produce demonstrable antagonism of a function mediated by physiologically released endorphin. But doses that are tenfold higher than that required for a clear demonstration of antagonism of the effects of morphine should be sufficient to produce some blockade of endorphin-mediated functions.

Naloxone binding to opiate receptors reaches an equilibrium fairly rapidly (403). Antagonism of the actions of an opiate drug occurs within minutes following the intravenous administration of naloxone, either in experimental animals in the laboratory or in the emergency room when the naloxone is used to reverse the potentially lethal effects of an opiate drug. Thus antagonism of a function normally mediated by endorphins should be apparent soon after naloxone administration. The drug has a relatively short half-life; antagonistic effects of a large dose of naloxone in humans therefore decline after about 2 hr (404). Effects of naloxone on physiological or pathological function that occur some time after drug administration, such as the observation that naloxone reduces the severity of some of the symptoms experienced by schizophrenic patients, with a maximum effect about 3 hr after naloxone administration (405), need to be interpreted with caution. While the effects could be dependent on the initial occupation of opiate receptors by the antagonist, the slow onset of clinical improvement makes it likely that secondary consequences of the blockade or other, opiate receptor-indepedent actions of naloxone are also necessary. It becomes less certain that endorphins are the causative agents of the symptoms reported to be alleviated by naloxone.

The following discussion is devoted to particular functions that the actions of opiate drugs suggest might be mediated by endorphins, and where sufficient experimental evidence, particularly concerning the effects of opiate antagonists, has accumulated to allow some preliminary conclusions to be drawn. Possible functions for endorphins in the mediation of reward or reinforcement, and in the control of motor activity, are considered in Chap. 7.

B. Endorphins and Hormonal Regulation

The most convincing evidence that endorphins are implicated in hormonal regulation comes from studies of prolactin (PRL) and growth hormone (GH). The release of GH from the anterior pituitary is thought to be suppressed by somatostatin liberated from tuberoinfundibular neurons with terminals in the median eminence. The somatostatin is transported from the median eminence to the anterior pituitary by the long portal vessels. In addition, there is evidence for the existence of an as yet uncharacterized GH releasing factor (406). Hypothalamic regulation of the anterior pituitary stores of PRL is also not completely understood. The existence of a release inhibiting factor has been postulated, but the relationship of this substance to dopamine, a potent suppressor of PRL release that is also present in tuberoinfundibular neurons and released into portal blood, is not clear (406). Dopamine suppression of PRL release can be reversed by dopamine receptor blocking agents (407). A specific releasing factor for PRL has not been identified, but thyrotropin releasing factor (TRF, pryo-Gly-His-Pro-NH_2) is a potent stimulator of release of both thyrotropin and PRL (406).

It has been known for several years that morphine and related drugs can stimulate the release of GH and PRL (407–409). These effects are produced by doses of morphine in rats of 10 mg/kg or more, and are clearly apparent within 30 min from drug injection. In humans, opiates seem to be more effective as PRL releasers than as releasers of GH (410). More recently it has been shown that Met- and Leu-enkephalin, several more stable synthetic analogs, and β-endorphin also release GH and PRL in rats (390, 411–415). The effectiveness of Met- and Leu-enkephalin after systemic injection suggests that a comparatively brief period of occupation of opiate receptors is adequate to stimulate release of the hormones. These peptides have a very short half-life in blood. In general, direct application of morphine (408, 412) or the opioid peptides (391, 412, 413) to anterior pituitary cells in culture does not cause release of GH or PRL, indicating that opiates effect hormone release by an action on the neuronal regulation of pituitary function. However, some release of PRL by direct application of enkephalin to pituitary cells in culture was reported by Lien et al.

(416). The in vivo release of GH and PRL by morphine and endorphins is antagonized by naloxone or naltrexone (390, 412, 414).

Since both enkephalins and β-endorphin cell bodies and nerve terminals are located in the hypothalamus (see Chap. 5), and it is also possible that β-endorphin in pituitary can gain access to brain via the hypothalamo-hypophysial vasculature (see Sec. IV. D), it is quite probable that the observed release of GH and PRL by exogenously administered opiates reflects a normal action of endorphins. This hypothesis receives support from the demonstration that naloxone, administered in the absence of any foreign opiate, lowers circulating levels of GH and PRL. Thus Bruni et al. (390) found that naloxone doses of 0.2 and 5 mg/kg in rats significantly reduced plasma GH and PRL levels, and Grandison and Guidotti (414) found that 1 mg/kg of naltrexone depressed plasma PRL levels. Shaar et al. (412) also observed significant reductions of plasma GH and PRL with naloxone doses of 0.1 to 0.4 mg/kg in rats, but failed to see a fall in plasma levels at higher doses, despite the demonstration of antagonism of morphine-provoked release by these higher doses. This anomaly remains unexplained.

The elevation of plasma PRL levels by estrogen administration, or by stresses such as footshock or exposure to ether and cardiac puncture, was also significantly reduced by naltrexone (414). Furthermore, in rats, naloxone has been shown to reduce the release of PRL provoked by 30 min of physical restraint, or by exposure to a temperature of 40°C (417). However, elevated PRL levels following administration of reserpine or haloperidol were not reduced by narcotic antagonists. These observations lead to the speculation that endorphins in the hypothalamus might provoke PRL release by suppressing the release of dopamine from the terminals of tuberoinfundibular neurons, thus reducing the dopamine-mediated inhibition of PRL release. Infusion of Met-enkephalin into the cerebral ventricles has been shown to affect the distribution of catecholamines within the terminals of tuberoinfundibular neurons within the hypothalamus under conditions in which an increase in plasma PRL level was provoked (418). β-Endorphin reduced dopamine concentration in the external layer of the median eminence (419). A presynaptic regulation of this type is characteristic of opiate action.

It is apparently also possible for PRL release to occur via a mechanism not requiring endorphins, since it has been reported that the surge of plasma PRL at proestrous in rats is not suppressed by naloxone (420). The proestrous increase in PRL is itself inhibited by morphine, and this inhibition can be blocked by naloxone (420).

GH release does not seem to be directly regulated by dopamine, but there are indications that monoamines may affect the release of somatostatin or GH releasing factor (421). The manner in which endorphins might be involved in this complex regulatory system is not understood. Cumulatively, however, these results provide fairly strong indirect support for a role for endorphins in the normal regulation of GH and PRL release.

There is increasing evidence suggesting a role for endorphins in the regulation of luteinizing hormone (LH) release by the pituitary. The ability of opiates to depress serum LH levels is well established (422, 423). Intraperitoneal administration of Met-enkephalin (5 mg/kg) is also reported to reduce plasma LH levels in male rats (390). Indication that this pharmacological action of opioids is mediated through receptors concerned in the normal regulation of LH is provided by the demonstration that naloxone in sexually mature male rats (390, 424), and naltexone in adult humans (425), given in the absence of any exogenous opioid agonist, substantially elevates serum LH levels. Naloxone does not affect the ability of luteinizing hormone releasing factor (LRF) to stimulate LH release from pituitary (424). It seems probable, therefore, that endogenous opioids exert a direct or indirect inhibitory control on LRF release. This hypothesis is supported by the observation that naloxone antagonizes the negative feedback inhibition of LH production induced by testosterone administration to castrated male rats (424). The elevation of serum LH by naloxone may be implicated in the increase in copulatory behavior induced by naloxone (2 mg/kg, i.p.) in sexually inactive adult male rats (426).

A recent study by Blank et al. (427) has demonstrated interesting developmental differences in the sensitivity of male and female rats to the ability of naloxone (2.5 mg/kg, s.c.) to increase serum LH levels. Male rats only showed sensitivity to naloxone at the onset of puberty (40-60 days), and as adults. In contrast, naloxone produced dramatic increases in serum LH at certain times during development in immature female rats, but failed to produce significant increases in adult females at any stages of the estrus cycle. The increase in serum LH produced by naloxone in 24-day-old (immature) females was shown to be completely suppressed by prior administration of estradiol, although this treatment had no effect on the reduction of serum PRL induced by naloxone in the same animals. The effect of estrogen is thus specific to the LH system. The authors suggest that estrogens (and perhaps testosterone in males) exert a regulatory effect on the control of LRF release by endogenous opioids. The apparent interaction between steroids and endorphins in the regulation of LH secretion and the onset of puberty requires confirmation, but present evidence clearly implies an important role for endorphins in this aspect of sexual function.

A role for endorphins in the regulation of other anterior pituitary hormones has not as yet been clearly demonstrated. However, Gibson et al. (428) have reported that Met-enkephalin administered intraventricularly to mice appears to inhibit one component of feedback regulation of corticosterone release. A possible role for endorphins in regulation of ACTH release is of particular interest in view of the common biosynthetic pathway shared by ACTH and β-endorphin in pituitary.

C. Endorphin Modulation of Pain Perception

Since the major therapeutic use of morphine is in the relief of pain, a similar function for endorphins should be considered. The location of both opiate receptors and enkephalins in structures located on the afferent pain pathway, such as the substantia gelatinosa of spinal cord and the midbrain periaqueductal gray region, support this hypothesis (see Chap. 5). The presence of β-endorphin-containing nerve fibers running from hypothalamus to the periaqueductal gray region is also compatible with an analgesic role for this peptide. Both enkephalins and β-endorphin have been shown to produce analgesia when administered into the cerebral ventricles. The effect of enkephalins is transient, and very large doses are required (47, 48), presumably because of the rapid degradation of these peptides. Analogs of enkephalin protected against peptidase attack are much more potent and produce longer-lasting effects (see Chap. 3). β-Endorphin is also a potent analgesic after intraventricular injection, with an action lasting for several hours (59, 429).

Many workers have attempted to provide evidence that endorphins are mobilized in response to the application of painful stimuli. The assumption has been made that endorphin will be released by the stimulus and partially attenuate the provoked response. Blockade of opiate receptors should therefore increase sensitivity to painful stimuli. Table 5 summarizes the results of experiments in which a direct effect of naloxone on pain threshold has been sought. A sensitizing effect of naloxone has not been consistently found (see Chap. 7).

In humans, naloxone has generally been ineffective in several varied experimental procedures. Thus naloxone did not affect subjective estimates of pain intensity in response to electrical stimulation of the arm (446), ischemic muscle pain (447), or pain resulting from immersion of the hand in cold water (450). In all except the first of these studies, the dose of naloxone administered was substantially above that required to reverse the effects of doses of opiate drugs producing severe respiratory depression. In a more detailed study of the effects of naloxone on electric shock pain, Buschbaum et al. (448) found different effects of naloxone depending on the initial pain sensitivity of the subject. Subjects who initially showed high sensitivity to pain generally showed reduced sensitivity after naloxone, while initially insensitive subjects found the electric shocks more painful after naloxone. It is therefore of intereset that naloxone also was reported to reduce the threshold of a nociceptive flexion reflex in a subject congenitally insenitive to pain while not affecting the threshold in normal subjects (451). Further studies of naloxone in congenital pain insensitivity are needed. Recently it has been reported that naloxone enhances pain following oral surgery (452). Interpretation of this result is complicated by the other drugs, including diazepam and nitrous oxide, that were given prior to naloxone, since naloxone has been shown to antagonize the analgesic effects of several drugs (see below).

In mice, naloxone has consistently reduced response latency in the hot plate test (430-434), when an escape jump was taken as the end point and the temperature of the hot plate adjusted so that the latency to jump was prolonged to 1 min or more. Naloxone had no effect on the much shorter pawlick latency (433) except in one study (435). It has been suggested that when the response has a short latency,

TABLE 5 Effects of Naloxone on Pain Thresholds

Species and method of measure of pain sensitivity	Dose of naloxone (mg/kg)	Effect of naloxone	References
Mouse			
Hot plate test	0.01–30	Reduction of response latency	430, 431
Hot plate test	0.5–4	Reduction of response latency	432, 433
Hot plate test	0.03–10	Reduction of response latency	434
Hot plate test	0.05–0.10	Reduction of response latency	435
Heat on nose; squeak response	0.9	Reduction of response latency	436
Formic acid or PGE_1-induced writing	1	No effect	437
Rat			
Shock escape threshold	12.5–100	No effect	438
Hot plate test	0.05–0.10	Reduction of response latency	435
Tail flick test (thermal stimulus)	2	Reduction of response latency	439
Tail flick test (thermal stimulus)	1, 10 or 20	No effect	440–442
Acetic acid-induced writhing	4	Increase frequency of writhing	443
Formalin-induced forepaw pain	10	No effect	444

Squirrel monkey			
Shock titration	0.3–10	No effect	445
Humans			
Electrical stimulation of arm (verbal report)	0.4 or 0.8	No effect	446
Ischemic muscle pain (verbal report)	2 or 10	No effect	447
Electrical stimulation of arm (verbal report) and measurement of evoked potentital from scalp	2	Threshold lowered in insensitive subjects, but raised in pain sensitive subjects	448
Electrical stimulation of arm; measurement of evoked potential from scalp	2	Increased potential during morning, but not in afternoon	449
Cold water pain (verbal report)	1 or 10	No effect	450
Nociceptive reflex of lower limb	Not stated	Reduced threshold in subject congenitally insensitive to pain	451
Clinical pain following oral surgery (subjective judgment)	9	Increase in pain severity	452

the elasped time is insufficient for mobilization of endorphin, but that longer latency responses allow time for release of endorphin which further prolongs the latency (431). Naloxone should therefore reduce the extended latency to its unmodulated level. This interpretation has not received support in recent studies by Grevert et al. (453). The latency to the escape jump response in mice was not reduced by hypophysectomy, indicating that pituitary endorphins are not concerned with setting the latency. However, naloxone no longer had an effect on the latency to jump in hypophysectomized animals. Thus, in this condition, there was no evidence for the participation of endorphins from any source in the determination of response latency. These experiments provide no explanation for the effects of naloxone on the jump response, but appear to refute the hypothesis that pain threshold in this test is modulated by endorphins. A recent study (454) has not confirmed the abolition of naloxone effect by hypophysectomy. The completeness of hypophysectomy and the possible occurence of hypothalamic damage may be critical factors, requiring evaluation in each experimental animal in future studies.

Naloxone also reduced the threshold for response to application of a thermal stimulation to the nose in mice (436). But when pain sensitivity was measured by the frequency of "writhing" or abdominal constriction induced by the intraperitoneal injection of an irritant substance, no hyperalgesic effect of naloxone was observed (437).

In rats, variable effects of naloxone on pain sensitivity have been reported. Naloxone had no effect on the shock escape threshold (438) or on the response to pressure applied to the tail (439). Three groups have failed to find any effect of naloxone on the latency of the tail flick response induced by a thermal stimulus (440–442), although a reduction in latency was reported in one study (439). Naloxone was also found to increase the frequency of writhing in rats after intraperitoneal injection of acetic acid (443). The writhing response to acetic acid continues up to 1 hr after injection of the irritant, and thus represents a prolonged stress for the animal. This procedure should therefore be considered in relation to stress associated analgesia, a phenomenon that has been shown to be antagonized by naloxone (see Table 6 and the discussion below).

In general, these experiemental studies of the direct effects of naloxone on pain threshold do not support the hypothesis that the direct application of all types of painful stimuli over short periods of time can provoke the release of endorphin to modulate the pain threshold. In some experiments, naloxone has appeared to reduce the threshold or latency of response to a thermal stimulus. However, naloxone was not universally effective in increasing sensitivity to a heat stimulus when behavioral measures of response were measured, and Duggan et al. (144) failed to find any effect of naloxone, injected systemically or applied iontophoretically into the substantia gelatinosa, on the responses of single spinal cord lamina V neurons to a noxious heat stimulus in cat, although antagonism of the depressent effects of morphine on the response to the noxious stimulus was clearly apparent. Two groups have failed to detect effects of naloxone on descending inhibitory pathways regulating nociceptive information transmission in brain stem (455) or spinal cord (456).

Naloxone has been shown to facilitate reflexes recorded from a ventral root in spinal cats (457, 458). The amplitude of both mono- and polysynaptic reflexes was increased (457). In doses as low as 5 μg/kg, i.v., naloxone increased the magnitude of the C-fiber reflex evoked by electrical stimulation of the ipsilateral superficial peroneal nerve or by the application of radiant heat to the footpad (458). A similar facilitation was seen with naltrexone and nalorphine. It is not clear whether the apparent differential sensitivity to naloxone of lamina V neurons and the ventral root potential indicates a specific regulatory role for endorphins on the efferent arm of some spinal C-fiber reflexes, or arises for purely technical reasons. In the chloralose-anesthetized cats used in the study of lamina V neuron sensitivity, activation of endorphin-containing neurons to release enkephalin might have been suppressed either by direct action of the anesthetic or by neuronally mediated inhibition.

An immediate attenuation of the perception of a noxious insult is of doubtful survival value to the animal, since it is important that potentially damaging painful stimuli should be rapidly and reliably detected so that avoiding action can be taken. However, once the appropriate action has been taken, severe prolonged pain can become incapacitating. In this situation, a system attenuating pain perception that was activated after the initial response to the noxious stimulus, and gave prolonged relief, might be useful.

There are indications that at least one physiological system exists for the long-term reduction of perceived pain. It has long been known that the severity of perceived pain resulting from significant wounds can be less in the stress of a battlefield (459). More recently, the analgesic efficacy of focal stimulation of specific brain regions (165, 167, 460, 461), of acupuncture (436, 462, 463), and of severe stress (464) have been experimentally demonstrated. Attempts have been made to evaluate the role of endorphins in these types of analgesia by assessing the ability of naloxone to reverse or block the analgesia. The results of such studies are summarized in Table 6.

Some interesting comparisons can be made. Thus careful studies of acupuncture analgesia or analgesia resulting from transcutaneous electrical stimulation in mice, rats, and humans have generally shown very significant antagonism by naloxone (436, 442, 463, 470). However, the relief of pain produced by transcutaneous electrical stimulation in patients with fractured ribs was not antagonized by naloxone (471). In other studies utilizing different modes of analgesia, naloxone antagonism has been partial or inconsistent, suggesting that perhaps both endorphin-mediated pathways and other systems have been activated. In two studies, the absence of any effect of naloxone on hypnosis analgesia has been very clear (472, 473). Variable effects of naloxone on analgesia produced by focal brain stimulation have been reported (440, 441, 465-470). It is probable that precise electrode placement is critical;

TABLE 6 Effects of Naloxone on Analgesia Produced by Various Experimental Procedures

Method of production of analgesia	Species and method of measure of pain sensitivity	Dose of naloxone	Naloxone antagonism	References
1. Stimulation of specific brain regions	Rat			
	Tail flick test	1 mg/kg	Partial	465, 466
	Tail flick test	1 or 10 mg/kg	Inconsistent	441
	Tail flick test	20 mg/kg	None	440
	Cat			
	Response to forceps pinch, or electrical tooth stimulation	0.3 mg/kg	Complete	467
	Humans			
	Pathological pain (verbal report)	0.05–0.2 mg (i.v.)	Complete	468
	Pathological pain (verbal report)	0.1–1 mg	Complete	469
2. Acupuncture analgesia	Mouse			
	Heat on nose; squeak response	0.9 mg/kg	Complete	436
	Humans			
	Electrical tooth stimulation (verbal report)	0.8 mg (i.v.)	Complete	463
2a. Transcutaneous electrical stimulation	Humans			
	Electrical tooth stimulation (verbal report)	0.4 mg (i.v.)	Partial	470
	Acute trauma pain (fractured ribs)	0.8 mg (i.v.)	None	471
	Rat			
	Tail flick test	1 mg/kg	Complete	442

3.	Hypnosis	Humans			
		Ischemic muscle pain (verbal report)	10 mg (i.v.)	None	472
		Humans			
		Electrical tooth stimulation (verbal report)	0.8 mg (i.v.)	None	473
4.	Vaginal stimulation	Rat			
		Electrical stimulation of tail –squeak response	1 or 10 mg/kg	None	474
5.	Cold water stress (or swim stress)	Rat			
		Flinch jump test	10 mg/kg	Partial	475
		Tail withdrawal from warm water	10 mg/kg	None	476
		Mouse			
		Tail flick test	10 mg/kg	None	476
		Phenylquinone writhing	10 mg/kg	None	476
6.	Footshock stress	Rat			
		Tail flick test	10 mg/kg	Partial	464
		Mouse			
		PGE_1-induced writhing frequency	1 mg/kg	Complete	437
7.	Nonopiate drugs	Mouse			
	(a) Nitrous oxide	Phenylbenzoquinone writhing	5 mg/kg	Complete	477
		Acetic acid-induced writhing	5 mg/kg	Complete	478
	(b) Aspirin and ethanol	Acetic acid-induced writhing	5–100 mg/kg	None	478
	(c) Substance P	Hot plate test	60 ng/mouse	Partial	216
		Hot plate test	0.2 mg/kg	Partial	219

the results suggest that, in the rat, at least two systems, only one of which is mediated by endorphins, can be activated by stimulation in the PAG region of midbrain.

Naloxone appears to be particularly effective in antagonizing analgesia of slow onset and prolonged action. Thus acupuncture analgesia, which has consistently been blocked by naloxone, develops slowly but outlasts the period of stimulation by many minutes or even hours. Focal brain stimulation can also produce very prolonged analgesia when appropriate electrode placements are made. It is noteworthy that in those studies where naloxone antagonisim of stimulation produced analgesia was not observed reliably, the duration of analgesia was comparatively brief (440, 441). The duration of hypnosis analgesia, which is not antagonized by naloxone, is largely determined by the directions of the hypnotist. Analgesia can be induced virtually instantaneously, and can be terminated immediately or allowed to persist for some time at the suggestion of the experimenter (473). Thus there is no indication here of an ongoing process outlasting the initial period of induction. Analgesia of long duration, however, is not an essential prerequisite for antagonism by naloxone, since footshock stress induced analgesia is of comparatively short duration but is reduced by naloxone (464). Even in these studies naloxone was more effective when several minutes elapsed between footshock and assessment of pain sensitivity. Naloxone did not affect pain thresholds in rats subjected to vaginal stimulation when measurements were made 1 min after commencement of vaginal probing (474).

Further evidence that stimulation produced analgesia is mediated by the release of endorphin to activate opiate receptors comes from studies of cross-tolerance with morphine. Rats tolerant to morphine are less sensitive to analgesia produced by focal brain stimulation than control rats (479). Recovery to initial levels of the analgesic response to brain stimulation occurred between 16 and 30 days after termination of the morphine treatment, a period similar to that required for recovery of the analgesic response to morphine after chronic treatment (480). Stimulation of the brain for 24 hr at sites producing analgesia resulted in a reduced sensitivity to subsequent brain stimulation, but this treatment did not cause tolerance to morphine (479), perhaps because morphine can act at many sites to produce analgesia, whereas repeated focal stimulation at any one site produces tolerance in only a select group of neurons.

The demonstration that morphine tolerance results in reduced sensitivity to stimulation-produced analgesia does not necessarily imply that the analgesia must be mediated by endorphin, although it does suggest that common neuronal pathways are involved in analgesia induced by morphine or by stimulation of the midbrain PAG region. Recent studies have shown that tolerance to opiates is accompanied by general changes in neuronal properties that can be demonstrated independently of the action of opiate drugs (481–483). These changes are reflected in a greater sensitivity to stimulatory agents and reduced sensitivity to inhibitory agents. The reduced sensitivity to focal brain stimulation in tolerant animals could therefore result from general changes in neuronal properties, and not specifically from the reduced effectiveness of endorphin acting on opiate receptors. However, morphine tolerance does not ubiquitously reduce the efficacy of analgesic procedures. Analgesia induced by vaginal stimulation was not reduced by a period of chronic morphine treatment (474).

The association of stimulation-produced analgesia and morphine analgesia is not entirely surprising since the areas in the brain in which stimulation evokes analgesia correspond strikingly with those regions in which microinjections of morphine are also effective (165-167). The midbrain PAG region has been most extensively studied, but additional sites are also known. Within the PAG, the precise localization giving most effective analgesia from morphine microinjection and electrical stimulation may not be identical (56, 57). These minor differences might reflect differences in the volume of neuronal substrate affected by electrical stimulation or injection of drug solution, or perhaps indicate that the electrically excitable components of endorphin-containing cells are separated from the morphine receptors. The specific neuronal pathways affected by focal brain stimulation and by morphine have not been completely elucidated, but there is evidence that pathways descending from the PAG through the brain stem to the spinal cord are implicated (165-167, 460, 461, 467). A role for a rostrally projecting catecholamine containing pathway, the dorsal periventricular bundle, has also been postulated (484).

The effect of naloxone on drug-induced analgesia is selective. The antagonism of opiate analgesia is well established (400). Analgesia induced by nitrous oxide (477, 478) and by low doses of substance P administered into the cerebral ventricles (216, 219) is also antagonized, suggesting the possibility that these agents might be releasers of endorphins in vivo. There is also evidence that the depressant effects of barbiturates and some general anesthetics are partially reduced by naloxone (485-487). However, the analgesic effects of aspirin and ethanol in the mouse writhing test were not modified by naloxone (478).

In summary, there is accumulating evidence to suggest that while the immediate response to painful stimuli is not normally regulated by endorphins, an endorphin system can be activated by procedures such as acupuncture, focal brain stimulation, prolonged stress, and some drugs, to raise the pain threshold. It has not yet been shown that this system is functional in severe pathological pain. Nor do endorphins appear to be implicated in the sometimes dramatic relief of severe prolonged pain that results from hypophysectomy in some patients, since naloxone does not provoke a resurgence of the pain (488).

The possible role of endorphins in the analgesic phenomena blocked by naloxone requires confirmation by other methods. Evidence directly supporting the hypothesis is lacking. It has been suggested that footshock stress mediated analgesia is accompanied by an increase in the brain level of endogenous opioids, assayed in crude aqueous buffer extracts of brain by a receptor binding assay (464). However, Fratta et al. (489) did not find any changes in brain levels of Met-enkephalin measured by radioimmunoassay after application of the same footshock stress. It is possible that the changes in opioid activity observed by Akil et al. (464) could be attributed to β-endorphin or to an as yet uncharacterized brain endorphin. Ultimately, measures of the rate of turnover of specific endorphins in discrete regions of brain, following application of analgesia provoking stimuli, will be required if the role of endorphins is to be elucidated more fully.

D. Endorphins in the Modulation of Body Temperature

A biphasic action of morphine on body temperature that parallels its action on motor activity is well established; low doses induce hyperthermia, while higher doses are hypothermic in rats (490). Since muscular activity, including shivering, is an important source of heat (491), the effects of opiates on motor activity (see Chap. 7) and on body temperature may be interrelated (492). Goldstein and Lowery (493) have considered the possiblity that endorphins might play a role in normal thermoregulation by sustaining body temperature in cool environments. In rats maintained at both 23°C and 2°C, naloxone (at 10 mg/kg) did cause a small but statistically significant reduction in body temperature. But since the rats held in a cool environment had a slightly higher body temperature than rats kept at 23°C, and naloxone did not produce a profound hypothermia in these animals, endorphins do not seem to be implicated in the mechanisms by which rats maintain their body temperature during exposure to cold.

It is possible that endorphins are implicated in hyperthermic responses to some kinds of stress. Bläsig et al. (337) have shown that the hyperthermia associated with the stress of transportation and handling in rats is antagonized by (–)-naloxone but not by (+)-naloxone, suggesting a probable role for endorphins. The same stress also elevated circulating plasma levels of β-endorphin about eightfold, to a level of approximately 1 nM. It has not as yet been shown that the presence of β-endorphin in plasma at this concentration is hyperthermic in rats. Nevertheless, the possibility that β-endorphin released from pituitary can gain access to hypothalamic thermoregulatory centers cannot be excluded. The demonstration by Lal et al. (494) that a conditioned hyperthermia is antagonized by naloxone in rats does suggest that some physiological temperature-regulating systems might be mediated by endorphins, but many possible sites of naloxone action between perception of the conditioning stimulus and elevation of body temperature can be envisaged.

E. Lack of Subjective Effects of Opiate Antagonists; Relevance to Endorphin Function

A number of experimental studies in animals utilizing opiate antagonists have provided some indications of specific physiological functions for endorphins. It is probable that careful analysis of other systems will reveal further effects of opiate antagonists, suggesting other functions for endorphins. Against these observations, the failure of naloxone, given as a single dose to normal human subjects, to produce subjective effects must be evaluated. Grevert and Goldstein (450) found that an intravenous dose of 10 mg of naloxone produced no effect on responses to a questionnaire evaluating mood (Profile of Mood State Questionnaire), furthermore, these subjects could not distinguish between naloxone and saline injections. It is likely that the moderately painful stimulus employed in the measurement of pain threshold in these studies did not provoke endorphin release. Short-term blockade of release of growth hormone or prolactin would not have been detected. There was no indication of impairment of motor function in any subject.

Since endorphin release is probably provoked under very specific circumstances, short-term studies with single doses of naloxone do not provide an adequate measure of the normal role of endorphins. Unfortunately, long-term administration of naloxone or naltrexone has only been studied in former heroin addicts. In these subjects the only consistently reported disturbance of normal function is abdominal discomfort (for a review of naltrexone effects in the treatment of heroin addicts, see Ref. 495). However, hormonal function, experimental analgesias, and other functions in which endorphins might be implicated have not been evaluated in detail in these subjects. Nevertheless, it is surprising that complaints of, for example, lack of pleasurable rewards, have not been voiced with sufficient frequency for the effect to have been identified as a drug-induced phenomenon. It could be argued that the use of former heroin addicts precludes the demonstration of antagonism of endorphins by naloxone or naltrexone, because the normal function of endorphins is suppressed in former addicts. Suppressed endorphin function could be a pathological defect in individiuals who subsequently become heroin addicts, or could arise as a result of the prolonged administration of exogenous opiates. This argument is not supported by the very limited data on endorphin function in opiate-dependent animals, where brain and pituitary stores of endorphins are essentially unaffected by chronic opiate administration or withdrawal (see Sec. VI). There is therefore a need for more critical studies of opiate antagonist effect on specific systems in humans.

VI. ENDORPHIN FUNCTION IN OPIATE TOLERANCE AND DEPENDENCE

Animals rendered tolerant to the analgesic action of morphine are also tolerant to the analgesic effects of intraventricularly administered β-endorphin (496). Repeated intraventricular administration of partially purified pituitary endorphin (497) or β-endorphin (498, 499) also produces tolerance to the analgesic actions of subsequently administered endorphins or morphine. Cross-tolerance between morphine and enkephalins has also been demonstrated in isolated preparations of guinea pig ileum and mouse vas deferens (500). In the guinea pig ileum preparation, quantitatively similar shifts of the position and slope of the dose-response curves for normorphine and pituitary endorphin were observed after morphine pretreatment (375). Continuous infusion of Met-enkephalin or β-endorphin into the PAG of rat brain over a period of 70 hr also induced a state of physical dependence. Systemic administration of naloxone in these animals provoked a typical morphinelike withdrawal syndrome (501).

These results make it clear that long periods of opiate receptor activation lead to the development of tolerance and physical dependence, irrespective of whether the activating ligand is an alkaloid, a synthetic opiate, or an endogenous opioid peptide. For this reason it is very unlikely that opiate receptors are normally activated by endogenous ligands over long periods of time. Functional effectiveness of receptor occupation requires that the periods of occupation be short and relatively infrequent. When morphine is administered by intravenous infusion, tolerance can be detected within 3-4 hr (502). Thus periods of physiologically induced receptor occupation might be expected to be significantly shorter than 3 hr.

It has been suggested that the repeated administration of exogenous opiates, in doses sufficient to produce significant activation of opiate receptors, will result in a compensatory reduction in the release of endogenous opiates (503, 504). This hypothesis has not been confirmed in a study of plasma and pituitary levels of β-endorphin in rats (338). Acute administration of morphine (10 or 50 mg/kg, i.p.) raised rather than lowered plasma β-endorphin levels two- to threefold. However, the levels returned to normal during chronic treatment with morphine. The effects of chronic exposure to morphine on the pituitary gland content of endorphins has also been measured. Although implantation of morphine pellets in rats for 3 days did not affect pituitary endorphin content as measured by bioassay (335), repeated implantations of morphine pellets over a period of 1 month resulted in a substantial decline in both anterior and posterior lobe β-endorphin-like immunoreactivity (338). This effect may be more related to the severity of the stress applied to the animals than to a specific response to the high levels of circulating exogenous opioid drug. Naloxone-precipitated withdrawal also depleted anterior (but not posterior) lobe β-endorphin-like immunoreactivity, and increased the levels of the peptide in plasma (338). Again, the stress of precipitated withdrawal may be implicated. The effect of chronic treatment with opiates on the brain levels of enkephalins has also been investigated. Thus Fratta et al. (489) did not find any changes in the Met-enkephalin content (measured by radioimmunoassay) of rat brain regions in morphine-pretreated animals or after precipitation of withdrawal by an opiate antagonist. Similar results were obtained by Wesche et al. (109). An early report of elevated levels of enkephalin in brains of morphine-pretreated rats (505) could not be substantiated. With more reliable extraction and assay procedures, the same laboratory now finds no difference in Met- and Leu-enkephalin levels in whole brain, or separated hypothalamus or striatum after morphine pretreatment or withdrawal (506).

An interesting recent development has been the characterization of membrane-bound enzyme capable of cleaving enkephalin at the Gly-Phe bond, thus abolishing its opioid activity (98). The high affinity for enkephalin of this enzyme, and its location in membrane fractions containing opiate receptors, suggests a significant role in the termination of action of physiologically released enkephalin (see Sec. II. C).

The report, therefore, that the activity of this enzyme in brain membrane is substantially increased following implantation of a morphine pellet for 3 days in mice, may be of considerable importance in understanding the adaptive responses of the nervous system to sustained exposure to opiates. The implication that the activity of an enkephalin-degrading enzyme might be regulated by the level of occupation of opiate receptors clearly requires further study.

The possibility that a deficiency of the endorphin system is an etiological factor in opiate addiction, and contributes to the high relapse rate of former heroin addicts after detoxification has been raised (503). This hypothesis is very difficult to test experimentally. Although tests of pituitary endorphin function in humans will probably be developed in the near future, measures of brain endorphin function in humans present a more difficult problem. Indirect tests based on the effects of opiate antagonists cannot be applied to heroin addicts. However, tests based on behavioral or biochemical response to specific stimuli, which can be validated as being measures of brain endorphin function by animal studies, might be developed in the future.

VII. OVERVIEW

Many questions remain to be resolved before physiological functions can be assigned with certainty to any of the endorphins. However, many relevant data have accumulated and some preliminary suggestions can be made.

Both Met- and Leu-enkephalin have been shown to be present within the terminals and cell bodies of some central and peripheral neurons. In most cases the enkephalin-containing neurons appear to be local neurons intrinsic to particular structures, but some longer enkephalin-containing tracts have been found. It now seems improbable that Met-enkephalin is synthesized by cleavage of larger peptides that are also precursors for β-endorphin and ACTH. The biosynthesis of Leu-enkephalin is also obscure. Large potential precursor peptides containing both the Met- and Leu-enkephalin sequences have been found in brain and adrenal medulla. Peptides with C-terminal extensions of Leu-enkephalin have been isolated from hypothalamus and pituitary. Since these peptides have considerable opioid potency, it is not certain that they function as Leu-enkephalin precursors.

Although release of enkephalin from slices of brain tissue in vitro in response to elevated potassium concentrations, or to veratridine, has been demonstrated, it has not yet been possible to show that these peptides are released from intact neurons in situ in response to either electrical stimulation or physiological activation of specific neuronal pathways. Microiontophoretically applied enkephalins have been shown to affect the firing rates of neurons in many brain regions in a manner similar to opiate drugs. However, correlations of the quantities of enkephalin released with concentrations required to affect neuronal activity have not been reported. Ultimately it will be necessary to show that the same postsynaptic events follow physiological activation of an enkephalin-containing neuron in synaptic contact with an enkephalin-sensitive cell, and the direct application of exogenous enkephalin to that cell. Released enkephalin is rapidly degraded by peptidases in brain; specific uptake of enkephalins into cells has not been reported. Thus, although rigorous proof is lacking, there are many indications that enkephalins function as neurtotransmitters in brain.

The presence of β-endorphin in a select group of hypothalamic neurons with fiber tracts running to several brain structures containing opiate receptors is now well established. These neurons are not dependent on the pituitary gland for a source of β-endorphin, but probably synthesize the peptide by the same mechanism as pituitary corticotroph cells, since β-LPH and ACTH are probably present in the same neurons. Release of β-endorphin from these fibers has not yet been demonstrated. The β-endorphin-containing neurons are distinctly different from the neurons shown to contain enkephalin by immunocytochemical techniques and have a different distribution within the brain.

Intraventricular injections of β-endorphin have been shown to produce analgesia and immobility, to promote hormone release, and to affect the rate of turnover of some putative neurotransmitter substances in some brain structures. Microiontophoretically applied β-endorphin produces effects on neuronal firing rate similar to those of the enkephalins and opiate drugs. Whereas the intraventricular administration of β-endorphin produces effects lasting several hours, changes in firing rate induced by microiontophoretically applied β-endorphin have not been shown to last very much longer than the changes induced by the enkephalins. Since β-endorphin is relatively stable to enzymatic degradation, diffusion from the receptor may limit the duration of action of this peptide after local release. Thus available data are consistent with the possibility that β-endorphin may function as a neurotransmitter in a discrete group of neurons in the hypothalamus. A release of β-endorphin from hypothalamic neurons into the third ventricle from whence it may diffuse to other brain regions to modulate neuronal activity, is also conceivable.

The functions of β-endorphin in pituitary remain obscure. The concentration of peptide released into the general circulation by the most potent stimuli so far discovered (adrenalectomy, a grossly unphysiological procedure) is inadequate to produce more than marginal effects on peripheral structures bearing opiate receptors. An intrapituitary role in the regulation of release of neurohypophysial peptides (e.g., vasopressin or oxytocin) is possible but has not yet been demonstrated. Recent anatomical studies suggest that retrograde transport of peptides from pituitary to brain might occur under some circumstances. A function of pituitary β-endorphin as a modulator of the activity of hypothalamic neurons, or other opiate-sensitive neurons in close proximity with the cerebral ventricles, is conceivable. When the peptide gains access to receptors from blood or CSF, its resistance to enzymatic degradation suggests that long-lasting changes in neuronal activity might result.

Functional studies utilizing narcotic antagonists indicate that endorphins play a role in the normal regulation of PRL, and less certainly, GH release. Endorphins may also be implicated in the control of release of other anterior pituitary hormones such as LH. The hypothalamus is a probable site of endorphin action in hormonal regulation. This region contains a high concentration of opiate receptors, of enkephalin and β-endorphin, and transport of β-endorphin from pituitary to hypothalamus is possible. There is no evidence to suggest that endorphins act in the anterior pituitary to effect hormonal release.

Despite intensive studies of opiate antagonist effects on response to painful stimuli, no clear demonstration of a normal physiological role for endorphins in the modulation of pain perception has emerged. Further studies are also needed to elucidate possible roles for endorphins in motor control and in temperature regulation. Major advances in our understanding of the role of endorphins in specific functions will probably require the development of methods for the estimation of turnover rate in discrete brain nuclei, thus enabling the correlation of endorphin utilization with specific biochemical, electrophysiological, or behavioral effects.

ACKNOWLEDGMENTS

The authors wish to express their gratitude to Drs. Avram Goldstein, Vartan Ghazarossian, Robert R. M. Dent, Frances Leslie, and Priscilla Grevert for helpful discussion and advice, and to Janice C. Jeffery for help in the preparation of the manuscript. Research by the authors was supported in part by Grants DA 01199 and DA 07063 awarded by the National Institute on Drug Abuse.

REFERENCES

1. J. Hughes, T. W. Smith, H. W. Kosterlitz, L. A. Fothergill, B. A. Morgan, and H. R. Morris, *Nature, 258*: 577 (1975).
2. C. H. Li and D. Chung, *Proc. Natl. Acad. Sci. U.S.A., 73*: 1145 (1976).
3. R. Werman, *Comp. Biochem. Physiol., 18*: 745 (1966).
4. R. Werman, *Annu. Rev. Physiol., 34*: 337 (1972).
5. J. R. Cooper, F. E. Bloom, and R. H. Roth, *The Biochemical Basis of Neuropharmacology*, 3rd ed., Oxford University Press, New York, 1978, pp. 9–46.
6. R. Hammerschlag and E. Roberts, in *Basic Neurochemistry*, 2nd ed. (G. J. Siegel, R. W. Albers, R. Katzman, and B. W. Agranoff, eds.), Little, Brown, Boston, 1976, pp. 167–179.
7. J. W. Phillis, *The Pharmacology of Synapses*, Pergamon Press, Elmsford, N.Y., 1970.
8. R. C. A. Frederickson, *Life Sci., 21*: 23 (1977).
9. L. Terenius, *Annu. Rev. Pharmacol. Toxicol., 18*: 189 (1978).
10. A. Beaumont and J. Hughes, *Annu. Rev. Pharmacol. Toxicol., 19*: 245 (1979).
11. S. H. Snyder and H. B. Innis, *Annu. Rev. Biochem., 48*: 755 (1979).
12. R. J. Miller and P. Cuatrecasas, *Vitam. and Horm., 36*: 297 (1978).
13. T. Hokfelt, R. Elde, C. Johansson, L. Terenius, and L. Stein, *Neurosci. Lett., 5*: 25 (1977).

14. R. Simantov, M. J. Kuhar, G. R. Uhl, and S. H. Snyder, *Proc. Natl. Acad. Sci. U.S.A.*, *74*: 2167 (1977).
15. S. Watson, J. D. Barchas, and C. H. Li, *Proc. Natl. Acad. Sci. U.S.A.*, *74*: 5155 (1977).
16. S. J. Watson, H. Akil, C. W. Richard, and J. D. Barchas, *Nature*, *275*: 266 (1978).
17. F. E. Bloom, E. Battenberg, J. Rossier, N. Ling, and R. Guillemin, *Proc. Natl. Acad. Sci. U.S.A.*, *75*: 1591 (1978).
18. M. Sar, W. E. Stumpf, R. J. Miller, K. J. Shang, and P. Cuatrecasas, *J. Comp. Neurol.*, *182*: 17 (1978).
19. G. R. Uhl, R. R. Goodman, M. J. Kuhar, S. R. Childers, and S. H. Snyder, *Brain Res.*, *166*: 75 (1979).
20. G. Tramu and J. Leonardelli, *Brain Res.*, *168*: 457 (1979).
21. J. Hughes, H. W. Kosterlitz, and T. W. Smith, *Br. J. Pharmacol.*, *61*: 639 (1977).
22. J. S. Hong, H. Y. T. Yang, W. Fratta, and E. Costa, *Brain Res.*, *134*: 383 (1977).
23. J. Rossier, T. M. Vargo, S. Minick, N. Ling, F. E. Bloom, and R. Guillemin, *Proc. Natl. Acad. Sci. U.S.A.*, *74*: 5162 (1977).
24. J. Rossier, A. Bayon, T. M. Vargo, N. Ling, R. Guillemin, and F. E. Bloom, *Life Sci.*, *21*: 847 (1977).
25. R. J. Miller, K. J. Chang, B. R. Cooper, and P. Cuatrecasas, *J. Biol. Chem.*, *253*: 531 (1978).
26. I. Lindberg, S. J. Smyth, and J. L. Dahl, *Brain Res.*, *168*: 200 (1979).
27. A. M. DiGiulio, E. M. Majane, and H. Y. T. Yang, *Br. J. Pharmacol.*, *66*: 297 (1979).
28. C. B. Pert and S. H. Snyder, *Science*, *179*: 1011 (1973).
29. J. M. Miller, J. Pearson, and E. J. Simon, *Res. Commun. Chem. Pathol. Pharmacol.*, *6*: 1052 (1973).
30. C. B. Pert, M. J. Kuhar, and S. H. Snyder, *Proc. Natl. Acad. Sci. U.S.A.*, *73*: 3729 (1976).
31. S. F. Atweh and M. J. Kuhar, *Brain Res.*, *124*: 53 (1977).
32. S. F. Atweh and M. J. Kuhar, *Brain Res.*, *129*: 1 (1977).
33. S. F. Atweh and M. J. Kuhar, *Brain Res.*, *134*: 393 (1977).
34. T. W. Smith, J. Hughes, H. W. Kosterlitz, and R. P. Sosa, in *Opiates and Endogenous Opioid Peptides* (H. W. Kosterlitz, ed.), Elsevier/North-Holland, Amsterdam, 1976, pp. 57–62.
35. I. Creese and S. H. Snyder, *J. Pharmacol. Exp. Ther.*, *194*: 205 (1975).
36. M. Schultzberg, T. Hokfelt, J. M. Lundberg, L. Terenius, L. G. Elfvin, and R. Elde, *Acta Physiol. Scand.*, *103*: 475 (1978).
37. A. M. DiGuilio, H. Y. T. Yang, B. Lutold, W. Fratta, J. Hong, and E. Costa, *Neuropharmacology*, *17*: 989 (1978).
38. M. Schultzberg, J. M. Lundberg, T. Hokfelt, L. Terenius, J. Brandt, R. Elde, and M. Goldstein, *Neuroscience*, *3*: 1169 (1978).
39. F. M. Leslie, C. Chavin, and B. M. Cox, in *Endogenous and Exogenous Opiate Agonists and Antagonists*, (E. L. Way, ed.), Pergamon Press, Elmsford, N.Y., 1980.

40. G. W. Pasternak, R. Goodman, S. H. Snyder, *Life Sci., 16*: 1765(1975).
41. C. B. Pert, A. M. Snowman, and S. H. Snyder, *Brain Res., 70*: 174 (1974).
42. R. Simantov, A. M. Snowman, and S. H. Snyder, *Brain Res., 107*: 650 (1976).
43. G. Queen, C. Pinsky, and F. LaBella, *Biochem. Biophys. Res. Commun., 72*: 1021 (1976).
44. H. Osborne, V. Hollt, and A. Herz, *Life Sci., 22*: 611 (1978).
45. V. M. Pickel, T. H. Joh, D. J. Reis, S. E. Leeman, and R. J. Miller, *Brain Res., 160*: 387 (1979).
46. E. Habermann, *Naunyn-Schmiedeberg's Arch. Pharmacol., 197* (Suppl. 1): 511 (1977).
47. J. D. Belluzzi, N. Grant. V. Garsky, D. Sarantakis, C. D. Wise, and L. Stein, *Nature, 260*: 625 (1976).
48. H. H. Buscher, R. C. Hill, D. Romer, F. Cardinaux, A. Closse, D. Hauser, and J. Pless, *Nature, 261*: 423 (1976).
49. J. K. Chang, B. T. W. Fong, A. Pert, and C. B. Pert, *Life Sci., 18*: 1473 (1976).
50. C. B. Pert, A. Pert. J. K. Chang, and B. T. W. Fong, *Science, 194*: 330 (1976).
51. L. Graf, J. I. Szekely, A. Z. Ronai, Z. Dunai-Kovacs, and S. Bajusz, *Nature, 263*: 240 (1976).
52. Y. Jacquet and N. Marks, *Science, 194*: 632 (1976).
53. L. G. Sharpe, J. E. Garnett, and T. J. Cicero, *Behav. Biol., 11*: 303 (1974).
54. A. Pert and T. Yaksh, *Brain Res., 80*: 135 (1975).
55. Y. F. Jacquet and A. Lajtha, *Science, 182*: 490 (1973).
56. T. L. Yaksh, J. C. Yeung, and T. A. Rudy, *Brain Res., 114*: 83 (1976).
57. V. A. Lewis and G. F. Gebhart, *Brain Res., 124*: 283 (1977).
58. E. Wei, L. F. Tseng, H. H. Loh and C. H. Li, *Life Sci., 21*: 321 (1977).
59. H. H. Loh, L. F. Tseng, E. Wei, and C. H. Li, *Proc. Natl. Acad. Sci. U.S.A., 73*: 2895 (1976).
60. A. Pert, in *Opiates and Endogenous Opioid Peptides* (H. W. Kosterlitz, ed.), Elsevier/North-Holland, Amsterdam, 1976, pp. 87–94.
61. C. B. Pert, D. L. Bowie, B. T. W. Fong, and J. K. Chang, in *Opiates and Endogenous Opioid Peptides* (H. W. Kosterlitz, ed.), Elsevier/North-Holland, Amsterdam, 1976. pp. 79–86.
62. F. Bloom, D. Segal, N. Ling, and R. Guillemin, *Science, 194:* 630(1976).
63. J. M. Hambrook, B. A. Morgan, M. J. Rance, and C. F. C. Smith, *Nature, 262*: 782 (1976).
64. R. J. Miller, K. J. Chang, P. Cuatrecasas, and S. Wilkinson, *Biochem. Biophys. Res. Commun., 74*: 1311 (1977).
65. J. L. Meek, H. Y. T. Yang, and E. Costa, *Neuropharmacology, 16*: 151 (1977).
66. M. M. Puig, P. Gascon, G. L. Craviso, R. A. Bjur, G. Matsueda, J. M. Stewart, and J. M. Musacchio, *Arch. Int. Pharmacodyn. Ther., 226*: 69 (1977).
67. N. Marks, A. Grynbaum, and A. Neidle, *Biochem. Biophys. Res. Commun., 74*: 1552 (1977).
68. A. Grynbaum. A. J. Kastin, D. H. Coy, and N. Marks, *Brain Res. Bull., 2*: 479 (1977).
69. A. Dupont, L. Cusan, M. Garon, G. A. Urbina, and F. Labrie, *Life Sci., 21*: 907(1977).

70. J. M. Musacchio, M. M. Puig, and G. L. Craviso, in *Endorphins in Mental Health Research* (E. Usdin, W. E. Bunney, Jr., and N. S. Kline, eds.), Oxford University Press, New York, 1979, pp. 219–234.
71. E. Hazum, K. J. Chang, and P. Cuatrecasas, *Life Sci., 24*: 137 (1979).
72. E. G. Erdos, A. R. Johnson, and N. J. Boyden, *Biochem. Pharmacol., 27*: 843 (1978).
73. A. J. Kastin, C. Nissen, A. V. Schally, and D. A. Coy, *Brain Res. Bull., 1:* 583 (1976).
74. C. R. Beddell, R. B. Clark, G. W. Hardy, L. A. Lowe , F. B. Ubatuba, J. R. Vane, S. Wilkinson, K. J. Chang, P. Cuatrecasas, and R. J. Miller, *Proc. Soc. Lond., 198*: 249 (1977).
75. P. F. Von Voightlander and R. A. Lewis, *Res. Commun. Chem. Pathol. Pharmacol., 20*: 265 (1978).
76. S. Bajusz, A Patthy, A. Kenessey, L. Graf, J. I. Szekely, and A. Z. Ronai, *Biochem. Biophys. Res. Commun., 84*: 1045 (1978).
77. F. B. Craves, P. Y. Law, C. A. Hunt, and H. H. Loh, *J. Pharmacol. Exp. Ther., 206*: 492 (1978).
78. R. Simantov and S. H. Snyder, *Mol. Pharmacol., 12*: 987 (1976).
79. N. Marks, in *Frontiers in Neuroendocrinology* (W. F. Ganong and L. Martin, eds.), Raven Press, New York, 1978, pp. 329–377.
80. R. K. Barclay and M. A. Phillips, *Biochem. Biophys. Res. Commun., 81*: 1119 (1978).
81. M. Knight and W. A. Klee, *J. Biol. Chem., 253*: 3843 (1978).
82. A. C. Lane, M. J. Rance, and D. S. Walter, *J. Biol. Chem., 269*: 75(1977).
83. B. Malfroy, J. P. Swerts, A. Guyon, B. P. Roques, and J. C. Schwartz, *Nature, 276*: 523 (1978).
84. A. F. Bradbury, D. G. Smyth, C. R. Snell, J. F. W. Deakin, and S. Wendlandt, *Biochem. Biophys. Res. Commun., 74*: 748 (1977).
85. B. Malfroy, J. P. Swerts, C. Llorens, and J. C. Schwartz, *Neurosci. Lett., 11*: 329 (1979).
86. J. P. Swerts, R. Perdrisot, B. Malfroy, and J. C. Schwartz, *Eur. J. Pharmacol., 53*: 209 (1979).
87. S. Sullivan, H. Akil, and J. D. Barchas, *Commun. Psycopharmacol., 2*: 525 (1978).
88. C. Raduoco-Thomas, F. Garcin, G. Mack, and S. Raduoco-Thomas, in *Opiates and Endogenous Opioid Peptides* (H. W. Kosterlitz, ed.), Elsevier/North-Holland, Amsterdam, 1976, pp. 111–119.
89. P. Bolme, K. Fuxe, L. F. Agnati, R. Bradley, and J. Smithies, *Eur. J. Pharmacol., 48*: 319 (1978).
90. J. Florez, A. Mediavilla, A. Pazos, in *Characteristics and Function of Opioids* (J. M. van Ree and L. Terneius, eds.), Elsevier/North-Holand, Amsterdam, 1978, pp. 167–168.
91. A. Cowan, J. Doxey, and G. Metcalf, in *Opiates and Endogenous Opioid Peptides* (H. W. Kosterlitz, ed.), Elsevier/North-Holland, Amsterdam, 1976, pp. 95–102.
92. E. Wei and H. H. Loh, *Science, 193*: 1262 (1976).

93. L. Lazarus, N. Ling, and R. Guillemin, *Proc. Natl. Acad. Sci. U.S.A.*, *73*: 2156 (1976).
94. R. V. Lewis, S. Stein, L. D. Gerber, M. Rubinstein, and S. Udenfriend, *Proc. Natl. Acad. Sci. U.S.A.*, *75*: 4021 (1978).
95. K. Kanagawa and H. Matsuo, *Biochem. Biophys. Res. Commun.*, *86*: 153 (1979).
96. S. R. Childers and S. H. Snyder, in *Central Nervous System Effects of Hypothalamic Hormones and Other Peptides* (R. Collu, J. R. Ducharme, A. Barbeau, and J. C. Rochefort, eds.), Raven Press, New York, 1979, pp. 253–260.
97. H. Y. T. Yang, W. Fratta, J. S. Hong, A. M. DiGiulio, and E. Costa, *Neuropharmacology*, *17*: 433 (1978).
98. H. Akil, S. J. Watson, R. M. Levy, and J. D. Barchas, in *Characteristics and Function of Opioids* (J. M. van Ree and L. Terenius, eds.), Elsevier/North-Holland, Amsterdam, 1978, pp. 123–134.
99. S. J. Watson, C. W. Richard, and J. D. Barchas, *Science*, *200*: 180 (1978).
100. E. Weber, R. Martin, and K. H. Voigt, *Life Sci.*, *25*: 1111(1979).
101. G. Pelletier, L. Desy, J. C. Lissitsky, F. Labrie, and C. H. Li, *Life Sci.*, *22*: 1799 (1978).
102. G. Pelletier, R. Leclerc, F. Labrie, J. Cote, M. Chretien, and M. Lis, *Endocrinology*, *100*: 770 (1977).
103. F. E. Bloom, E. O. Battenberg, J. Rossier, N. Ling, J. Leppaluoto, T. M. Vargo, and R. Guillemin, *Life Sci.*, *20*: 43 (1977).
104. R. E. Mains, B. A. Eipper, and N. Ling, *Proc. Natl. Acad. Sci. U.S.A.*, *74*: 3014 (1977).
105. J. L. Roberts and E. Herbert, *Proc. Natl. Acad. Sci. U.S.A.*, *74*: 4826 (1977).
106. S. Nakanishi, A. Inoue, T. Kita, M. Nakamura, A. C. Y. Chang, S. N. Cohen, and S. Numa, *Nature*, *278*: 423 (1979).
107. P. Crine, C. Gianoulakis, N. G. Seidah, F. Gossard, P. D. Pezalla, M. Lis, and M. Chrétien, *Proc. Natl. Acad. Sci. U.S.A.*, *75*: 4719 (1978).
108. A. L. Cheung and A. Goldstein, *Life Sci.*, *19*: 1005 (1976).
109. D. Wesche, V. Hollt, and A. Herz, *Naunyn-Schmiedeberg's Arch Pharmacol.*, *301*: 79 (1978).
110. R. M. Kobayashi, M. Palkovits, R. J. Miller, K. J. Chang, and P. Cuatrecasas, *Life Sci.*, *22*: 527 (1978).
111. J. M. Lundberg, B. Hamberger, M. Schultzberg, T. Hokfelt, P. O. Granberg, S. Efendic, L. Terenius, M. Goldstein, and R. Luft, *Proc. Natl. Acad. Sci. U.S.A.*, *76*: 4079 (1979).
112. J. Rossier, R. V. Lewis, S. Stein, and S. Udenfriend, *Soc. Neurosci.* (abstr.), *5*: 538 (1979).
113. D. Clouet and M. Ratner, in *Opiates and Endogenous Opioid Peptides*, Elsevier/North-Holland, Amsterdam, 1976, pp. 71–78.
114. H. Y. T. Yang, J. S. Hong, W. Fratta, and E. Costa, *Adv. Biochem. Psychopharmacol.*, *18*: 149 (1978).
115. A. T. McKnight, R. P. Sosa, J. Hughes, and H. W. Kosterlitz, in *Characteristics and Function of Opioids* (J. M. van Ree and L. Terenius, eds.), Elsevier/North-Holland, Amsterdam, 1978, pp. 259–269.

116. A. A. Waterfield, R. W. J. Smokcum, J. Hughes, H. W. Kosterlitz, and G. Henderson, *Eur. J. Pharmacol., 43*: 107 (1977).
117. A. A. Waterfield and H. W. Kosterlitz, *Life Sci., 16*: 1787 (1975).
118. M. M. Puig, P. Gascon, G. L. Craviso, and J. M. Musacchio, *Science, 195*: 419 (1977).
119. M. M. Puig, P. Gascon, and J. M. Musacchio, *Eur. J. Pharmacol., 45*: 205 (1977).
120. J. M. Van Nueten, P. A. J. Janssen, and J. Fontaine, *Life Sci., 18*: 803 (1976).
121. I. J. Bodycote and G. B. Chesher, *Eur. J. Pharmacol., 57*: 259 (1979).
122. R. Schulz, M. Wuster, R. Simantov, S. Snyder, and A. Herz, *Eur. J. Pharmacol., 41*: 347 (1977).
123. G. Henderson, J. Hughes, and H. W. Kosterlitz, *Nature, 271*: 677 (1978).
124. J. A. Richter, D. L. Wesche, and R. C. A. Frederickson, *Eur. J. Pharmacol., 56*: 105 (1979).
125. H. Osborne, V. Hollt, and A. Herz, *Eur. J. Pharmacol., 48:* 219(1978).
126. L. L. Iversen, S. D. Iversen, F. E. Bloom, T. Vargo, and R. Guillemin, *Nature, 271*: 679 (1978).
127. A. Bayon, J. Rossier, A. Mauss, F. E. Bloom, L. L. Iversen, N. Ling, and E. Guillemin, *Proc. Natl. Acad. Sci. U.S.A., 75*: 3503 (1978).
128. R. R. Llinas and J. E. Heuser, eds., *Neurosci. Res. Program Bull., 15* (4); 557 (1977).
129. T. M. Jessel, L. L. Iversen, and I. Kanazawa, *Nature, 264*: 81 (1976).
130. A. Wahlstrom, L. Johansson, and L. Terenius, in *Opiates and Endogenous Opioid Peptides* (H. W. Kosterlitz, ed.), Elsevier/North-Holland, Amsterdam, 1976, pp. 49–56.
131. R. A. North, *Life Sci., 24*: 1527 (1979).
132. J. P. Gent and J. H. Wolstencroft, in *Opiates and Endogenous Opioid Peptides* (H. W. Kosterlitz, ed.), Elsevier/North-Holland, Amsterdam, 1976, pp. 217–224.
133. J. P. Gent and J. H. Wolstencroft, *Nature, 261*: 426 (1976).
134. P. B. Bradley, I. Briggs, R. J. Gayton, and L. A. Lambert, *Nature, 261*: 425 (1976).
135. P. B. Bradley, R. J. Gayton, and L. A. Lambert, *Br. J. Pharmacol., 61*: 147 (1977).
136. R. G. Hill, C. M. Pepper, and J. F. Mitchell, *Nature, 262*: 604 (1976).
137. R. G. Hill and C. M. Pepper, *Br. J. Pharmacol., 58*: 459P (1976).
138. R. G. Hill, C. M. Pepper, and J. F. Mitchell, in *Opiates and Endogenous Opioid Peptides* (H. W. Kosterlitz, ed.), Elsevier/North-Holland, Amsterdam, 1976, pp. 225–238.
139. W. Zieglgansberger, J. P. Fry, A. Herz, L. Moroder, and E. Wunsch, *Brain Res., 115*: 160 (1976).
140. R. C. A. Frederickson and F. H. Norris, *Science, 194*: 440 (1976).
141. P. S. McCarthy, R. J. Walker, and G. N. Woodruff, *J. Physiol. (Lond.), 267*: 40P (1977).
142. W. S. Young, S. J. Bird, and M. J. Kuhar, *Brain Res., 129:* 366 (1977).
143. R. A. North and J. T. Williams, *Nature, 264*: 460 (1976).
144. A. W. Dugan, J. G. Hall, and P. M. Headley, *Nature, 264*: 456 (1976).
145. A. W. Dugan, J. G. Hall, and P. M. Headley, *Br. J. Pharmacol., 61*: 399 (1977).
146. J. Davies and A. Dray, *Br. J. Pharmacol., 58*: 458P (1976).

147. R. A. Nicoll, G. R. Siggins, N. Ling, F. E. Bloom, and R. Guillemin, *Proc. Natl. Acad. Sci. U.S.A.*, *74*: 2584 (1977).
148. J. Davies and A. Dray, *Nature*, *262*: 603 (1976).
149. J. Davies and A. Dray, *Br. J. Pharmacol.*, *63*: 87 (1978).
150. R. G. Hill, J. F. Mitchell, and C. M. Pepper, *J. Physiol. (Lond.)*, *272*: 50P (1977).
151. W. Zieglgansberger, G. R. Siggins, E. French, and F. E. Bloom, in *Characteristics and Function of Opioids* (J. M. Van Ree and L. Terenius, eds.), Elsevier/North-Holland, Amsterdam, 1978, pp. 75–86.
152. D. Taylor, B. Hoffer, W. Zieglgansberger, G. Siggins, N. Ling, A. Seiger, and L. Olson, *Brain Res.*, *176*: 135 (1979).
153. W. Zieglgansberger, E. D. French, G. R. Siggins, and F. E. Bloom, *Science*, *205*: 415 (1979).
154. P. B. Bradley and G. J. Bramwell, *Neuropharmacology*, *16*: 519 (1977).
155. S. J. Bird and M. J. Kuhar, *Brain Res.*, *122*: 523 (1977).
156. M. Satoh, W. Zieglgansberger, and A. Herz, *Brain Res.*, *115*: 99 (1976).
157. M. R. Palmer, D. H. Morris, D. A. Taylor, J. M. Stewart, and B. J. Hoffer, *Life Sci.*, *23*: 851 (1978).
158. R. Dingledine and A. Goldstein, *J. Pharmacol. Exp. Ther.*, *196*: 97 (1976).
159. R. A. North and M. Tonini, *Br. J. Pharmacol.*, *61*: 541 (1977).
160. R. A. North, Y. Katayama, and J. T. Williams, *Brain Res.*, *165*: 67 (1979).
161. R. K. Anderson, J. P. Lund, and E. Puil, *Can. J. Physiol. Pharmacol.*, *56*: 216 (1978).
162. M. Satoh, A. Akaike, and H. Takagi, *Brain Res.*, *169*: 406 (1979).
163. H. Takagi, M. Satoh, A. Akaike, T. Shibata, H. Yajima, and H. Ogawa, *Eur. J. Pharmacol.*, *49*: 113 (1978).
164. A. I. Basbaum, C. H. Clanton, and H. L. Fields, *J. Comp. Neurol.*, *178*: 209 (1978).
165. D. J. Mayer and D. D. Price, *Pain*, *2*: 379 (1976).
166. F. W. L. Kerr and K. L. Casey, eds., *Neurosci. Res. Program Bull.*, *16*: 1 (1978).
167. T. L. Yaksh and T. A. Rudy, *Pain*, *4*: 299 (1978).
168. H. L. Fields and A. I. Basbaum, *Annu. Rev. Physiol.*, *40*: 217 (1978).
169. C. Lamotte, C. B. Pert, and S. H. Snyder, *Brain Res.*, *112*: 407 (1976).
170. R. G. Hill and C. M. Pepper, *Eur. J. Pharmacol.*, *47*: 223 (1978).
171. B. M. Cox and and M. Weinstock, *Br. J. Pharmacol.*, *27*: 81 (1966).
172. G. Henderson, J. Hughes, and H. W. Kosterlitz, *Br. J. Pharmacol.*, *46*: 764 (1972).
173. J. T. Williams and R. North, *Brain Res.*, *165*: 57 (1979).
174. E. A. North and W. Zieglgansberger, *Brain Res.*, *144*: 208 (1978).
175. W. Zieglgansberger and I. F. Tulloch, *Brain Res.*, *167*: 53 (1979).
176. J. L. Barker, T. G. Smith, Jr., and J. H. Neale, *Brain Res.*, *154*: 153 (1978).
177. J. L. Barker, J. H. Neale, T. G. Smith, Jr., and R. L. Macdonald, *Science*, *199*: 1451 (1978).
178. J. M. Hiller, E. J. Simon, S. M. Crain, and E. R. Peterson, *Brain Res.*, *145*: 396 (1978).

179. A. W. Mudge, S. E. Leeman, and G. D. Fishbach, *Proc. Natl. Acad. Sci. U.S.A.*, *76*: 526 (1979).
180. S. J. Henriksen. F. E. Bloom, F. McCoy, N. Ling and R. Guillemin, *Proc.Natl. Acd. Sci. U.S.A.*, *75*: 5221 (1978).
181. H. Frenk, G. Urca, and J. C. Liebeskind, *Brain Res.*, *147*: 327 (1978).
182. G. Henderson, *Eur. J. Pharmacol.*, *39*: 409 (1976).
183. T. Segawa, H. Murakami, H. Ogawa, and H. Yajima, *Jpn. J. Pharmacol.*, *28*: 13 (1978).
184. K. Jhamandas and M. Sutak, *Br. J. Pharmacol.*, *58*: 101 (1976).
185. K. Jhamandas, J. Sawynok, and M. Sutak, *Nature*, *269*: 433 (1977).
186. L. J. Botticelli and R. J. Wurtman, *Life Sci.*, *24*: 1799 (1979).
187. H. D. Taube, E. Borowski, T. Endo, and K. Starke, *Eur. J. Pharmacol.*, *38*: 377 (1976).
188. E. S. Vizi, L. G. Harsing, and J. Knoll, *Neuroscience*, *2*: 953 (1977).
189. S. Algeri, A. Consolazione, G. Calderini, G. Achilli, E. P. Canas, and S. Garattini, *Experientia*, *34*: 1488 (1978).
190. S. Algeri, G. Calderini, A. Consolazione, and G. Lomuscio, in *Characteristics and Function of Opioids* (J. M. van Ree and L. Terenius, eds.), Elsevier/North-Holland, Amsterdam, 1978, pp. 347–349.
191. N. Subramanian, P. Mitznegg, W. Sprugel, W. Domschke, S. Domschke, E. Wunsch, and L. Demling, *Naunyn-Schmiedeberg's Arch. Pharmacol.*, *299*: 163 (1977).
192. H. Pollard, C. Llorens, J. J. Bonnet, J. Costentin, and J. C. Schwartz, *Neurosci. Lett.*, *7*: 295 (1977).
193. A. Czlonkowski, V. Hollt, and A. Herz, *Life Sci.*, *22*: 953 (1978).
194. K. Kuschinsky, *Arzneim.-Forsch.*, *26*: 563 (1976).
195. S. Berney and O. Hornykiewicz, *Commun. Psychopharmacol.*, *1*: 597 (1977).
196. K. Izumi, T. Motomatsu, M. Chretien, R. F. Butterworth, M. Lis, N. Seidah, and A. Barbeau, *Life Sci.*, *20*: 1149 (1977).
197. J. S. Hong, H. Y. T. Yang, W. Fratta, and E. Costa, *J. Pharmacol. Exp. Ther.*, *205*: 141 (1978).
198. A. Pert, in *Characteristics and Function of Opioids* (J. M. van Ree and L. Terenius, eds.), Elsevier/North-Holland, Amsterdam, 1978, pp. 389–401.
199. A. Pert, L. A. DeWald, H. Liao, and C. Sivit, in *Endorphins in Mental Health Research* (W. E. Bunney, E. Usdin, and N. S. Kline, eds.), Oxford University Press, New York, 1979, pp. 45–61.
200. R. G. Browne, D. C. Derrington, and D. S. Segal, *Life Sci.*, *24*: 933 (1979).
201. S. Algeri, G. Calderini, A. Consolazione, and S. Garattini, *Eur. J. Pharmacol.*, *45*: 207 (1977).
202. G. Biggio, M. Casu, M. G. Corda, C. DiBello, and G. L. Gessa, *Science*, *200*: 552 (1978).
203. C. L. E. Broekkamp, A. G. Phillips, and A. R. Cools, *Nature*, *278*: 561 (1979).
204. F. Moroni, E. Peralta, D. L. Cheney, and E. Costa, *J. Pharmacol. Exp. Ther.*, *208*: 190 (1979).
205. F. Moroni, D. L. Cheney, E. Peralta, and E. Costa, *J. Pharmacol. Exp. Ther.*, *207*: 870 (1978).

206. J. S. Hong, H. Y. Yang, and E. Costa, *Neuropharmacology*, *16*: 451 (1977).
207. A. C. Cuello and G. Paxinos, *Nature*, *271*: 178 (1978).
208. M. Otsuka and T. Takahashi, *Annu. Rev. Pharmacol.*, *17*: 425 (1977).
209. S. Leeman and E. A. Mroz, *Life Sci.*, *15*: 2033 (1974).
210. T. M. Jessel and L. L. Iversen, *Nature*, *268*: 549 (1977).
211. T. Hokfelt, A. Ljungdahl, L. Terenius, R. Elde, and G. Nilsson, *Proc. Natl. Acad. Sci. U.S.A.*, *74*: 3081 (1977).
212. T. Jessel, A. Tsunoo, I. Kanazawa, and M. Otsuka, *Brain Res.*, *168*: 247 (1979).
213. Y. Nakata, Y. Kusaka, and T. Segawa, *Life Sci.*, *24*: 1651 (1979).
214. M. Otsuka and S. Konishi, *Nature*, *264*: 83 (1976).
215. J. L. Henry, *Brain Res.*, *114*: 439 (1976).
216. J. M. Stewert, C. J. Getto, K. Nelder, E. B. Reeve, W. A. Krivoy, and E. Zimmerman, *Nature*, *262*: 784 (1976).
217. J. B. Malick and J. M. Goldstein, *Life Sci.*, *23*: 835 (1978).
218. P. Oehme, J. Bergmann, M. Bienert, H. Hilse, L. Piesche, P. Minh Thu, and E. Scheer, in *Substance P* (U.S. Von Euler and B. Pernow, eds.), Raven Press, New York, 1977, p. 327.
219. R. C. A. Frederickson, V. Burgis, C. E. Harrel, and J. D. Edwards, *Science*, *199*: 1359 (1978).
220. M. S. Starr, T. H. James, and D. Gaytten, *Eur. J. Pharmacol.*, *48*: 203(1978).
221. L. Terenius, *J. Pharm. Pharmacol.*, *27*: 450 (1975).
222. R. Melzack and P. D. Wall, *Science*, *150*: 971 (1965).
223. P. Greengard, in *Advances in Cyclic Nucleotide Research*, Vol. 5 (G. I. Drummond, P. Greengard, and G. A. Robison, eds.), Raven Press, New York, 1975, p. 585.
224. H. O. J. Collier and A. C. Roy, *Nature*, *248*: 24 (1974).
225. W. A. Klee and M. Nirenberg, *Proc. Natl. Acad. Sci. U.S.A.*, *71*: 3474 (1974).
226. S. K. Sharma, M. Nirenberg, and W. A. Klee, *Proc. Natl. Acad. Sci. U.S.A.*, *72*: 590 (1975).
227. J. Traber, R. J. Gullis, and B. Hamprecht, *Life Sci.*, *16*: 63 (1975).
228. S. K. Sharma, W. A. Klee, and M. Nirenberg, *Proc. Natl. Acad. Sci. U.S.A.*, *72*: 3092 (1975).
229. J. Traber, K. Fischer, S. Latzin, and B. Hamprecht, *Nature*, *253*: 120 (1975).
230. W. A. Klee, S. K. Sharma, and M. Nirenberg, *Life Sci.*, *16*: 69 (1975).
231. M. Brandt, R. Gullis, K. Fischer, C. Buchen, B. Hamprecht, L. Moroder, and E. Wunsch, *Nature*, *262*: 311 (1976).
232. W. A. Klee and M. Nirenberg, *Nature*, *263*: 609 (1976).
233. A. Lampert, M. Nirenberg, and W. A. Klee, *Proc. Natl. Acad. Sci. U.S.A.*, *73*: 3165 (1976).
234. M. Brandt, C. Buchen, and B. Hamprecht, *FEBS Lett.*, *80*: 251 (1977).
235. S. A. Walczak, D. Wilkening, and M. H. Makman, *Brain Res.*, *160*: 105 (1979).
236. G. Biggio, M. G. Corda, M. Casu, and G. L. Gessa, *Life Sci.*, *23*: 335 (1978).
237. A. J. Blume, *Proc. Natl. Acad. Sci. U.S.A.*, *75*: 1713 (1978).
238. S. R. Childers and S. H. Snyder, *Life Sci.*, *23*: 759 (1978).
239. A. J. Blume, *Life Sci.*, *22*: 1843 (1978).
240. P. J. Karras and R. A. North, *Br. J. Pharmacol.*, *65*: 647 (1979).

241. W. R. Martin, C. G. Eades, J. A. Thompson, R. E. Huppler, and P. E. Gilbert, *J. Pharmacol. Exp. Ther., 197*: 517 (1976).
242. P. E. Gilbert and W. R. Martin, *J. Pharmacol. Exp. Ther., 198*: 66 (1976).
243. J. A. H. Lord, A. A. Waterfield, J. Hughes, and H. W. Kosterlitz, in *Opiates and Endogenous Opioid Peptides* (H. W. Kosterlitz, ed.), Elsevier/North-Holland, Amsterdam, 1976, pp. 275–280.
244. J. A. H. Lord, A. A. Waterfield, J. Hughes, and H. W. Kosterlitz, *Nature, 267*: 495 (1977).
245. A. A. Waterfield, J. A. H. Lord, J. Hughes, and H. W. Kosterlitz, *Eur. J. Pharmacol., 47*: 249 (1978).
246. J. C. Szerb and M. M. Vohra, *Life Sci., 24*: 1983 (1979).
247. W. B. Pickworth and L. G. Sharp, *Neuropharmacology, 18*: 617 (1979).
248. T. L. Yaksh, R. C. A. Frederickson, S. P. Huang, and T. A. Rudy, *Brain Res., 148*: 516 (1978).
249. J. I. Szekely, Z. Dunai-Kovacs, E. Miglecz, A. Z. Ronai, and S. Bajusz, *J. Pharmacol. Exp. Ther., 207*: 878 (1978).
250. H. W. Kosterlitz and F. M. Leslie, *Br. J. Pharmacol., 64*: 607 (1978).
251. F. M. Leslie and H. W. Kosterlitz, *Eur. J. Pharmacol., 56*: 379 (1979).
252. K. J. Chang and P. Cuatrecasas, *J. Biol. Chem., 254*: 2610 (1979).
253. K. J. Chang, R. J. Miller, and P. Cuatrecasas, *Mol. Pharmacol., 14*: 961 (1978).
254. K. J. Chang, B. R. Cooper, E. Hazum, and P. Cuatrecasas, *Mol. Pharmacol., 16*: 91 (1979).
255. P. Y. Law and H. H. Loh, *Res. Commun. Chem. Pathol. Pharmacol., 21*: 409 (1978).
256. R. Simantov, S. R. Childers, and S. H. Snyder, *Eur. J. Pharmacol., 47*: 319 (1978).
257. S. R. Childers, I. Creese, A. M. Snowman, and S. H. Snyder, *Eur. J. Pharmacol., 55*: 11 (1979).
258. H. Frenk, B. C. McCarty, and J. C. Liebeskind, *Science, 200*: 335 (1978).
259. H. Teschemacher, K. E. Opheim, B. M. Cox, and A. Goldstein, *Life Sci., 16*: 1771 (1975).
260. B. M. Cox, K. E. Opheim, H. Teschemacher, and A. Goldstein, *Life Sci., 16*: 1777 (1975).
261. B. M. Cox, S. Gentleman, T. P. Su, and A. Goldstein, *Brain Res., 115*: 285 (1976).
262. S. Gentleman, M. Ross, L. I. Lowney, B. M. Cox, and A. Goldstein, in *Opiates and Endogenous Opioid Peptides* (H. W. Kosterlitz, ed.), Elsevier/North-Holland, Amsterdam, 1976, pp. 27–34.
263. C. H. Li, *Nature, 201*: 924 (1964).
264. A. F. Bradbury, W. F. Feldberg, D. G. Smyth, and C. R. Snell, in *Opiates and Endogenous Opioid Peptides* (H. W. Kosterlitz, ed.), Elsevier/North-Holland, Amsterdam, 1976, pp. 9–17.
265. B. M. Cox, A. Goldstein, and C. H. Li, *Proc. Natl. Acad. Sci. U.S.A., 73*: 1821 (1976).
266. N. Ling and R. Guillemin, *Proc. Natl. Acad. Sci. U.S.A., 73*: 3308 (1976).

267. C. H. Li, D. Chung, and B. A. Doneen, *Biochem. Biophys. Res. Commun., 72*: 1542 (1976).
268. D. T. Krieger, A. Liotta, T. Suda, M. Palkovits, and M. J. Brownstein, *Biochem. Biophys. Res. Commun., 76*: 930 (1977).
269. E. A. Zimmerman, A. Liotta, and D. T. Krieger, *Cell Tissue Res., 186*: 393 (1978).
270. F. LaBella, G. Queen, J. Senshyn, M. Lis, and M. Chretien, *Biochem. Biophys. Res. Commun., 75*: 350 (1977).
271. D. T. Krieger and A. Liotta, *Science, 205*: 366 (1979).
272. M. Rubinstein, S. Stein, and S. Udenfriend, *Proc. Natl. Acad. Sci. U.S.A., 75*: 669 (1978).
273. B. M. Austen, D. G. Smyth, and C. R. Snell, *Nature, 269*: 619 (1977).
274. D. G. Smyth and C. R. Snell, *FEBS Lett., 78*: 225 (1977).
275. B. M. Austen and D. G. Smyth, *Biochem. Biophys. Res. Commun., 77*: 86 (1977).
276. B. M. Austen, D. G. Smyth, and C. R. Snell, *Nature, 269*: 619 (1977).
277. A. Patthy, L. Graf, A. Kenessey, J. I. Szekely, and S. Bajusz, *Biochem. Biophys. Res. Commun., 79*: 254 (1977).
278. M. J. Geisow and D. G. Smyth, *Biochem. Biophys. Res. Commun., 75*: 625 (1977).
279. B. M. Austen and D. G. Smyth, *Biochem. Biophys. Res. Commun., 76*: 477 (1977).
280. M. J. Geisow, J. F. W. Deakin, J. D. Dostrovsky, and D. G. Smyth, *Nature, 269*: 167 (1977).
281. C. S. Wu, N. Lee, H. H. Loh, J. T. Yang, and C. H. Li, *Proc. Natl. Acad. Sci U.S.A., 76*: 3656 (1979).
282. R. M. Palmour, F. R. Ervin, J. K. Chang, and B. Fong, in *Characteristics and Function of Opioids* (J. M. van Ree and L. Terenius, eds.), Elsevier/North Holland, Amsterdam, 1978, pp. 283–284.
283. W. C. Chang, A. J. Rao, and C. H. Li, *J. Peptide Protein, Res., 11*: 93 (1978).
284. D. G. Smyth, D. E. Massey, S. Zakarian, and M. Finnie, *Nature, 279*: 252 (1979).
285. A. Kenessey, L. Graf, and M. Palkovits, *Brain Res. Bull., 2*: 247 (1977).
286. H. Osborne, R. Przewlocki, V. Hollt, and A. Herz, *Eur. J. Pharmacol., 55*: 425 (1979).
287. H. Akil, D. E. Richardson, J. D. Barchas, and C. H. Li, *Proc. Natl. Acad. Sci. U.S.A., 75*: 5170 (1978).
288. Y. Hosobuchi, J. Rossier, F. E. Bloom, and R. Guillemin, *Science, 203*: 279 (1979).
289. D. V. Reynolds, *Science, 164*: 444 (1969).
290. D. E. Richardson and H. Akil, *J. Neurosurg., 47*: 184 (1977).
291. D. Taylor, B. Hoffer, W. Zieglgansberger, G. Siggins, N. Ling, A. Seiger, and L. Olson, *Brain Res., 176*: 135 (1979).
292. S. Arbilla and S. Z. Langer, *Nature, 271*: 559 (1978).
293. H. H. Loh, D. A. Brase, S. Sampath-Khanna, J. Mar, E. L. Way, and C. H. Li, *Nature, 264*: 567 (1976).

294. F. Moroni, E. Peralta, D. L. Cheney, and E. Costa, *J. Pharmacol. Exp. Ther.*, *208*: 190 (1979).
295. F. Moroni, D. L. Cheney, E. Peralta, and E. Costa, *J. Pharmacol. Exp. Ther.*, *207*: 870 (1978).
296. T. Motomatsu, M. Lis, N. Seidah, and M. Chretien, *Can. J. Neurol. Sci.*, *1*: 49 (1977).
297. F. Moroni, D. L. Cheney, and E. Costa, *Nature*, *267*: 267 (1977).
298. F. Moroni, D. L. Cheney, and E. Costa, *Neuropharmacology*, *17*: 191 (1978).
299. A. Goldstein, B. M. Cox, W. A. Klee, and M. Nirenberg, *Nature*, *265*: 362 (1977).
300. A. Wahlstrom, M. Brandt, L. Moroder, E. Wunsch, G. Lindeberg, U. Ragnarsson, L. Terenius, and B. Hamprecht, *FEBS Lett.*, *77*: 28 (1977).
301. M. Rubinstein, S. Stein, and S. Udenfriend, *Proc. Natl. Acad. Sci. U.S.A.*, *74*: 4969 (1977).
302. M. Ross, R. Dingledine, B. M. Cox, and A. Goldstein, *Brain Res.*, *124*: 523 (1977).
303. L. I. Lowney, S. B. Gentleman, and A. Goldstein, *Life Sci.*, *24*: 2377 (1979).
304. E. R. Baizman and B. M. Cox, *Life Sci.*, *22*: 519 (1978).
305. R. Guillemin, N. Ling, and T. Vargo, *Biochem. Biophys. Res. Commun.*, *77*: 361 (1977).
306. M. Ross, V. Ghazarossian, B. M. Cox, and A. Goldstein, *Life Sci.*, *22*: 1123 (1978).
307. A. Howe and A. J. Thody, *J. Physiol.*, *203*: 159 (1969).
308. A. J. Thody, *Neuroendocrinology*, *16*: 323 (1974).
309. S. Taleisnik, J. De Olmos, R. Orías, and M. E. Tomatis, *J. Endocrinol.*, *39*: 485 (1967).
310. C. W. Jones and B. T. Pickering, *J. Physiol.*, *203*: 449 (1969).
311. A. J. Kastin, *Fed. Proc.*, *26*: 255 (1967).
312. A. Howe and A. J. Thody, *J. Endocrinol.*, *46*: 201 (1970).
313. S. Taleisnik, M. E. Tomatis, and M. E. Celis, *Neuroendocrinology*, *10*: 235 (1972).
314. H. Sachs, P. Fawcett, Y. Takabatake, and D. Portanova, *Recent Prog. Horm. Res.*, *25*: 447 (1969).
315. E. R. Baizman, B. M. Cox, and A. Goldstein, *Neuroendocrinology*, *28*: 402 (1972).
316. M. M. Mata, H. Gainer, and W. A. Klee, *Life Sci.*, *21*: 1159 (1977).
317. A. Howe, *J. Endocrinol.*, *59*: 385 (1973).
318. J. Rossier, E. Battenberg, Q. Pittman, A. Bayon, L. Koda, R. Miller, R. Guillemin, and F. Bloom, *Nature*, *277*: 653 (1979).
319. R. Guillemin, T. M. Vargo, J. Rossier, S. Minick, N. Ling, C. Rivier, W.Vale, and F. E. Bloom, *Science*, *197*: 1367 (1977).
320. J. Rossier, E. D. French, C. Rivier, N. Ling, R. Guillemin, and F. E. Bloom, *Nature,* 270*: 618 (1977).*
321. S. W. Smith and R. R. Gala, *J. Endocrinol.*, *74*: 303 (1977).
322. R. Przewlocki, V. Hollt, and A. Herz, *Eur. J. Pharmacol.*, *51*: 179 (1978).
323. R. Przewlocki, V. Hollt, K. H. Voigt, and A. Herz, *Life Sci.*, *24*: 1601 (1979).

324. W. Vale, C. Rivier, L. Yang, S. Minick, and R. Guillemin, *Endocrinology*, *103*: 1910 (1978).
325. V. Raymond, L. Ferland, J. Lepine, J. C. Lissitsky, and F. Labrie, in *Characteristics and Function of Opioids* (J. M. van Ree and L. Terenius, eds.), Elsevier/North-Holland, Amsterdam, 1978, pp. 287-288.
326. R. G. Allen, E. Herbert, M. Hinman, H. Shibuya, and C. B. Pert, *Proc. Natl. Acad. Sci. U.S.A.*, *75*: 4972 (1978).
327. R. Przewlocki, V. Holt, and A. Herz, in *Characteristics and Function of Opioids* (J. M. van Ree and L. Terenius, eds.), Elsevier/North-Holland, Amsterdam, 1978, pp. 285–286.
328. J. Kraicer and A. R. Morris, *Neuroendocrinology*, *20*: 79 (1976).
329. W. W. Douglas and P. S. Taraskevich, *J. Physiol.*, *285*: 171 (1978).
330. J. C. Lissitsky, O. Morin, A. Dupont, F. Labrie, N. G. Seidah, M. Chretien, M. Lis, and D. H. Coy, *Life Sci.*, *22*: 1715 (1978).
331. C. M. Moriaty and G. C. Moriaty, *Endocrinology*, *96*: 1419 (1975).
332. J. Kraicer, G. Berand, and D. W. Lywood, *Neuroendocrinology*, *23*: 352 (1977).
333. C. B. Pert, A. Pert, and J. F. Tallman, *Proc. Natl. Acad. Sci. U.S.A.*, *73*' 2226 (1976).
334. R. Schulz, M. Wüster, and A. Herz, *Life Sci.*, *21*: 105 (1977).
335. B. M. Cox, E. R. Baizman, T. P. Su, O. H. Osman, and A. Goldstein, *Adv. Biochem. Psychopharmacol.*, *18*: 183 (1978).
336. H. S. Tager and D. S. Steiner, *Annu. Rev. Biochem.*, *43*: 509 (1974).
337. J. Bläsig, V. Höllt, U. Bäuerle, and A. Herz, *Life Sci.*, *23*: 2525 (1978).
338. V. Hollt, R. Przewlocki, and A. Herz, *Life Sci.*, *23*: 1057 (1978).
339. D. T. Krieger, A. Liotta, and C. H. Li, *Life Sci.*, *21*: 1771 (1978).
340. E. Weidremann, T. Saito, J. A. Linfoot, and C. H. Li, *J. Clin. Endocrinol. Metab.*, *45*: 1108 (1977).
341. J. J. H. Gilkes, G. A. Bloomfield, A. P. Scott, P. J. Lowry, J. G. Ratcliffe, J. Landon, and L. H. Rees, *J. Clin. Endocrinol. Metab.*, *40*: 450 (1975).
342. L. H. Rees, D. M. Cook, J. W. Kendall, R. M. Kramer, J. G. Ratcliffe, R. A. Knight, *Endocrinology*, *89*: 254 (1971).
343. S. A. Berson and R. S. Yalow, *J. Clin. Invest.*, *47*: 2725 (1968).
344. T. Suda, A. S. Liotta, and D. T. Krieger, *Science*, *202*: 221 (1978).
345. K. Nakao, Y. Nakai, S. Oki, K. Horii, and H. Imura, *J. Clin. Invest.*, *62*: 1395 (1978).
346. S. L. Wardlaw and A. G. Frantz, *J. Clin. Endocrinol. Metab.*, *48*: 176 (1979).
347. N. Aronin, B. Schickmanter, A. S. Liotta, and D. T. Krieger, *Abstr. 61st Meet. Endocr. Soc.*, 129 (1979).
348. V. E. Ghazarossian. R. R. Dent, K. Otsu, M. Ross, B. M. Cox, and A. Goldstein, *Anal. Biochem.*, *102*: 80 (1980).
349. Y. Nakai, K. Nakao, S. Oki, H. Imura, and C. H. Li, *Life Sci.*, *23*: 2293 (1978).
350. I. Bachelot, A. R. Wolfsen, and W. D. Odell, *J. Clin. Endocrinol. Metab.*, *44*: 939 (1977).
351. R. M. Palmour, F. R. Ervin, H. Wagemaker, and R. Cade, in *Endorphins in Mental Health Research* (E. Usdin, W. E. Bunney, Jr., and N. S. Kline, eds.), Oxford University Press, New York, 1979, p. 581.

352. B. M. Cox, M. Ross, A. Goldstein, and R. Palmour, *Brain Res., 165*: 311 (1979).
353. J. J. H. Gilkes, R. A. J. Eady, L. H. Rees, D. D. Munro, and J. F. Moorhead, *Br. Med. J., 1*: 656 (1975).
354. M. Ross, P. A. Berger, and A. Goldstein, *Science, 205*: 1163 (1979).
355. J. Hughes, *Brain Res., 88*: 295 (1975).
356. R. Guillemin, N. Ling, and R. Burgus, *C. R. Hebd. Seances Acad. Sci., Ser. D., 282*: 783 (1976).
357. W. D. M. Paton, *Br. J. Pharmacol., 12*: 119 (1957).
358. H. W. Kosterlitz, J. A. H. Lord, and A. J. Watt, in *Agonist and Antagonist Actions of Narcotic Analgesic Drugs* (H. W. Kosterlitz, H. O. J. Collier, and J. E. Villarreal, eds.), University Park Press, Baltimore, 1973, pp. 45–61.
359. J. Hughes, H. W. Kosterlitz, and F. M. Leslie, *Br. J. Pharmacol., 53*: 371 (1975).
360. R. Elde, T. Hokfelt, O. Johansson, and L. Terenius, *Neuroscience, 1*: 349 (1976).
361. J. Hughes, H. W. Kosterlitz, and T. W. Smith, *Br. J. Pharmacol., 61*: 639 (1977).
362. W. Schaumann, *Br. J. Pharmacol., 10*: 456 (1955).
363. J. C. Szerb, *Br. J. Pharmacol., 16*: 23 (1961).
364. T. F. Burks, *J. Pharmacol. Exp. Ther., 185*: 530 (1973).
365. H. W. Kosterlitz and D. W. Taylor, *Br. J. Pharmacol., 14*: 209 (1959).
366. U. Trendelenburg, *Br. J. Pharmacol., 12*: 79 (1957).
367. A. B. Cairnie, H. W. Kosterlitz, and D. W. Taylor, *Br. J. Pharmacol., 17*: 539 (1961).
368. S. Lemaire, J. Magnan, and D. Regoli, *Br. J. Pharmacol., 64*: 327 (1978).
369. R. Shulz, E. Faase, M. Wüster, and A. Herz, *Life Sci., 24*: 843 (1979).
370. B. T. Altura, A. Gebrewald, and B. M. Altura, *Fed. Proc., 37*: 471 (1978).
371. B. M. Cox, F. M. Leslie, and C. Charkin, *Adv. Biochem. Psychopharmacol., 22*: 353 (1980).
372. R. Schulz, M. Wuster, R. Simantov, S. Snyder, and A. Herz, *Eur. J. Pharmacol., 41*: 347 (1977).
373. R. Simantov, S. R. Childers, and S. H. Snyder, *Mol. Pharmacol., 14*: 69 (1978).
374. C. Charkin, B. M. Cox, and A. Goldstein, *Mol. Pharmacol., 15*: 751 (1979).
375. B. M. Cox and R. Padhya, *Br. J. Pharmacol., 61*: 271 (1977).
376. B. A. Doneen, D. Chung, D. Yamashiro, P. Y. Law, H. H. Loh, and C. H. Li, *Biochem, Biophys, Res. Commun., 74*: 656 (1977).
377. B. M. Cox, unpublished observation.
378. M. Chrétein, N. G. Seidah, S. Benjannet, N. Dragon, R. Routhier, T. Motomatsu, P. Crine, and M. Lis, *Annu. N. Y. Acad. Sci., 297*: 84 (1977).
379. H. H. Loh and C. H. Li, *Annu. N. Y. Acad. Sci., 297*: 115 (1977).
380. H. N. Duke, M. Pickford, and J. A. Watt, *Q. J. Exp. Physiol. Cogn. Med. Sci., 36*: 149 (1951).
381. R. E. Weitzman, D. A. Fisher, S. Minick, N. Ling, and R. Guillemin, *Endocrinology, 101*: 1643 (1977).
382. D. Pearson, A. Shainberg, S. Malamud, and H. Sachs, *Endocrinology, 96*: 994 (1975).

383. T. B. van Wimersma Griedanus, T. J. Thody, H. Verspaget, G. A. de Rotte, H. J. H. Goedamans, G. Croiset, and J. M. van Ree, *Life Sci.*, *24*: 579 (1979).
384. G. W. Bisset, H. S. Chowdrey, and W. Feldberg, *Br. J. Pharmacol.*, *62*: 370 (1978).
385. L. F. Tseng, H. H. Loh, and C. H. Li, *Int. J. Peptide Protein Res.*, *12*: 173 (1978).
386. J. P. Huidobro-Toro, F. Huidobro, and R. Croxatto, *Life Sci.*, *24*: 697 (1979).
387. J. Haldas and W. H. Sawyer, *Proc. Soc. Exp. Biol. Med.*, *157*: 476 (1978).
388. R. Simantov and S. H. Snyder, *Brain Res.*, *124*: 178 (1977).
389. R. P. Maickel, M. C. Braude, and J. E. Zabik, *Neuropharmacology*, *16*: 863 (1977).
390. T. F. Bruni, D. Van Vugt, S. Marshall, and J. Meites, *Life Sci.*, *21*: 461 (1977).
391. R. Guillemin, N. Ling, L. Lazarus, R. Burgus, S. Minick, F. E. Bloom, R. Nicoll, G. Siggins, and D. Segal, *Annu. N. Y. Acad. Sci.*, *297*: 131 (1977).
392. G. B. Wislocki and L. S. King, *Am. J. Anat.*, *58*: 428 (1936).
393. J. D. Green, *Am. J. Anat.*, *88*: 225 (1951).
394. B. Török, *Acta Morphol. Acad. Sci. Hung.*, *4*: 83 (1954).
395. G. Oliver, R. S. Mical, and J. C. Porter, *Endocrinology*, *101*: 598 (1977).
396. R. B. Page, B. L. Munger, and R. M. Bergland, *Am. J. Anat.*, *146*: 273 (1976).
397. R. B. Page and R. M. Bergland, *Am. J. Anat.*, *148*: 345 (1977).
398. R. M. Bergland, S. L. Davis, and R. B. Page, *Lancet*, *2* (8032): 276 (1977).
399. N. Ogawa, A. E. Panerai, G. Forsbach, V. Havlicek, and H. G. Friesen, *Proc. Can. Soc. Endocrinol. (Abstr.)*, *25*: 683 (1977).
400. H. Blumberg and H. B. Dayton, in *Agonist and Antagonist Actions of Narcotic Analgesic Drugs* (H. W. Kosterlitz, H. O. J. Collier, and J. E. Villarreal, eds.), University Park Press, Baltimore, 1973, pp. 110–119.
401. R. Dingledine, L. L. Iversen, and E. Breuker, *Eur. J. Pharmacol.*, *47*: 19 (1978).
402. A. Z. Rónai, I. Berzétei, and S. Bajasz, *Eur. J. Pharmacol.*, *49*: 393 (1977).
403. S. H. Snyder, G. W. Pasternak, and C. B. Pert, in *Handbook of Psychopharmacology*, Vol. 5 (L. L. Iversen, S. D. Iverson, and S. H. Snyder, eds.), Plenum Press, New York, 1975, p. 329.
404. D. R. Jasinski, W. R. Martin, and C. A. Haertzen, *J. Pharmacol. Exp. Ther.*, *157*: 420 (1967).
405. H. M. Emrich, C. Cording, S. Piree, A. Kolling, D. Uzerssen, and A. Herz, *Pharmakopsychiatr. Neuro-pharmakol.*, *10*: 265 (1977).
406. W. Vale and C. Rivier, in *Handbook of Psychopharmacology*, Vol. 5 (L. L. Iversen, S. D. Iverson, and S. H. Snyder, eds.), Plenum Press, New York, 1975, p. 195.
407. S. M. McCann, S. R. Ojeda, C. Libertan, P. G. Harms, and L. Krulich, in *Narcotics and the Hypothalamus* (E. Zimmerman, and R. George, eds.), Raven Press, New York, 1974, pp. 121–135.
408. P. Brazeu, W. Vale, and R. Guillemin, in *Narcotics and the Hypothalamus* (E. Zimmerman and R. George, eds.) Raven Press, New York, 1974, pp. 109–117.
409. N. Kokka and R. George, in *Narcotics and the Hypothalamus* (E. Zimmerman and R. George, eds.), Raven Press, New York, 1974, pp. 137–157.

410. A. Tolis, J. Hickey, and H. Guyda, *J. Clin. Endocrinol. Metab.*, *41*: 797 (1975).
411. L. Cusan, A. Dupont, G. S. Kledzik, F. Labrie, D. H. Coy, and A. V. Schally, *Nature*, *268*: 544 (1977).
412. C. J. Shaar, R. C. A. Frederickson, N. B. Dininger, and L. Jackson, *Life Sci.*, *21*: 853 (1977).
413. C. Rivier, W. Vale, N. Ling, M. Brown, and R. Guillemin, *Endocrinology*, *100*: 238 (1977).
414. L. Grandison and A. Guidotti, *Nature*, *270*: 357 (1977).
415. K. Chihara, A. Arimura, D. H. Coy, and A. V. Schally, *Endocrinology*, *102*: 281 (1978).
416. E. L. Lien, R. L. Feinchel, V. Garsky, D. Sarantakis, and N. H. Grant, *Life Sci.*, *19*: 837 (1976).
417. D. A. Van Vugt, J. F. Bruni, and J. Meites, *Life Sci.*, *22*: 85 (1975).
418. L. Ferland, K. Fuxe, P. Eneroth, J. A. Gustafsson, and P. Skett, *Eur. J. Pharmacol.*, *43*: 89 (1977).
419. K. Fuxe, L. Ferland, L. F. Agnati, P. Eneroth, J. A. Gustafsson, F. Labrie, and P. Skett, *Acta Pharmacol. Scand.*, *41*: 48 (1977).
420. T. Muraki, Y. Tokunaga, and T. Makuro, *Endocrinol. Jpn.*, *24*: 313 (1977).
421. J. B. Martin, S. Reichlin, and G. M. Brown, in *Clinical Neuroendocrinology*, Davis, Philadelphia, 1977, pp. 147–178.
422. T. J. Cicero, T. M. Badger, C. R. Wilcox, R. D. Bell, and E. R. Meyer, *J. Pharmacol. Exp. Ther.*, *203*: 548 (1977).
423. J. H. Mendelson, R. E. Meyer, J. Ellingboe, S. M. Mirin, and M. McDougle, *J. Pharmacol. Exp. Ther.*, *195*: 296 (1975).
424. T. J. Cicero, B. A. Schanker, and E. R. Meyer, *Endocrinology*, *104*: 1286 (1979).
425. S. M. Mirin, J. H. Mendelson, J. Ellingboe, and R. E. Meyer, *Psychoneuroendocrinology*, *1*: 359 (1976).
426. G. L. Gessa, E. Pagliatti, and B. Quarantotti Pellegrini, *Science*, *204*: 203 (1979).
427. M. S. Blank, A. E. Panerai, and H. G. Freissen, *Science*, *203*: 1129 (1979).
428. A. Gibson, M. Ginsburg, M. Hall, and S. L. Hart, *Br. J. Pharmacol.*, *66*: 164 (1979).
429. W. F. Feldberg and D. G. Smyth, *Br. J. Pharmacol.*, *60*: 445 (1977).
430. J. J. Jacob, E. C. Tremblay, and M. C. Colombel, *Psychopharmacologia*, *37*: 217(1977).
431. J. J. Jacob and K. Ramabadran, *Eur. J. Pharmacol.*, *46*: 393 (1977).
432. R. C. A. Frederickson, R. Nickander, E. L. Smithwick, R. Shuman, and F. H. Norris, in *Opiatres and Endogenous Opioids* (H. W. Kosterlitz, ed.), Elsevier/North-Holland, Amsterdam, 1976, pp. 239–246.
433. R. C. A. Frederickson, V. Burgis, and J. D. Edwards, *Science*, *198*: 756 (1977).
434. P. Grevert and A. Goldstein, *Psychopharmacology*, *53*: 111 (1977).
435. J. J. Carmody, P. R. Carroll, and D. Morgans, *Life Sci.*, *24*: 1149 (1979).
436. B. Pomeranz and D. Chiu, *Life Sci.*, *19*: 1757 (1976).
437. G. B. Chesher and B. Chan, *Life Sci.*, *21*: 1569 (1977).
438. A. Goldstein, G. T. Pryor, L. S. Otis, and F. Larsen, *Life Sci.*, *18*: 599 (1976).
439. G. C. Berntson and J. M. Walker, *Brain Res. Bull.*, *2*: 157 (1977).
440. T. L. Yaksh, J. C. Yeung, and T. A. Rudy, *Life Sci.*, *18*: 1193 (1976).

441. A. Pert and M. Walter, *Life Sci.*, *19*: 1023 (1976).
442. C. J. Woolf, G. D. Barratt, D. Mitchell, and R. A. Myers, *Eur. J. Pharmacol.*, *45*: 311 (1977).
443. N. Kokka and A. S. Fairhurst, *Life Sci.*, *21*: 975 (1977).
444. R. A. North, *Life Sci.*, *22*: 295 (1978).
445. L. A. Dykstra and D. E. McMillan, *J. Pharmacol. Exp. Ther.*, *202*: 660 (1977).
446. A. El-Sobky, J. O. Dostrovsky, and P. D. Wall, *Nature*, *263*: 783 (1976).
447. P. Grevert and A. Goldstein, *Proc. Natl. Acad. Sci. U.S.A.*, *74*: 1291 (1977).
448. M. S. Buschbaum, G. C. Davis, and W. E. Bunney, Jr., *Nature*, *270*: 620 (1977).
449. G. C. Davis, M. S. Buschbaum, and W. E. Bunney, Jr., *Life Sci.*, *23*: 1449 (1978).
450. P. Grevert and A. Goldstein, *Science*, *199*: 1093 (1978).
451. H. Dehen, J. C. Willer, F. Boureau, and J. Cambier, *Lancet*, *2*: 293 (1977).
452. J. D. Levine, N. C. Gordon, R. T. Jones, and H. L. Fields, *Nature*, *272*: 826 (1978).
453. P. Grevert, E. R. Baizman, and A. Goldstein, *Life Sci.*, *23*: 723 (1978).
454. R. C. A. Frederickson, D. L. Wesche, and J. A. Richter, in *Characteristics and Functions of Opioids* (J. van Ree and L. Terenius, eds.), Elsevier/North-Holland, Amsterdam, 1978, p. 169.
455. J. W. Hu, J. O. Dostrovsky, and B. J. Sessle, *Nature*, *276*: 283 (1978).
456. E. Carstens, D. Klumpp, and M. Zimmerman, *Neurosci. Lett.*, *11*: 323 (1979).
457. J. Goldfarb and J. W. Wu, *Neuropharmacology*, *15*: 785 (1976).
458. J. A. Bell and W. R. Martin, *Eur. J. Pharmacol.*, *42*: 147 (1977).
459. H. K. Beecher, *Ann. Surg.*, *123*: 96 (1946).
460. A. I. Basbaum, C. H. Clanton, and H. L. Fields, *Proc. Natl. Acad. Sci. U.S.A.*, *73*: 4685 (1976).
461. A. I. Basbaum, N. J. E. Marley, J. O'Keefe, and C. H. Clanton, *Pain*, *3*: 43 (1977).
462. B. Pomeranz, R. Cheng, and P. Law, *Exp. Neurol.*, *54*: 172 (1978).
463. D. J. Mayer, D. D. Price, and A. Rafic, *Brain Res.*, *121*: 368 (1977).
464. H. Akil, J. Madden, R. L. Patrick, and J. D. Barchas, in *Opiates and Endogenous Opioid Peptides* (H. W. Kosterlitz, ed.), Elsevier/North-Holland, Amsterdam, 1976, pp. 63–70.
465. H. Akil, D. J. Mayer, and J. C. Liebeskind, *C. R. Hebd. Seances Acad. Sci., Ser. D.*, *274*: 3603 (1972).
466. H. Akil, D. J. Mayer, and J. C. Liebeskind, *Science*, *191*: 961 (1976).
467. J. L. Oliveras, Y. Hosobuchi, F. Redjemi, G. Guilband, and J. M. Besson, *Brain Res.*, *120*: 221 (1977).
468. J. E. Adams, *Pain*, *2*: 161 (1976).
469. Y. Hosobuchi, J. E. Adams, and R. Linchitz, *Science*, *197*: 183 (1977).
470. C. R. Chapman and C. Benedetti, *Life Sci.*, *21*: 1645 (1977).
471. C. J. Woolf, D. Mitchell, R. A. Myers, and G. D. Barrett, *S. Afr. Med. J.*, *53*: 179 (1978).
472. A. Goldstein and E. R. Hilgard, *Proc. Natl. Acad. Sci. U.S.A.*, *72*: 2041 (1975).
473. J. Barber and D. Mayer, *Pain*, *4*: 41 (1977).
474. W. R. Crowley, J. F. Rodriguez-Sierra, and B. R. Komisaruk, *Psychopharacologia*, *54*: 223 (1977).

475. R. J. Bodnar, D. D. Kelley, A. Spiagga, and M. Glisman, *Fed. Proc., 36*: 1010 (1977).
476. H. Lal, T. Spaulding, and S. Fielding, *Commun. Psychopharmacol., 2*: 263 (1978).
477. B. A. Berkowitz, D. A. Finck, and S. H. Ngai, *Science, 194*: 967 (1976).
478. B. A. Berkowitz, D. A. Finck, and S. H. Ngai, *J. Pharmacol. Exp. Ther., 203*: 539 (1977).
479. D. J. Mayer and R. L. Hayes, *Science, 188*: 941 (1975).
480. B. M. Cox, M. Ginsburg, and J. Willis, *Br. J. Pharmacol., 53*: 383 (1975).
481. R. Schulz and A. Goldstein, *Nature, 244*: 168 (1973).
482. R. Schulz and A. Herz, *Life Sci., 19*: 1117 (1976).
483. B. M. Cox, *Life Sci., 24*: 1503 (1979).
484. S. J. Watson, H. Akil, and J. D. Barchas, *Brain Res., 130*: 335 (1977).
485. A. B. Finck, S. H. Ngai, and B. A. Berkowitz, *Anesthesiology, 46*: 241 (1977).
486. Z. Fürst, F. F. Foldes, and J. Knoll, *Life Sci., 20*: 921 (1977).
487. P. E. Gilbert and W. R. Martin, *Life Sci., 20*: 1401 (1977).
488. D. S. Missfeldt and A. Goldstein, *N. Engl. J. Med., 297*: 1236 (1977).
489. W. Fratta, H. Y. T. Yang, J. Hong, and E. Costa, *Nature, 268*: 452 (1977).
490. L. M. Gunne, Arch. Int. Pharmacodyn. Ther., 129: 416 (1960).
491. J. S. Hart, in *Comparative Physiology of Thermoregulation*, Vol. 2 (G. C. Whittow, ed.), Academic Press, New York, 1971, pp. 2–151.
492. J. W. Sloan, J. W. Brooks, A. J. Eisenman, and W. R. Martin, *Psychopharmacologia, 3*: 291 (1962).
493. A. Goldstein and P. Lowery, *Life Sci., 17*: 927 (1975).
494. H. Lal, S. Miksic, and N. Smith, *Life Sci., 18*: 971 (1975).
495. D. Julius and P. Renaud, eds., *Natl. Inst. Drug Abuse Monogr., No. 9, U.S.* Dept. of Health, Education and Welfare, Washington, D. C., 1976.
496. L. F. Tseng, H. H. Loh, and C. H. Li, *Proc. Natl. Acad. Sci. U.S.A., 73*: 4187 (1976).
497. J. Bläsig and A. Herz, *Naunyn-Schmiedeberg's Arch. Pharmacol., 294*: 297 (1976).
498. J. M. van Ree, D. DeWied, A. F. Bradbury, E. C. Hulme, D. G. Smyth, and C. R. Snell, *Nature, 264*: 792 (1976).
499. Y. Hosobuchi, M. Meglio, J. E. Adams, and C. H. Li, *Proc. Natl. Acad. Sci. U.S.A., 74*: 4017 (1977).
500. A. A. Waterfield, J. Hughes, and H. W. Kosterlitz, *Nature, 260*: 624 (1976).
501. E. Wei and H. H. Loh, *Science, 193*: 1262 (1976).
502. B. M. Cox, M. Ginsburg, and O. H. Osman, *Br. J. Pharmacol., 33*: 245 (1968).
503. A. Goldstein, *Science, 193*: 1081 (1976).
504. J. Hughes, *Br. J. Addict., 71*: 199 (1976).
505. R. Simantov and S. H. Snyder, *Nature, 262*: 505 (1976).
506. S. R. Childers, R. Simantov, and S. H. Snyder, *Eur. J. Pharmacol., 46*: 289 (1977).
507. J. C. Lissitsky, P. Giraud, R. L. Eskay, and C. Oliver, *Acta Endocrinol., 91* (Suppl. 225): 73 (1979).

chapter 7

Animal Pharmacology of Endorphins

Jeffrey B. Malick and Jeffrey M. Goldstein

Stuart Pharmaceuticals
Division of ICI Americas Inc.
Wilmington, Delaware

I. INTRODUCTION

The development of a method for detecting opiate receptors in mouse brain by Goldstein and coworkers (1) in 1971 and the subsequent demonstration of the occurrence of sterospecific opiate binding sites in brain (2-4) triggered an explosive research effort designed to discover the endogenous opiate ligands for these receptors. Shortly thereafter (1975), Hughes and coworkers (5) identified two pentapeptides, methionine- and leucine-enkephalin, that exhibited morphinomimetic activity when tested on the guinea pig ileum and mouse vas deferens preparations. Since these initial discoveries, many other naturally occurring opiatelike substances (endorphins) have been discovered.

In addition to its analgesic activity, Jaffe (6) described the activities of morphine on the central nervous system as drowsiness, alterations in mood and mental clouding. Therefore, if abnormally high levels of endorphins were to occur for any reason, it is conceivable that similar effects would be observed. In contrast, abnormally low levels of endorphins would be expected to result in significant alterations in pain sensitivity, mood, and behavior.

Quite naturally, the initial pharmacological evaluations of the endorphins centered on their potential analgesic activity. However, subsequent studies have explored their potential in numerous areas (e.g., memory, reinforcement, aggression, sexual behavior, etc.). The purpose of this chapter is to summarize and discuss the results of many of the pertinent pharmacological evaluations that have been performed with the endorphins.

II. ROLE OF ENDORPHINS IN PAIN PERCEPTION

A. Activity of Endorphins in Laboratory Tests Predictive of Analgesic Activity

A summary of the many studies reported in the literature to assess the analgesic potential of the naturally occurring opiatelike substances (endorphins) is presented; no discussion of the many synthetic endorphins, several of which appear to be extremely potent antinociceptive agents in animals, is given in this chapter (some of these are discussed elsewhere in this volume).

Most of the results discussed concern the activities of Met-enkephalin, Leu-enkephalin, and β-endorphin; however, brief mention will be made of the activity of β-lipotropin and several of the other endorphins (e.g., α-endorphin, γ-endorphin) which have been discovered in animals and humans and that could play a significant role in the modulation of pain.

Methionine-Enkephalin The results of the analgesic studies performed on Met-enkephalin in various laboratories are summarized in Table 1. A few months after the discovery of the enkephalins, Belluzzi and coworkers (7) first reported analgesic activity following the central administration of enkephalins to rats. In this study, rats were implanted stereotaxically with permanently indwelling cannulae, the tips of which were located in the lateral ventricle. One week after surgery, the rats were tested in the tail flick test (8) for analgesic activity following the intracerebroventricular infusion of Met-enkephalin. The tail flick test has been used frequently to evaluate the analgesic potential of the endorphins since it is a test that readily detects opiate drugs (e.g., morphine) (9). Following the administration of Met-enkephalin (100 and 200 μg per rat, i.c.v.), statistically significant, dose-related increases in tail flick latencies (i.e., the time from initial exposure to the noxious stimulus, a focused radiant heat source, to the tail flick response) were observed. The analgesia produced by the highest dose (200 μg per rat) of Met-enkephalin appeared to be equivalent to that produced by a 10 μg per rat dose of morphine sulfate; thus, although Met-enkephalin produced significant analgesia, it was approximately 20 times less potent than morphine when administered into the ventricles. Met-enkephalin exhibited a rapid onset (2-6 min) of analgesic activity, which also rapidly disappeared by 10–12 min post-drug infusion. The delay between time of administration and onset of activity was most likely attributable to diffusion time to the active sites and the short duration of activity was probably due to the rapid catabolism of enkephalins by brain enzymes. Since pretreatment with naloxone (2 mg/kg,s.c.), a pure narcotic antagonist, significantly antagonized the analgesic activity produced by Met-enkephalin, it appeared to produce this activity by an interaction with opiate receptors.

Shortly thereafter, Malick and Goldstein reported the results of their studies (10, 11), in which, for the first time, complete dose-response curves were generated in order to compare the analgesic potencies of Met-enkephalin and morphine via the potency ratio analysis of Litchfield and Wilcoxon (12). The methodology used in this study is discussed briefly as an example of the procedures utilized commonly in many of the studies reported in this chapter.

Rats were stereotaxically implanted with cannulae located in the dorsal border of the raphe nucleus in the midbrain periaqueductal gray (PAG). This site was chosen since it had been shown to be one of the primary sites in the brain at which morphine exhibited potent analgesic activity. Rats were allowed at least 1 week to recover fully from the trauma associated with the surgical implantation of the guide cannula prior to the initiation of drug studies. All rats were then tested for their responsiveness to the noxious stimulus, which in the case of the tail flick procedure is radiant heat, following the infusion of the vehicle (sterile water) in which the test drugs were dissolved; such evaluations are used as control baselines and are absolutely necessary to assure that the rat does not respond to vehicle alone. Any animal that exhibited a significant alteration from control baselines following control (vehicle) infusion was eliminated from the study. In fact, in the study detailed below, none of the subjects exhibited a significant change following vehicle infusion. Infusions were accomplished by inserting an internal cannula into the permanently implanted guide cannula; the internal cannula extended 2 mm beyond the tip of the guide cannula. An infusion pump was used to deliver a small volume (1 μl or less into tissue) relatively slowly and at a constant rate; in the present study drugs were infused in a 1 μl volume over 24 sec (infusion rate = 0.04 μl/sec). The internal cannula should be left in place for a short period of time (e.g., 25 sec) in an attempt to prevent the infused fluid form immediately flowing back up the guide cannula. Rats were then placed in a standard Plexiglas restrainer so that only the tail protruded. Control sessions were performed on the morning of each day of drug testing and consisted of infusion of sterile water and testing for tail flick responses (latency to respond) at 1, 3, and 7 min postinfusion. After establishing same-day control thresholds for each rat, drugs were infused and tail flick latencies were measured once again at the same intervals postinfusion. Thus each rat served as its own control. Any rat exhibiting a 50% or greater increase in response latency as compared to its own same-day control values was considered to have exhibited a significant analgesic response. The heat source was terminated if the rat did not respond within 20 sec, to prevent tissue damage. When animals were used more than once, at least 7 days was allowed between drug administration in an attempt to avoid the development of tolerance. Animals were sacrificed at the end of the experiments and cannulae were confirmed to be in the PAG. The results of this study are summarized in Table 2.

Both morphine and Met-enkephalin exhibited potent, dose-related analgesic activity following infusion into the PAG (Table 2). Met-enkephalin was found to be approximately four times less potent than morphine on a weight basis; however, on a molar basis the potency of Met-enkephalin would be increased by a factor of 2 relative to morphine (i.e., molar ED_{50} values: Met-enkephalin = 0.27 μmol; morphine = 0.13 μmol). Thus Malick and Goldstein (11) reported that Met-enkephalin was

TABLE 1 Effects of Met-Enkephalin in Various Tests Predictive of Analgesic Activity in Animals

Species	Analgesic model	Route of administration	Dose (μg)	Injection volume (μl)	Analgesic activity	References
Rat	Tail flick	I.c.v.[a]	100,200	10	Significant analgesia at both doses; onset (2–6) min); duration (10–12 min)	7
Rat	Tail flick	I.c. (PAG)[b]	30–360	3	Significant analgesia only at 120 μg/rat; duration < 3 min	15
Rat	Tail flick	I.c. (PAG)	4.8–48	1	ED_{50} = 15.5 (9.9–24.2) μg/rat; peak activity (1 min); short duration (dropping off by 7 min)	10,11
Rat	Tail flick	I.c.v.	400	20	Moderate prolongation of reaction times; duration: 4–6 min	18
Rat	Tail flick	I.c.v.	Several[c]	20	Weak analgesic activity; impossible to calculate an ED_{50} as high as 6.7×10^{-7} mol/rat	19
Rat	Tail flick	I.c.v.	200	10	8 of 13 drug-naive rats exhibited significant analgesia; duration 1–40 min (median = 4 min)	20
Rat	Tail flick	I.c.v.	200	10	Slight, significant analgesia; maximum increase in latency = 2.0 sec; duration = 4 min	21
Rat	Tail flick	I.c.v.	670 nmol	20	Slight analgesia; duration = 8 min	17

Rat	Hot plate (44.5°C)	I.c.v.	100	10	No analgesia; apparent increase in pain perception (increased paw licking)	31
Rat	Hot plate (55.5°C)	I.c.v.	100	10	Transient analgesia; 10 min duration; N = 1	30
Mouse	Tail flick; hot plate; acetic acid writhing	I.c.v.	50	5	Weak analgesic activity; duration duration < 10 min	22
Mouse	Tail flick	I.v.[d]	Several[c]	—[e]	ED_{50} = 170 mg/kg; 15 sec duration	16
Mouse	Tail flick	I.c.v.	56–180	10–30	ED_{50} = 75 (52–100); peak activity (2 min); duration (5 min)	16
Mouse	Tail flick	I.c.v.	Several[c]	—[e]	ED_{50} = 68 μg/mouse at 2 min post-infusion	23
Cat	Tail pinch	I.c.v.	50–400	40	No analgesic activity	35
Cat	Tail pinch	I.v.	1 mg/kg	—[e]	No analgesic activity	35
Cat	Pinch test (tail, limbs, ears)	I.c.v.	100–400	500	No analgesic activity	36
Cat	Tooth pulp	I.c.v.	100–400	500	No analgesic activity	36

[a]Intracerebroventricular.
[b]Intracerebral; periaqueductal gray.
[c]Actual doses not reported.
[d]Intravenous.
[e]Not reported.

TABLE 2 Analgesic Activity of Met-Enkephalin and Morphine in the Tail Flick Test in Rats Following Intracerebral Administration

Treatment	Dose (μg/rat)	N[a]	Rats exhibiting a significant increase in response latency (%)[b]	ED_{50} (μg/rat) (95% C.L.)[c]
Sterile water	1 μl	133	0.0	–
Morphine SO_4	1.7	7	28.6	3.7
(7 min)[d]	3.0	7	28.6	(2.2–6.1)
	10.0	10	80.0	
		9	100.0	
Met-enkephalin	4.8	19	21.1	15.5
(1 min)[d]	9.6	17	35.3	(9.9–24.2)
	16.0	19	47.4	
	48.0	16	81.3	

[a]Number of rats tested.
[b]Any rat exhibiting a 50% or greater increase latency was considered to be significantly affected.
[c]ED_{50} and 95% confidence limits were calculated by the method of Litchfield and Wilcoxon (12).
[d]Data from time of peak activity.
Source: Data from Ref. 11, reprinted with permission from *Life Sciences*, *20*: 827–832, J.B. Malick and J.M. Goldstein, Analgesic activity of enkephalins following intracerebral administration in the rat, copyright 1977, Pergamon Press, Ltd.

considerably more potent than indicated by Belluzzi and associates (7). This difference in potency can probably be attributed to the fact that Belluzzi and coworkers (7) utilized the intraventricular route of administration, which required diffusion to the site(s) of action; this could have markedly reduced the activity of the peptide since enkephalins have been shown to be rapidly deactivated by peptidases in brain and other tissue (13). Following intracerebral infusion (PAG), the analgesic activity of Met-enkephalin peaked by 1-min postinfusion but had a very short duration of activity (its activity had significantly diminished by 7 min postinfusion); this is in agreement with the short duration of activity reported by Belluzzi and coworkers (7). In contrast, the activity of morphine did not peak until the 7-min observation time but persisted for as long as several hours postinfusion, which is consistent with previous observations (14). The analgesic activity of Met-enkephalin was completely antagonized by pretreatment with the narcotic receptor antagonist, naloxone (see Table 3). The high dose of naloxone (20 mg/kg, i.p.) used in this antagonism study was chosen since previous studies had demonstrated that although much lower doses will antagonize parenteral doses of morphine, relatively high doses of the antagonist were necessary to antagonize morphine-induced analgesia following direct infusion into the PAG.

In contrast to the studies of Malick and Goldstein (11), Chang and coworkers (15) reported that Met-enkephalin was at least 20 times less potent than morphine in the tail flick test in rats following infusion into the PAG; however, in their study, no dose-response relationship was observed (significant activity was exhibited at 120 μg per rat but not at 30 or 360 μg per rat). In the studies of Büscher and associates (16), Met-enkephalin was also shown to be markedly less potent than morphine following intraventricular administration in the tail flick procedure in mice; although morphine was 75 times more potent than Met-enkephalin, the potency ratio could have been biased once again in favor of morphine because of the route of administration. This would make compounds that were rapidly degraded appear less potent than those which are not when administered at locations that were not the sites of such activity. Büscher and coworkers (16) also reported analgesic activity in the mouse tail flick model following intravenous administration (ED_{50} = 170 mg/kg, i.v.); however, the analgesic activity only lasted for 15 sec (see Table 1).

Several additional laboratories have also shown that Met-enkephalin produced significant, although frequently weak analgesic activity in the tail flick test following intraventricular administration in both rats (17-21) and mice (22,23) (see Table 1 for details).

The hot plate procedure (24-27) is another analgesia model in rodents which has been routinely used to evaluate opiate analgesics. In the original version of the

TABLE 3 Inhibition of Analgesic Activity by Pretreatment with Naloxone

Treatment	Dose (μg/rat)	Number of rats significantly affected[a]/number of rats tested (mean % change in response latency[b]): Drug alone	Drug + naloxone[c]	P-value[d]
Sterile water	1 μl	0/28 (—)	0/28 (—)	–
Morphine SO_4	10	9/9 (201.55)	3/9 (30.84)	<0.001
Met-enkephalin	48	10/10 (168.01)	0/10 (5.59)	<0.001

[a]Data from time to peak activity.
[b]Mean percent change in response latency =

$$\frac{\text{mean predrug threshold - mean postdrug threshold}}{\text{mean pre-drug threshold}} \times 100$$

[c]Naloxone HC1 (20 mg/kg, i.p.) 30 min prior to drug infusion.
[d]Paired Student's t-test comparing mean percent change in response latency for drug + naloxone to drug alone.
Source: Data from Ref. 11, reprinted with permission from *Life Sciences, 20*: 827-832, J.B. Malick and J.M. Goldstein, Analgesic activity of enkephalins following intracerebral administration in the rat, copyright 1977, Pergamon Press, Ltd.

hot plate procedure, the temperature of the surface of the plate was maintained at 54-56°C by the vapors of a boiling solvent, usually pure acetone or a mixture of solvents (26, 28). However, with the advent of modern technology, it is now possible to electronically maintain the platform surface very accurately at any desired termperature (29). Briefly, rodents are placed on the surface of the test platform within the confines of a bell jar or other container and are observed for reactions to the heat-induced pain; the end points vary from laboratory to laboratory but usually consist of licking of the paws, rapid lifting of a paw, or an attempt to escape from the area. A cutoff time (standardly 30 or 60 sec) is used to prevent tissue damage, which is especially critical if the animals are to be tested more than once.

Bradbury and associates (30), using the hot plate test, demonstrated a transient analgesic response (approximately 10 min in duration) following a total dose of 100 μg intraventricularly in the only rat tested when the temperature of the plate was 55.5°C. However, Leybin and coworkers (31) administered the identical dose (100 μg per rat, i.c.v.) with the plate temperature at 44.5°C and failed to observe any analgesic response; in fact, they apparently observed hyperalgesia (an increase in paw licking). Surprisingly, they (31) reported that the animals that received Met-enkephalin exhibited signs of narcotic withdrawal (e.g., wet dog shakes, restlessness, stereotypy, defecation, etc.) between 1 and 3 min after the initiation of drug infusion. The differences in these results cannot be easily reconciled. In mice, intraventricular administration of Met-enkephalin (50 μg per mouse) resulted in a significant analgesic response which lasted for less than 10 min (22).

Chemically induced writhing (abdominal constriction) in mice has been used frequently to assess analgesic potential; these models detect analgesic activity with both narcotic and nonnarcotic analgesics (32-34). Loh and coworkers (22) demonstrated weak antinociceptive activity following Met-enkephalin (50 μg per mouse, i.c.v.) in the acetic acid-induced writhing test (Table 1).

Feldberg and Smyth (35) failed to demonstrate analgesia with Met-enkephalin in the tail pinch test in cats following either intraventricular (50-400 μg) or intravenous (1 mg/kg) administration. Meglio and associates (36) also failed to observe analgesic activity in cats utilizing pinch procedures (pinching tail, limbs, or ears) following intraventricular administration of Met-enkephalin over a wide range of doses (100-400 μg per cat, i.c.v.). Furthermore, Met-enkephalin was also found to be ineffective in cats over a wide range of doses (100-400 μg per cat, i.c.v.) in the electrically stimulated tooth pulp procedure (36). Thus to date, Met-enkephalin has not been shown to be an analgesic in the cat utilizing tooth pulp or pinch procedures. This may either be due to species differences or to the different types of analgesic methodologies that have been used in cats thus far, none of which has been utilized to assess the analgesic potential of Met-enkephalin in rodents.

In summary, Met-enkephalin has been shown to produce significant analgesic activity in rodents in several different types of analgesic procedures (i.e., hot plate, tail flick, writhing) following intraventricular administration. When it was infused (intracutaneously) directly into the site at which morphine was active (e.g., PAG), activity almost comparable to that observed with morphine was observed (10, 11); however, if Met-enkephalin was placed into the ventricles, where it had to diffuse to the site of action, it appeared to be much less potent than morphine, but this was probably due to rapid catabolism prior to the peptide reaching its receptor site. In one study (16), Met-enkephalin exhibited weak activity in the mouse tail flick procedure following intravenous administration.

Leucine-Enkephalin Whereas Met-enkephalin has been investigated extensively for its analgesic potential, only a handful of investigators have evaluated Leu-enkephalin as an analgesic. The results of these studies are summarized in Table 4.

As with Met-enkephalin, Belluzzi and coworkers (7) were the first to report that Leu-enkephalin produced a statistically significant analgesic response when infused directly into the brain of rats (see Table 4). Following intraventricular administration of Leu-enkephalin (100 and 200 μg per rat, i.c.v.), a significant prolongation of tail flick latencies was observed; the onset of this activity occurred at 2-6 min postdrug infusion and the duration of the analgesic activity was very short (10-12 min). In this study, intraventricular administration of a dose of 10 μg of morphine produced an equivalent analgesic response to that observed after the highest dose (200 μg per rat) of Leu-enkephalin tested; the duration of morphine's activity was also considerably longer (> 1 hr) than that observed with Leu-enkephalin. As was the case with Met-enkephalin, the analgesic activity of Leu-enkephalin was also reversed by treatment with a narcotic antagonist, naloxone (2 mg/kg, s.c.) (7).

Malick and Goldstein (10,11) also reported that Leu-enkephalin exhibited analgesic activity in the rat tail flick test. However, in their study they administered the drugs intracerebrally directly into one of the sites of action of morphine, the PAG. The major reason for infusing the drugs directly into the PAG rather than into the ventricles was to overcome the problems associated with diffusion: for example, since these pentapeptides are rapidly catabolized, most of their activity would be lost before they actually reached the appropriate receptor sites. Malick and Goldstein (11) were the first to generate a complete dose-response curve and establish an ED_{50} dose for producing significant analgesia with Leu-enkephalin; it exhibited an ED_{50} of 14.8 μg per rat, i.c. as compared to 2.7 μg per rat for morphine. Leu-enkephalin exhibited peak activity by 3 min postinfusion and its activity had significantly diminished by 7 min postdrug. On a molar basis, Leu-enkephalin was only two times less potent than morphine when given in the PAG; molar ED_{50} values were 0.27 and 0.13 μmol for Leu-enkephalin and morphine, respectively. Once again, pretreatment (30 min prior to Leu-enkephalin) with naloxone (20 mg/kg, i.p.) prevented the analgesic activity of Leu-enkephalin (7).

Leybin and coworkers (31) reported that Leu-enkephalin (100 μg per rat, i.c.v.) produced a significant analgesic response that lasted for at least 10 min after infusion into the lateral ventricle when tested in the hot plate test (44.5°C).

TABLE 4 Effects of Leu-Enkephalin in Laboratory Tests Predictive of Analgesic Activity

Species	Analgesic model	Route of administration	Dose (μg)	Injection volume (μl)	Analgesic activity	References
Rat	Tail flick	I.c.v.[a]	100,200	10	Significant analgesia at both doses; onset (2–6 min); duration: 10–12 min	7
Rat	Tail Flick	I.c. (PAG)	6–24	1	ED_{50} = 14.8 (9.4–23.2) μg/rat; peak activity (3 min); activity dropping off by 7 min but still significant	10, 11
Rat	Tail flick	I.c. (PAG)[b]	30–360	3	No analgesic activity	15
Rat	Hot plate (44.5°C)	I.c.v.	100	10	Significant analgesia for at least 10 min	31
Mouse	Tail flick	I.v.[c]	320 mg/kg	—[d]	Weakly active in 4 of 10 mice	16
Mouse	Tail flick	I.c.v.	180–420	10–30	ED_{50} = 240 (159–363) μg/mouse; peak activity at 2 min; duration = 5 min	16

[a]Intracerebroventricular.
[b]Intracerebral; periaqueductal gray.
[c]Intravenous.
[d]Not reported.

Büscher and associates (16) evaluated Leu-enkephalin in the tail flick test in mice and found that it exhibited weak but significant analgesic activity (ED_{50} = 240 μg per mouse) following intraventricular administration; the activity peaked rapidly and also disappeared very quickly (see Table 4). In the same studies Leu-enkephalin also produced significant but weak analgesia in 40% of the mice tested following intravenous (320 mg/kg) dosing (16). These investigators also found Met-enkephalin to be approximately three times as potent as Leu-enkephalin following intraventricular administration (16). Another interesting observation in their studies was that it required a significantly higher dose of naloxone to antagonize the analgesic response of Leu-enkephalin compared to the amount necessary to antagonize the effects of either Met-enkephalin or morphine; a dose of naloxone as low as 0.1 mg/kg, s.c. could inhibit the analgesic activity of both Met-enkephalin and morphine, whereas 10 mg/kg, s.c. was necessary to inhibit the actions of Leu-enkephalin (16). They suggested that the different susceptibilities of the two enkephalins to inhibition by naloxone might indicate that the leucine form might have partial agonist (i.e., both agonist and antagonist) activity at opiate receptor sites, whereas Met-enkephalin may be more of a true narcotic agonist. This is in contrast to the findings of Chang and coworkers (15), in which they predict, on the basis of the sodium shift on opiate receptor binding [when binding is performed in the presence and absence of sodium, antagonists exhibit one- to threefold losses, and partial agonists have intermediate sodium response ratios (37)], that Met-enkephalin is a partial agonist and Leu-enkephalin is a pure agonist.

Leu-enkephalin failed to produce significant changes in tail flick latencies over a wide range of doses (30–360 μg per rat) when infused into the PAG in rats in a study performed by Chang and coworkers (15). It is difficult to understand the lack of activity in this study, especially since the peptide was injected into one of the sites of morphine action (PAG); this finding with Leu-enkephalin is in contrast to previous reports of analgesic activity following both intracerebral administration in the PAG (11) and intraventricular infusion (7) in the rat tail flick test.

In summary, Leu-enkephalin has generally been shown to be an analgesic following both infusion into various areas of the brain, and in one case it even produced a weak, short-lasting antinociceptive response following intravenous administration. In general, with the exception of the results of Malick and Goldstein (11), in which Leu- and Met-enkephalin were essentially equipotent, most investigators have reported that Leu-enkephalin is less potent than the methionine form of enkephalin as an analgesic.

Beta-Endorphin β-Endorphin, the 31-amino acid fraction of β-lipotropin that contains within it the exact sequence of Met-enkephalin (β-LPH 61–65), was first shown to be a potent analgesic by Loh and coworkers (22). In mice, doses of 0.5 and 1.0 μg intraventricularly produced a dose-related analgesic response in both the hot plate and tail flick procedures; the analgesic action lasted from 60–90 min postinfusion and closely resembled the duration observed with morphine under similar conditions. β-Endorphin (0.5 μg/mouse, i.c.v.) also produced a significant antinociceptive response in the acetic acid-induced writhing test; the duration of this action was also 60-90 min (22). In addition, in this original report (22), the investigators also reported that β-endorphin (0.25 and 1.0 μg per rat, i.c.) produced a significant dose-related analgesic response in the ice water-induced shaking test in rats following infusion into the PAG (Table 5); in this test, repetitive shaking movements are induced by immersion of anesthetized rats into ice water. Although the latter model certainly measures central opiatelike activity, it is difficult to see how it is a measure of analgesic activity if the animals are anesthetized. All the aforementioned analgesic responses were readily antagonized by pretreatment with naloxone. The ED_{50} doses for β-endorphin were calculated to be 0.92, 1.52, and 2.32 nmol/kg, i.c. in the writhing, tail flick, and hot plate tests, respectively; thus on a molar basis β-endorphin was approximately 18-33 times as potent as morphine in the mouse (22).

Numerous investigators have reported that β-endorphin was a potent, long-acting analgesic in both mice and rats in the tail flick and hot plate procedures, and in the acetic acid-induced writhing test in mice (see Table 5) following infusion into the brain.

Several authors have also evaluated the analgesic potential of β-endorphin following intravenous administration: potent analgesic activity was observed in the tail flick test (38, 39) and in the hot plate procedure (38) in mice. In the tail flick test, β-endorphin exhibited an ED_{50} of 3.3 μmol/kg, i.v. and it was 3.4 times as potent as morphine (39); the duration of β-endorphin's analgesic activity following intravenous infusion was between 20 and 30 min. In the studies by Tseng and associates (38), the duration of activity with β-endorphin was between 30 and 60 min postintravenous infusion (see Table 5).

In the cat, Feldberg and Smyth (35) demonstrated significant analgesic activity following infusion (i.c.v.) into the third ventricle; the activity was reported to last in excess of 2 hr postinfusion as measured by a tail pinch procedure (35). Doses of β-endorphin as low as 2.5 μg, i.c.v. produced a weak but statistically significant analgesic response, whereas at higher doses (10-20 μg; 2.9-5.7 nmol), potent long-lasting analgesia was observed (35). In these studies, β-endorphin was estimated to be 100-200 times as potent as morphine.

Meglio and coworkers (36) also evaluated β-endorphin as an analgesic in cats. In their pinch test, they evaluated the responses of cats to pinching of the tail, ears, and limbs with forceps and to electrical stimulation of the tooth pulp prior to and following intraventricular infusion of drugs. Following infusion of 6.25 μg of β-endorphin, no significant alterations in behavior or responses to pain were observed. Although the 12.5-μg dose also failed to elicit analgesia, behavioral alterations (e.g., fine tremors, mild excitation) were seen. Significant analgesic activity was observed in both the pinch procedure and the tooth pulp test at both higher doses (25 and 50 μg, i.c.v.) of β-endorphin (36). The duration of the analgesia produced by β-endorphin was shown to be 2–3 hr. In their procedures, morphine sulfate failed to exhibit significant alterations in pain thresholds until doses of 150 and 200 μg were infused intraventricularly; thus β-endorphin was approximately six times as potent as morphine (36).

Because of its potent, long-lasting analgesic activity in animals, β-endorphin has been evaluated as an analgesic in humans. Catlin and associates (40) were the first to evaluate the analgesic potential of β-endorphin in humans in a very preliminary manner in patients suffering with chronic pain due to advanced cancer. Of the three subjects evaluated, two exhibited a good analgesic response to β-endorphin (one each at doses of 6.3 and 180 μg/kg, i.v.) and one subject reported a slight reduction in pain following 100 μg/kg i.v. Morphine (125 μg/kg, i.v.) produced good to excellent analgesic responses in all three subjects. As a result of this open trial, β-endorphin clearly appeared to be an analgesic in humans.

Hosobuchi and Li (41) evaluated the analgesic potential of β-endorphin following intraventricular infusion in patients who had been implanted with electrodes for producing electrical brain stimulation-induced analgesia from the central gray. They administered total doses of 100, 200, and 400 μg, i.c.v. to three patients suffering from intractable pain which had been managed only with opiate analgesics. The minimal effective dose for producing a significant analgesic response was found to be 200 μg. Alterations of acute pain thresholds as measured by thermal dolorimetry was also observed; however, clinical pain relief occurred much sooner than and outlived the elevation of acute pain thresholds by 4–6 hr. The pain relief produced by β-endorphin was antagonized by intravenous infusion of 0.8 mg of naloxone (41). This study, once again in a very small patient population, indicated that β-endorphin could produce a powerful, long-lasting analgesic action following intraventricular administration; no adverse side effects were noted. Additional clinical trials with strict double-blind controls are necessary to fully evaluate the analgesic potential of β-endorphin in humans.

In summary, β-endorphin has been shown to be a potent, long-acting analgesic in rodents, cats, and humans. In comparison to morphine, β-endorphin was found to be approximately 18–33 times as potent as this poppy alkaloid following intracerebroventricular administration in rodents and approximately three to four times as potent following intravenous infusion.

Beta-Lipotropin β-Lipotropin (β-LPH), a 91-amino acid peptide which may be a prohormone (42) for some of the morphinomimetic peptides (e.g., β-endorphin, Met-enkephalin) also has been shown to possess analgesic activity (18). Ronai and associates (18) reported that β-LPH was approximately two times weaker than morphine as an analgesic (calculated on a molar basis) following intraventricular administration in the tail flick test in rats; ED_{50} values were 7.7 and 17.0 nmol per rat for morphine and β-LPH, respectively. In this study, the analgesic activity of both β-LPH and morphine peaked between 30 and 60 min and at the highest doses lasted up to

TABLE 5 Effects of β-Endorphin in Laboratory Analgesic Tests

Species	Analgesic model	Route of administration	Dose (μg)	Injection volume (μl)	Analgesic activity	Reference
Rat	Tail flick	I.c.v.[a]	0.8 nmol	20	Potent analgesic activity; onset (15–30 min); duration (60–90 min)	17
Rat	Tail flick	I.c.v.	Several[b]	5	Significant analgesia between 0.6–1.6 nmol/rat	47
Rat	Tail flick	I.c.v.	Several[b]	20	ED_{50} = 0.59 nmol/rat; duration = 60–120 min	48
Rat	Hot plate (54.2°)	I.c.v.	0.3–4.5	3	Significant analgesia only at 4.5 μg/rat; onset (20 min); duration (40–60 min)	46
Rat	Hot plate (55.5°)	I.c.v.	0.0015 μmol	10	Potent analgesic activity; duration up to 100 min	30
Rat	Ice water-induced shaking	I.c.v.[c]	Several[b]	1	Dose-related analgesia; ED_{50} = 0.4 nmol/rat	49
Rat	Ice water-induced shaking	I.c. (PAG)[d]	0.25, 1	0.5	Dose-related analgesia	22
Mouse	Tail flick	I.c.v.	Several[b]	5	ED_{50} = 0.03 nmol/mouse; 34.7 times as potent as morphine	49
Mouse	Tail flick	I.c.v.	Several[b]	5	ED_{50} = 0.11 μg/mouse	50
Mouse	Tail flick; hot plate	I.c.v.	Several[b]	5	ED_{50} = 0.15 μg/mouse; duration > 60 min	45

Mouse	Tail flick	I.v.[e]	8–20 mg/kg	—[f]	ED_{50} = 9.4 (6.9–12.8) mg/kg; duration (30–60 min)	38
Mouse	Tail flick	I.c.v.	Several[b]	—[f]	ED_{50} = 0.3 μg/mouse	23
Mouse	Tail flick	I.c.v.	Several[b]	—[f]	ED_{50} = 0.03 (0.02–0.04) nmol/mouse; duration = 30–60 min; 48.4 times as potent as morphine	39
Mouse	Tail flick	I.v.	Several[b]	—[f]	ED_{50} = 3.32 (1.86–5.69) μmol/kg; 3.4 times as potent as morphine; duration = 20–30 min	39
Mouse	Tail flick; hot plate; acetic acid writhing	I.c.v.	0.5, 1	5	Dose-related analgesia; duration (60–90 min)	22
Mouse	Hot plate	I.c.v.	Several[b]	20	ED_{50} = 0.17 nmol/mouse	48
Mouse	Hot plate	I.v.	8–20 mg/kg	—	ED_{50} = 12.0 (8.0–18.0) mg/kg; duration (30–60) min)	38
Mouse	Hot plate	I.c.v.	Several[b]	—[f]	ED_{50} = 0.03 (0.02–0.04) nmol/mouse; 32.8 times as potent as morphine	39

TABLE 5 (Continued)

Species	Analgesic model	Route of administration	Dose (μg)	Injection volume (μl)	Analgesic activity	Reference
Mouse	Acetic acid writhing	I.c.v.	Several[b]	—[f]	ED_{50} = 0.03 (0.02–0.04) nmol/mouse; 17.3 times as potent as morphine	39
Cat	Tail pinch	I.c.v.	2.5–20	40	Significant analgesia at all doses; duration > 2 hr	35
Cat	Pinch (tail, limbs, ears); tooth pulp stimulation	I.c.v.	6.25–50	0.5 ml	Minimal effective dose = 25 μg; duration = 120–180 min	36
Humans	Cancer pain	I.v.	6.3, 100, 180 $\mu g/kg$	—[f]	One subject at each dose; significant analgesia at 6.3 and 180 $\mu g/kg$; very preliminary evaluation	40
Humans	Heat	I.c.v.	100–400	2 ml	Pain relief for as long as 6 hr	41

[a]Intracerebroventricular.
[b]Actual doses not reported.
[c]Periaqueductal gray fourth ventricular space.
[d]Intracerebral; periaqueductal gray.
[e]Intravenous.
[f]Not reported.

120 min post infusion. Subcutaneous administration of naloxone (2 mg/kg) antagonized the analgesic effects of both morphine and β-LPH. β-LPH was completely inactive as an analgesic when administered intravenously in doses up to 130 mg/kg.

In contrast, Feldberg and Smyth (43) failed to demonstrate any analgesic activity with β-LPH (150 μg, i.c.v.) in the cat using the tail pinch method of Russell and Tate (44). In fact, they failed to observe any morphinelike behavioral effects following the infusion of β-LPH. In this same study, doses of 10 and 20 μg of β-endorphin produced a potent, long-lasting analgesic response.

B. Tolerance Studies

Tseng and coworkers (51) attempted to determine whether the analgesic actions of β-endorphin would be likely to tolerate on repeated administration by determining whether it would exhibit cross-tolerance in rodents that had received chronic morphine. In this study, mice were rendered tolerant to morphine by subcutaneously implanting them with morphine pellets for 3 days; controls were implanted with placebo pellets. The pellets were removed 72 hr after implantation and the mice were injected intracerebroventricularly with either β-endorphin or morphine using the method of Haley and McCormick (52). Analgesic activity was then assessed utilizing both the tail flick and hot plate procedures. In placebo-implanted mice, β-endorphin (1 μg per mouse, i.c.v.) produced a significant analgesic response in 80–100% of the mice tested in both analgesic models. However, in the morphine pellet-implanted groups, β-endorphin produced a significantly diminished analgesic response. When median antinociceptive doses were calculated, β-endorphin exhibited an eight- to ninefold increase in AD_{50} values in the morphine-implanted mice as compared to controls; morphine exhibited similar tolerance effects. Thus β-endorphin clearly exhibited analgesic cross-tolerance to morphine in mice.

In another study, subacute administration of β-endorphin (4.5 μg per rat, i.c.v.; twice daily for 2 days and once on the test day) resulted in the development of tolerance to its analgesic effects in the tail flick procedure in rats (46). In addition, in rats treated repeatedly with β-endorphin, there was some evidence for cross-tolerance to intracerebroventricularly administered morphine. However, when morphine was administered intraperitoneally to animals that had received the same β-endorphin treatment for 3 days, no signs of cross-tolerance were evident. The only explanation given by the authors for this discrepancy was that perhaps "the population of receptors involved in mediating the antinociceptive effects of relatively low peripheral doses of morphine may not be identical to that occupied after intracerebral injection" (46).

In cats, acute tolerance was observed to the analgesic effects of β-endorphin if a second administration (i.c.v.) was given within 24 hr of the initial treatment (36, 53); if the second administration of β-endorphin was given 48 hr or more after initial exposure, no tolerance was observed (53). Although tolerance to the analgesic actions of β-endorphin occurred very rapidly, the behavioral syndrome (e.g., tremor, excitation, stereotypy) persisted (53). Hosobuchi and coworkers (53) reported that intraperitoneal injection of 5-hydroxytryptophan (10 mg/kg) could both reverse the tolerance to the analgesic activity of β-endorphin as well as potentiate the analgesic effects of a subliminal dose of β-endorphin; the results suggested that perhaps β-endorphin produced its analgesic effect by activation of serotonergic pathways. Earlier reports (54) demonstrated similar interactions between morphine and 5-hydroxytryptophan, in that the latter both reduced the development of tolerance to morphine and potentiated its analgesic actions in mice.

In rats that have been made dependent on and tolerant to morphine (pellet implantation for 5 days), Simantov and Snyder (55) observed significantly elevated brain enkephalin levels. In addition, when these rats were treated with naloxone (1 mg/kg, i.p.), enkephalin levels dropped to control levels within 1 hr. Thus there appears to be an excellent correlation between the development of tolerance to the analgesic effects of morphine and elevated enkephalin levels.

Tolerance has also been observed at the neuronal level in electrophysiological studies. Briefly, opiates and endorphins have been shown to decrease the sensitivity of single neurons to putative excitatory transmitters, and tolerance to these inhibitory actions appears to develop following repeated exposure (56).

In summary, tolerance to the analgesic actions of β-endorphin develops rapidly upon repeated administration, and although the results are not as consistent, there also appears to be a cross-tolerance between endorphins and morphine.

C. Electrical Stimulation-Induced Analgesia

The demonstration that electrical stimulation of the mesencephalic gray in rats produced a profound analgesic response was one of the earliest reports providing experimental evidence suggestive of the presence of endogenous morphinelike substances in the brain (57). The analgesia produced by the electrical brain stimulation was sufficient to permit a laparotomy to be performed (57). Subsequent reports have demonstrated that electrical stimulation of medial brainstem regions, especially the periaqueductal gray (PAG), resulted in potent analgesic activity in the rat (58, 59), cat (60, 61), rhesus monkey (62), and humans (63, 64); Mayer and Price (65) have written an excellent review on brain stimulation-induced analgesia.

Brain stimulation-induced analgesia is significantly antagonized by naloxone, a narcotic antagonist (63, 66). In addition, microinjection of morphine into the PAG resulted in marked naloxone-reversible analgesic activity (67, 68), and brain stimulation-induced analgesia exhibited both tolerance (69) and cross-tolerance to morphine administered at the same brain site (69, 70). Therefore, it was believed that the electrical stimulation caused the release of some endogenous substance which resulted in an opiatelike analgesic response; today we have good evidence that the substances being released are endorphins.

D. Acupuncture Analgesia

Acupuncture has been reported to produce potent analgesic activity in humans. Several reports (71-73) have provided evidence that acupuncture significantly increases experimental pain thresholds in humans. The consistent observation that acupuncture analgesia takes some time to reach its maximal effectiveness and that clinical pain relief lasts long after the needles have been removed suggests a possible neurohumoral mechanism of action. Acupuncture-induced analgesia in humans has been significantly antagonized by the narcotic antagonist, naloxone (73). Thus it has been proposed that acupuncture induces the release of endorphins, which then produce the elevations in pain thresholds observed after this treatment.

In mice, electroacupuncture also produces profound analgesia to pain induced by heat sources (74); furthermore, naloxone also blocked this response. Naloxone has also been shown to produce hyperalgesia under certain circumstances in mice (75). Further evidence in support of the mediation of acupuncture analgesia by endorphins comes form the report that removal of the pituitary in rats, a probable site for endorphin production, prevents this response (76); in addition, only a poor analgesic response could be obtained in the CBXK mouse, a strain that has few opiate receptors (77). Acupuncture has been shown to cause a release of endorphins (78). Therefore, the evidence is in favor of acupuncture analgesia being mediated by endorphins released as a result of this stimulation.

E. Stress-Induced Analgesia

Stress, in the form of inescapable footshock, has been shown to produce profound analgesia in rats (79) and mice (80); this response can be prevented or reversed by naloxone (79, 80). In addition, similar receptor systems may mediate both stress-induced and narcotic analgesia since footshock-induced analgesia could not be elicited in mice that had been made tolerant to morphine (80). Analgesia can also be induced by other types of stress, such as restraint (81) or forced cold water swimming (82). Not all types of stress-induced analgesic responses may be mediated totally by endorphins since swim stress analgesia is only partially reversed by naloxone (82), and although naloxone usually antagonizes footshock-induced analgesia, it does not do it under all circumstances (79). Footshock-induced stress has been shown to produce increased β-endorphin levels in blood but not in the brain of rats (83); however, increased brain levels of endorphins have been observed in at least one study (84). Therefore, further studies will be necessary to determine the role of released endorphins in stress-induced analgesia.

III. PHYSICAL DEPENDENCE AND ABUSE POTENTIAL

Wei and Loh (85) were the first to demonstrate that the endorphins could cause physical dependence. Since it would be extremely difficult to demonstrate the development of physical dependence with substances that are catabolized very rapidly (e.g., Met-enkephalin), they used osmotic minipumps for chronic drug delivery directly into the brain of rats via chronically indwelling cannulae (PAG, fourth ventricular space) to overcome this problem. When rats that had been infused for 70 hr with Met-enkephalin or β-endorphin were challenged with naloxone, they manifested a morphinelike withdrawal syndrome characterized primarily by shaking, teeth chattering, and repeated attempts to escape (22, 85). Wei (86) evaluated seven enkephalin analogs and found an excellent correlation between potency as an analgesic and physical dependency liability; that is, the greater the antinociceptive activity, the greater the potential for producing physical dependence. Thus endorphins clearly demonstrated physical dependence liability in rats following subacute infusion directly into the brain. Further evidence that the endorphins are likely to produce dependence liability comes from a report that Met-enkephalin (3.5 and 7.0 μmol/kg, i.c.v.) inhibited naloxone-induced withdrawal syndrome in mice rendered dependent by the pellet implantation method (87).

Using an in vitro model, the isolate guinea pig ileum, Schulz and Herz (88) claimed to be able to predict dependence liability with opiates. In their preparation, myenteric plexus-longitudinal muscle strips taken from morphine-tolerant/dependent guinea pigs which were kept in continuous contact with normorphine after removal exhibited tonic contracture upon naloxone challenge ("withdrawal response"). As a result of their evaluation in this model, it was predicted that both Leu- and Met-enkephalin would exhibit morphinelike physical dependence.

At the neuronal level, physical dependence liability can be demonstrated by the naloxone-induced increases in spontaneous and/or L-glutamate- and acetylcholine-induced activity observed in single-cell preparations from morphine-tolerant/dependent rats (56); these enhanced responses appear to represent specific withdrawal effects at the single neuron level.

Tseng and coworkers (51) used a modification of the mouse jump test (89) to determine the physical dependence liability of β-endorphin. In this procedure, mice were rendered morphine dependent by pellet implantation; 72 hr later the pellets were removed and the mice were challenged with naloxone and observed for the precipitation of withdrawal jumping. β-Endorphin caused a dose-related inhibition of naloxone-induced jumping in morphine-tolerant mice; on a molar basis, β-endorphin was 10 times more potent than morphine as a suppressant of jumping. In contrast to β-endorphin, Met-enkephalin failed to inhibit jumping at doses up to 200 μg/mouse, i.c.v. Thus β-endorphin exhibited clear-cut physical dependence liability in the mouse jump test, a procedure considered to be a reliable predictor of such activity.

Self-administration procedures are used as a means of predicting substance abuse liability in humans. Belluzzi and Stein (90) found that both Met- and Leu-enkephalin were self-administered by the rat; in these studies, each lever press delivered 1 μl of the drug solution into the lateral ventricle via a chronically indwelling cannula. A subsequent study in rhesus monkeys clearly demonstrated that a potent, long-lasting synthetic enkephalin analog, FK 33–824, was intravenously self-administered in both drug-naive and morphine-dependent animals (91). Thus all the naturally occurring and synthetic endorphins that have been evaluated thus far would be predicted to possess significant abuse potential in humans.

Elevated brain enkephalin levels were observed in rats treated chronically with morphine (55); however, no significant alteration in narcotic receptors, either in affinity or number of binding sites (ligands: [^{3}H] etorphine and [^{3}H] naltrexone), were observed in any brain area studied from rats that were implanted with morphine pellets for several days to yield a physically dependent/tolerant state (92). Thus the tolerance and physical dependence that occurs after chronic administration of opiates does not appear to be due to obvious changes in opiate receptors in brain.

IV. EFFECTS OF ENDORPHINS ON BEHAVIOR

In addition to their analgesic activity and dependence-producing properties, the endorphins also influence a wide range of behavior. The following are areas that have been investigated.

A. Reinforcement Mechanisms

Animals and humans will electrically stimulate their brains (self-stimulatory behavior) and the reinforcement system within the brain has been thoroughly mapped. Belluzzi and Stein (90) reported that lever-press responses reinforced by electrical stimulation of the medial forebrain bundle were significantly suppressed following intraventricular administration of the highest dose of Leu-enkephalin (200 μg per rat) that was tested but not after Met-enkephalin (100 and 200 μg per rat). The finding that Leu-enkephalin was a more potent suppressant of self-stimulatory behavior then Met-enkephalin correlates with the fact that Leu-enkephalin was self-administered to a greater extent than the methionine form (90).

Goldstein and Malick (93) reported that morphine selectively antagonized self-stimulatory behavior when infused at the site of stimulation via an electrode cannula into the medial forebrain bundle at the level of the lateral hypothalamus in rats (Table 6). In a subsequent study, a significant reduction in self-stimulation rates was observed following infusion of Leu-enkephalin (120 μg per rat) into this same lateral hypothalamic site (Table 6); the peak time of this activity was 20 min post-drug infusion, which was the same time of peak effect for morphine (93). Since the lowest dose of morphine producing a significant suppression of self-stimulation was 5 μg per rat, it was considerably more potent than Leu-enkephalin as a depressant of reinforcement mechanisms (Table 6).

Stein and Belluzzi (94) hypothesized that self-stimulation in brain regions that contain relatively high concentrations of enkephalins [e.g., lateral hypothalamus,

TABLE 6 Effects of Intracerebral Administration of Leu-Enkephalin and Morphine on Brain-Stimulated Reinforcement

Treatment	Dose (μg/rat)	N[a]	Mean response rates ± S.E.M. Predrug	Post-drug	P-value[b]
Sterile water	—	20	556 ± 32	562 ± 28	N.S.[c]
Leu-enkephalin	30	3	599 ± 35	619 ± 121	N.S.
	60	5	538 ± 85	472 ± 139	N.S.
	120	10	551 ± 59	309 ± 89	<0.01
Morphine	1	6	586 ± 41	516 ± 167	N.S.
	5	4	520 ± 100	280 ± 128	<0.05

[a]Number of rats tested.
[b]Student's t-test comparing predrug to postdrug response rates.
[c]N.S., not significant.
Source: From Ref. 93.

PAG (95)] may depend, at least in part, on the release of endorphins, which would then activate "opiate reward receptors." In support of this hypothesis, they had previously shown that naloxone was a potent antagonist of self-stimulatory behavior in rats (90,94). Of the five self-stimulation sites that they have tested, the substantia nigra appeared to be most sensitive to the effects of naloxone (50% suppression dose = 0.48 mg/kg, s.c.) (94). However, in contrast, other authors (96) have found that self-stimulatory responses were attenuated in the caudate and lateral hypothalamus only after very high doses of naloxone (40 mg/kg, i.p.); we have confirmed this finding in the lateral hypothalamus (unpublished results). Intraventricular administration of both Leu- and Met-enkephalin also produced a significant suppression of operant behavior maintained by food reinforcement (90); thus endorphins may regulate biological drives. Stein and Belluzzi (94) proposed that while the incentive for goal-directed behavior (drive-inducing effect) may be mediated by catecholamines, the satisfaction or feeling of well-being attained by the reward (drive-reducing effect) may be mediated by opiate receptors. Since the endorphins are self-administered and may modulate or control self-stimulatory behavior, it has been proposed that an endorphin(s) may act as an endogenous euphorigen or a reward transmitter (94).

B. Learning and Memory

Many studies with opiates have implied that they may play a significant role in memory processes. For example, mice injected with opiates (e.g., heroin, morphine) exhibited poor retention of a discriminative avoidance task 24 hr post-drug administration (97). In addition, injection of levorphanol into the amygdala of rats produced time-dependent and dose-related decrements in retention of passive avoidance conditioning (98); this effect was stereospecific and reversible with naloxone.

Recently, Stein and Belluzzi (94) studied the effects of Leu- and Met-enkephalin on memory formation in rats. In a one-trial learning procedure, rats received a mildly painful electric shock after stepping down from a shelf to a grid floor. Immediately after the initial trial, rats were given either placebo, morphine, or one of the enkephalins intraventricularly via permanently indwelling cannulae. All rats were then retested 3 days later (retention test) to evaluate long-term memory of the shock. The longer the retest step-down latencies, the better the long-term memory of the shock. The rats that received morphine (20 μg) or Met-enkephalin (200 μg) exhibited a significant facilitation of the learned response; animals treated with Leu-enkephalin (200 μg) exhibited step-down latencies that were not significantly different from the placebo-treated control group (94). If the morphine administration was delayed for 15 min after the first trial, presumably beyond the time necessary for memory consolidation, the memory-enhancing effect was completely abolished. These results suggest that posttrial activation of endorphin receptors may facilitate memory consolidation.

Rigter and coworkers (99) also evaluated enkephalins in a one-trial situation in which rats were punished (footshock) for entering a dark chamber. In their procedure, if carbon dioxide was administered immediately after the acquisition trial, amnesia was produced, as evidenced by the relative lack of avoidance on the retest trial. They reported that both Met- and Leu-enkephalin (3 μg per rat, s.c.) attenuated carbon dioxide-induced amnesia when administered before the retrieval test. Naloxone failed to alter the amnesia by itself and it failed to block the anti-amnesia effects of the pentapeptides. Thus this action of the enkephalins does not appear to be mediated by opiate receptors. In a subsequent study, Met-enkephalin, but not Leu-enkephalin, decreased amnesia in a dose-related manner when given prior to the acquisition trial (100); this result suggests that the two pentapeptides may possess different pharmacological properties. Thus the endorphins may directly or indirectly influence memory processes.

Kastin and coworkers (101) administered Met-enkephalin intraperitoneally (80 μg/kg) and found that it facilitated the ability of rats to run a complex maze for food reward; in contrast, morphine-treated rats ran the maze much slower and exhibited a greater number of errors than vehicle-treated controls. In addition, rats treated with an enkephalin analog, D-Phe^4-Met-enkephalin, which has essentially no opiate activity, also performed the maze task significantly better than controls; thus the behavioral effects of the enkephalins in this study are probably not due to actions at opiate receptors.

β-Endorphin was found to increase response latencies in an avoidance task in rats following intravenous administration (102). Olsen and coworkers (103) also found that several enkephalin and endorphin analogs increased the response latencies for fear habituation in goldfish; however, this effect may not have been related to influences on learning since the fish appeared immobilized. Rigter and associates (104) reported that administration of Leu-enkephalin (400 μg/kg, i.p.) to rats impaired acquisition of a one-way active avoidance response, facilitated acquisition of an inhibitory avoidance response, and had no effect on acquisition of a swim escape response. Thus endorphins may strengthen the tendency to suppress behavior in the presence of cues that previously had been associated with aversive stimulation.

DeWied and associates (105) studied the influence of endorphins on extinction behavior in aversively motivated tasks. Whereas the majority of the peptides tested [e.g., Met-enkephalin, α-endorphin, β-endorphin, ACTH 4–10 (β-LPH 47–53)] inhibited the extinction of a pole jump avoidance response following subcutaneous administration, γ-endorphin was unique in that it facilitated extinction (106). LeMoal and coworkers (107) confirmed the observation that α- and γ-endorphin have opposite effects on pole jump avoidance, the former inhibiting and the latter facilitating extinction; however, when water-deprived rats were tested in a runway task for water reinforcement, both α- and γ-endorphin inhibited extinction of this response (107). Therefore, the effects of these peptides may be situation dependent.

Whereas nanogram quantities of endorphins (e.g., α-endorphin) significantly delayed extinction of a pole jump avoidance response, microgram quantities of β-endorphin were required to produce analgesia in the rat. This suggests that the primary physiological function(s) of these peptides is not the modulation of pain thresholds.

C. Sexual Behavior

Heroin addicts and chronic users of narcotic analgesics frequently complain about sexual dysfunction (e.g., frigidity, impotence) (108). In addition, it has been reported that when heroin addicts undergo methadone maintenance, they often report that their erectional insufficiency, delayed time for ejaculation, and reduced libido improve (108).

The influence of β-endorphin on male sexual behavior in rats has been studied by Meyerson and coworkers (109, 110). They reported that intraventricularly administered β-endorphin (1 μg) inhibited mounting behavior or caused it to occur in an abnormal way (no real clasp and thrust); consequently, very few intromissions were achieved (109, 110). In these studies, β-endorphin did not produce other effects (e.g., catalepsy, rigidity) that would prevent mounting, and the effects were antagonized by naltrexone pretreatment. In another study (111), D-Ala^{2}-Met-enkephalinamide (6 μg, i.c.v.) completely suppressed copulatory behavior in rats. In contrast, D-Ala^{2}-γ-endorphin appeared to enhance sexual arounsal in male rats (112).

Although the influence of endorphins on sexual performance has not been studied in humans to date, Goldstein and Hanstein reported that naloxone failed to influence masturbation variables in the male (113). Thus endorphin systems may or may not modulate sexual behavior.

D. Locomotor Activity

When the influence of endorphins on spontaneous locomotor activity was studied, the vast majority of investigators reported that they significantly reduced activity.

Although low doses (1 μg, i.c.v.) of β-endorphin, which altered sexual behavior, failed to influence exploratory activities (ambulation, rearing) in male rats (110), higher doses (5 μg, i.c.v.) produced a profund decrease in motor activity (114). In another study, Bhargava (115) reported that both morphine and Met-enkephalin were equipotent as suppressors of motor actiivty in rats following intracerebroventricular infusion; doses of both as low as 7.0 μmol/kg, i.c.v. produced a profound decrease in motor activity that was readily antagonized by pretreatment with naloxone (1 mg/kg, s.c.). In mice, Frigeni and coworkers (116) reported that Met-enkephalin failed to significantly alter motor activity in two strains of mice (DBA and C57) at a dose (200 μg, i.c.v.) that produce significant analgesic activity as measured in the hot plate test. Thus, once again, endorphins did not influence motor activity at doses influencing other behavioral responses.

Amir and coworkers (117) found that chronic naltrexone (10 mg/kg, s.c. for 8 consecutive days) treatment resulted in a significant elevation in locomotor activity after drug treatment was terminated, the most pronounced increase occurring 7 days after the last naltrexone treatment. These results suggest that chronic opiate receptor blockade leads to supersensitivity of dopaminergic systems mediating motor activity (e.g., nucleus accumbens); thus endorphins may modulate neuronal activity in pathways that control motor movement (e.g., ambulation) in the brain.

E. Miscellaneous Behavior Actions

Morphine has been shown to produce a significant increase in grooming behavior in rats (118). β-Endorphin has also been shown to enhance grooming in rats (112, 119); the grooming effects were reversed by naloxone. In contrast, α-endorphin produced little (119) or no increase in grooming (112) and Leu- and Met-enkephalin (119) and γ-endorphin (112) failed to elicit any alterations in grooming behavior. Thus β-endorphin more closely resembles morphine in regard to its effects on this behavior than do the other endorphins evaluated thus far.

Catalepsy produced by β-endorphin has been observed by many investigators. Jacquet and Marks (120) reported that microinjection of 4 μg of β-endorphin into the periaqueductal gray of the rat resulted in profound sedation and catalepsy, whereas Met- and Leu-enkephalin produced an attenuated form of this behavior. Bloom and coworkers (121) also reported that β-endorphin (50 μg) injected into the lateral ventricle of rats produced marked and prolonged muscular rigidity and immobility which appeared similar to the catatonic state. These effects of β-endorphin in rats where antagonized by naloxone (121, 122). Feldberg and Smyth (43) showed that infusion of β-endorphin into the third ventricle of the cat also resulted in a naloxone-reversible cataleptic state. Although at least part of the cataleptic response to β-endorphin is mediated through effects at narcotic receptor sites, part of its activity appears to be mediated by dopaminergic mechanisms. Izumi and associates (122) have shown that intraventricularly administered β-endorphin (13 μmol; 43 μg) produced akinesia in the rat; pretreatment with apomorphine (20 mg/kg, s.c.), a dopaminergic agonist, prevented the akinesia, whereas pretreatment with α-methyl-p-tyrosine (250 mg/kg, i.p.) potentiated the muscle rigidity induced by β-endorphin. The cataleptic effect of β-endorphin was shown to be prevented by the injection of 1-dihydroxyphenylalanine (L-dopa), whereas 1-5-hydroxytryptophan (5-HTP) potentiated the cataleptic effect of this peptide (123).

Further evidence suggestive of the fact that dopaminergic mechanisms may account for some of the behavioral effects of the endorphins comes from the studies of Plotnikoff and coworkers (124); in these studies, systemic injections of Met-enkephalin markedly potentiated dopa-induced behavioral hyperactivity but had no activity in a serotonin potentiation model. Furthermore, several enkephalin analogs have been shown to produce a syndrome characterized by stereotyped motor activity following intraventricular administration in mice (125, 126); this activation syndrome was significantly antagonizd by dopamine receptor antagonists (e.g., pimozide, fluspirolene).

The endorphins have been implicated in the control of feeding behavior. Elevated concentrations of β-endorphin were found in the plasma and pituitary of obese rats (127) and the pituitaries of obese mice (128); in addition, rats that were fasted for 2–3 days exhibitied a significant decrease in hypothalamic, but not pituitary, β-endorphin (129). β-Endorphin has been shown to stimulate food intake when administered intraventricularly (130), whereas naloxone suppresses spontaneous food intake in normal rats (131) and abolished overeating in genetically obese rats (132). Naloxone also awakens hibernating animals (133) and thus may act to signal that food reserves are low. Leu- and Met-enkephalin (100–200 μg per rat, i.c.v.) also inhibited drinking induced by either water deprivation or intracerebroventricularly administered angiotensin II (134).

Endorphin systems may also play an important role in the organism's response to stressful situations. Arrigo-Reina and Ferri (135) reported that naloxone increased the intensity of gastric ulceration following restraint/cold exposure-induced stress in rats; in contrast, morphine (10 mg/kg, s.c.) completely abolished stress-induced ulceration in their experiments (135). Stress and anxiety are closely interrelated, and a few studies have been performed to assess the role of endorphins in anxiety. Grevert and Goldstein (136) reported that naloxone (10 mg/kg, i.v.) produced a significant increase in tension-anxiety scores in humans. In rats, Billingsley and Kubena (137) reported that naloxone pretreatment could significantly antagonize tha anxiolytic effects of chlordiazepoxide in the shock-induced suppression of drinking test (138) in rats. In addition, Malick (unpublished observations) found that morphine produced a dose-related disinhibitory (antianxiety effect) in the neophobic suppression of drinking test in rats (139); this effect was naloxone reversible.

V. OTHER PHARMACOLOGICAL EFFECTS OF ENDORPHINS

Endorphins have been shown to be present along the entire length of the gastrointestinal tract. Using the guinea pig ileum preparation made famous by Kosterlitz and coworkers (5), Mitznegg and associates (140) demonstrated that enkephalins could inhibit contractions elicited by a wide range of agents (e.g., barium chloride, acetylcholine, histamine). Morphine and other opiates have long been known for their pronounced effects on gastric motility; they inhibit gastric emptying, decrease gastric contractile activity, and inhibit intestinal contractions. Konturek (141) reported that the enkephalins will mimic all the actions of morphine on the gut of the dog. Thus endorphins may play a role in the local regulation of gut smooth muscle motility in addition to other physiological function in the gastrointestinal tract.

Met-enkephalin (120 μg) produced seizures following infusion into the forebrain dorsomedial nucleus of the thalamus (142); however, no electroencephalogram changes were noted at several other brain sites. Subsequently, Leu-enkephalin was also shown to produce seizures, and, in fact, the duration of such seizures appeared to be longer than following Met-enkephalin. Although naloxone was capable of blocking these seizures in most studies (142, 143), at least one group claimed they were not reversed by narcotic antagonists (144). However, Met-enkephalin was shown to cause slight reductions in audiogenic seizures following parenteral administration in mice (124).

Numerous other actions of endorphins have been observed. In cats, intraventricular administration of Met-enkephalin induced emesis and hyperthermia (145); hyperthermia was also produced by α-endorphin in rats (121). β-Endorphin was reported to cause insomnia in cats (146) and shifts in hippocampal theta rhythm indicative of increased arousal states in rats (105). Copious salivation was observed following β-endorphin in rodents (147). Endorphins have also been shown to exhibit profound depressent effects on the respiratory and cardiovascular system (148, 149).

VI. SUMMARY AND CONCLUSIONS

The endorphins exhibit profound effects on numerous systems of the body. As expected, they certainly exhibit potent analgesic activitiy in a wide variety of procedures and in a great number of species, including humans. However, the modulation of pain mechanisms within the body may not be the primary function of the endorphins; this is suggested by the fact that the potency of the endorphins for producing other behavioral changes (e.g., influences on extinction of avoidance responses) is greater than their analgesic potency.

The other effects of the endorphins are so varied that it would be too time consuming to mention them all again. However, strong evidence exists to indicate that they may play an important modulatory or homeostatic function in almost every major organ system in the body in addition to their important role in the central nervous system. We have only begun to scratch the surface of this new field and it remains one of the most explosive and exciting areas for future discovery.

REFERENCES

1. A. Goldstein, L. I. Lowney, and B. K. Pal, *Proc. Natl. Acad. Sci. U.S.A., 68:* 1742 (1971).

2. C. B. Pert and S. H. Snyder, *Science, 179*: 1011 (1973).
3. E. J. Simon, J. M. Hiller, and I. Edelman, *Proc. Natl. Acad. Sci. U.S.A., 70*: 1947 (1973).
4. L. Terenius, *Acta Pharmacol. Toxicol., 32*: 317 (1973).
5. J. Hughes, T. W. Smith, H. W. Kosterlitz, L. A. Fothergill, B. A. Morgan, and H. R. Morris, *Nature, 258*: 577 (1975).
6. J. H. Jaffe, in *The Pharmacological Basis of Therapeutics* (L. S. Goodman and A. Gilman, eds.), Macmillan, New York, 1975, p. 284.
7. J. D. Belluzzi, N. Grant, V. Garsky, D. Sarantakis, C. D. Wise, and L. Stein, *Nature, 260*: 625 (1976).
8. F. E. D'Amour and D. L. Smith, *J. Pharmacol. Exp. Ther., 72*: 74 (1941).
9. A. S. Bloom, W. L. Dewey, L. S. Harris, and K. K. Brosius, *J. Pharmacol. Exp. Ther., 198*: 33 (1976).
10. J. B. Malick and J. M. Goldstein, *Pharmacologist, 18*: 120 (1976).
11. J. B. Malick and J. M. Goldstein, *Life Sci., 20*: 827 (1977).
12. J. T. Litchfield, Jr. and F. Wilcoxon, *J. Pharmacol. Exp. Ther., 96*: 99 (1949).
13. J. M. Hambrook, F. A. Morgan, M. J. Rance, and C. F. C. Smith, *Nature, 262*: 782 (1976).
14. T. L. Yaksh, J. C. DuChateau, and T. A. Rudy, *Brain Res., 104*: 367 (1976).
15. J. K. Chang, B. T. W. Fong, A. Pert, and C. B. Pert, *Life Sci., 18*: 1473 (1976).
16. H. H. Büscher, R. C. Hill, D. Romer, F. Cardinaux, A. Closse, D. Hauser, and J. Pless, *Nature, 261*: 423 (1976).
17. L. Graf, J. I. Szekely, A. Z. Ronai, Z. Dunai-Kovacs, and S. Bajusz, *Nature, 263*: 240 (1976).
18. A. Z. Ronai, J. I. Szekely, L. Graf, Z. Dunai-Kovacs, and S. Bajusz, *Life Sci., 19*: 733 (1976).
19. J. I. Szekely, A. Z. Ronai, Z. Dunai-Kovacs, L. Graf, and S. Bajusz, *Experientia, 33*: 54 (1977).
20. G. Urca, H. Frenk, J. C. Liebeskind, and A. Taylor, *Science, 197*: 83 (1977).
21. J. M. Walker, G. G. Bernston, C. A. Sandman, D. H. Coy, A. V. Schally, and A. J. Kastin, *Science, 196*: 85 (1977).
22. H. H. Loh, L. F. Tseng, E. Wei, and C. H. Li, *Proc. Natl. Acad. Sci. U.S.A., 73*: 2895 (1976).
23. D. Romer, H. H. Büscher, R.C. Hill, J. Pless, W. Bauer, F. Cardinaux, A. Closse, D. Hauser, and R. Huguenin, *Nature, 268*: 547 (1977).
24. N. B. Eddy and D. Leimbach, *J. Pharmacol. Exp. Ther., 107*: 385 (1953).
25. H. F. Fraser and L. S. Harris, *Annu. Rev. Pharmacol., 7*: 277 (1967).
26. J. Cochin, in *Selected Pharmacological Testing Methods*, Vol. 3 (A. Burger, ed.), Marcel Dekker, New York, 1968, p. 121.
27. W. L. Dewey and L. S. Harris, *J. Pharmacol. Exp. Ther., 179*: 652 (1971).
28. T. Johannesson and L. A. Woods, *Acta Pharmacol. Toxicol., 21*: 381 (1964).
29. J. M. Goldstein and J. B. Malick, *Life Sci., 25*: 431 (1979).
30. A. F. Bradbury, D. G. Smyth, C. R. Snell, J. F. W. Deakin, and S. Wendlandt, *Biochem. Biophys. Res. Commun., 74*: 748 (1977).
31. L. Leybin, C. Pinsky, F. S. LaBella, V. Havlicek, and M. Rezek, *Nature, 264*: 458 (1976).

32. R. T. Brittain, D. N. Lehrer, and P. S. Spencer, *Nature, 200*: 895 (1963).
33. H. I. Chernov, D. E. Wilson, F. Fowler, and A. J. Plummer, *Arch. Int. Pharmacodyn. Ther., 167*: 171 (1967).
34. R. I. Taber, D. D. Greenhouse, J. K. Rendell, and S. Irwin, *J. Pharmacol. Exp. Ther., 169*: 29 (1969).
35. W. Feldberg and D. G. Smyth, *J. Physiol., 260*: 30P (1976).
36. M. Meglio, Y. Hosobuchi, H. H. Loh, J. E. Adams, and C. H. Li, *Proc. Natl. Acad. Sci. U.S.A., 74*: 774 (1977).
37. C. B. Pert and S. H. Snyder, *Mol. Pharmacol., 10*: 868 (1974).
38. L. F. Tseng, H. H. Loh, and C. H. Li, *Nature, 263*: 239 (1976).
39. C. H. Li, D. Yamashiro, L. F. Tseng, and H. H. Loh, *J. Med. Chem., 20*: 325 (1977).
40. D. H. Catlin, K. K. Hui, H. H. Loh, and C. H. Li, *Commun. Psychopharmacol., 1*: 493 (1977).
41. Y. Hosobuchi and C. H. Li, *Commun. Psychopharmacol., 2*: 33 (1978).
42. L. H. Lazarus, N. Ling, and R. Guillemin, *Proc. Natl. Acad. Sci. U.S.A., 73*: 2156 (1976).
43. W. Feldberg and D. G. Smyth, *Br. J. Pharmacol., 60*: 445 (1977).
44. W. J. Russell and M. A. Tate, *J. Physiol. (Lond.), 248*: 5 (1975).
45. L. F. Tseng, H. H. Loh, and C. H. Li, *Nature, 263*: 239 (1976).
46. J. M. vanRee, D. DeWied, A. F. Bradbury, E. Hulme, D. G. Smyth, and C. R. Snell, *Nature, 264*: 792 (1976).
47. M. J. Geisow, J. F. W. Deakin, J. O. Dostrovsky, and D. G. Smyth, *Nature, 269*: 167 (1977).
48. J. I. Szekely, A. Z. Ronai, Z. Dunai-Kovacs, E. Miglecz, I. Berzetri, S. Bajusz, and L. Graf, *Eur. J. Pharmacol., 43*: 293 (1977).
49. E. J. Wei, L. F. Tseng, H. H. Loh, and C. H. Li, *Life Sci., 21*: 321 (1977).
50. D. Yamishiro, L. F. Tseng, B. A. Doneen, H. H. Loh, and C. H. Li, *Int. J. Peptide Protein Res., 10*: 159 (1977).
51. L. Tseng, H. H. Loh, and C. H. Li, *Proc. Natl. Acad. Sci. U.S.A., 73*: 4187 (1976).
52. T. J. Haley and W. G. McCormick, *Br. J. Pharmacol., 12*: 12 (1957).
53. Y. Hosobuchi, M. Meglio, J. E. Adams, and C. H. Li, *Proc. Natl. Acad. Sci. U.S.A., 74*: 4017 (1977).
54. E. Contreras, L. Tomayo, L. Quijada, and E. Silva, *Eur. J. Pharmacol., 22*: 339 (1973).
55. R. Simantov and S. H. Snyder, *Nature, 262*: 505 (1976).
56. J. P. Fry, W. Zieglgansberger, and A. Herz, in *Characteristics and Functions of Opioids* (J. M. vanRee and L. Terenius, eds.), Elsevier/North-Holland, New York, 1978, p. 99.
57. D. V. Reynolds, *Science, 164*: 444 (1969).
58. S. Balagura and T. Ralph, *Brain Res., 60*: 369 (1973).
59. D. J. Mayer and J. C. Liebeskind, *Brain Res., 68*: 73 (1974).
60. J. C. Liebeskind, G. Guilbaud, J. M. Besson, and J. L. Oliveras, *Brain Res., 50*: 441 (1973).
61. J. L. Oliveras, J. M. Besson, G. Guilbaud, and J. C. Liebeskind, *Exp. Brain Res.,*

20: 32 (1974).
62. S. J. Goodman and V. Holcombe, in *Advances in Pain Research and Therapy,* Vol. 1 (J. J. Bonica and D. G. Albe-Fessard, eds.), Raven Press, New York, 1976, p. 495.
63. J. E. Adams, *Pain, 2*: 161 (1976).
64. D. E. Richardson and H. Akil, paper presented at Annu. Meet. Am. Assoc., Neurol. Surg., 1973.
65. D. J. Mayer and D. D. Price, *Pain, 2*: 379 (1976).
66. H. Akil, D. J. Mayer, and J. C. Liebeskind, *Science, 191*: 961 (1976).
67. A. Herz, K. Albus, J. Metys, P. Schubert, and H. Teschemacher, *Neuropharmacology*, *9*: 539 (1970).
68. A. Pert and T. Yaksh, *Brain Res., 80*: 135 (1974).
69. D. J. Mayer and R. Hayes, *Science, 188*: 941 (1975).
70. D. J. Mayer and R. Murphin, *Fed. Proc., 35*: 385 (1976).
71. S. A. Anderson, T. Ericson, E. Holmgren, and G. Lindqvist, *Brain Res., 63:* 393 (1973).
72. S. A. Anderson and E. Holmgren, *J. Chin. Med., 3*: 311 (1975).
73. D. J. Mayer, D. D. Price, and A. Rafii, *Brain Res., 121*: 368 (1977).
74. B. R. Pomeranz and D. Chin, *Life Sci., 19*: 1757 (1976).
75. L. Leybin, C. Pinsky, F. S. LaBella, V. Havlicek, and M. Rezek, *Nature, 264*: 458 (1976).
76. B. Pomeranz, in *The Endorphins* (E. Costa and M. Trabucchi, eds.), Raven Press, New York, 1978, p. 351.
77. J. M. Peets and B. Pomeranz, *Nature, 273*: 675 (1978).
78. C. H. L. Peng, M. P. Yang, S. H. Kok, and Y. K. Woo, *Comp. Med. East West, 6*: 57 (1978).
79. J. W. Lewis, J. T. Cannon, and J. C. Liebeskind, *Science, 208*: 623 (1980).
80. G. B. Chesher and B. Chan, *Life Sci., 21*: 1569 (1977).
81. S. K. Bhattachary, P. R. Keshary, and A. K. Sanyal, *Eur. J. Pharmacol., 50*: 83 (1978).
82. R. J. Bodnar, D. D. Kelley, A. Spiaggia, C. Pavlides, and M. Glussman, *Bull. Psychon. Soc., 12:* 125(1978).
83. J. Rossier, E. D. French, C. Rivier, N. Ling, R. Guillemin, and F. E. Bloom, *Nature, 270*: 618 (1977).
84. I. V. J. Madden, H. Akil, R. L. Patrick, and I. D. Barchas, *Nature, 265*: 358 (1977).
85. E. Wei and H. Loh, in *Opiates and Endogenous Opioid Peptides* (H. W. Kosterlitz, ed.), Elsevier/North-Holland, New York, 1976, p. 303.
86. E. Wei, in *Characteristics and Functions of Opioids* (J. M. van Ree and L. T. Terenius, eds.), Elsevier/North-Holland, New York, 1978, p. 445.
87. H. N. Bhargava, *Eur. J. Pharmacol., 41*: 81 (1977).
88. R. Schutz and A. Herz, in *Opiates and Endogenous Opioid Peptides* (H. Kosterlitz, ed.), Elsevier/North-Holland, New York, 1976, p. 319).
89. E. L. Way, H. H. Loh, and F. H. Shen, *J. Pharmacol. Exp. Ther., 167*: 1 (1969).
90. J. D. Belluzzi and L. Stein, *Nature, 266*: 556 (1977).
91. N. K. Mello and J. H. Mendelson, *Pharmacol. Biochem. Behav., 9*: 579 (1978).

92. K. A. Bonnet, J. M. Hiller, and E. J. Simon, in *Opiates and Endogenous Opioid Peptides* (H. Kosterlitz, ed.), Elsevier/North-Holland, New York, 1976, p. 335.
93. J. M. Goldstein and J. B. Malick, *Pharmacol. Biochem. Behav.*, *7*: 475 (1977).
94. L. Stein and J. D. Belluzzi, in *The Endorphins* (E. Costa and M. Trabucchi, eds.), Raven Press, New York, 1978, p. 299.
95. H. Y. T. Yang, J. S. Hong, W. Fratta, and E. Costa, in *The Endorphins* (E. Costa and M. Trabucchi, eds.), Raven Press, New York, 1978, p. 149.
96. D. vanderKooy, F. G. LePiane, and A. G. Phillips, *Life Sci.*, *20*: 981 (1977).
97. B. S. Kapp and M. Gallagher, *Trends Neurosci.*, July, 177 (1979).
98. M. Gallagher and B. S. Kapp, *Life Sci.*, *23*: 1973 (1978).
99. H. Rigter, H. Greven, and H. vanRiezen, *Neuropharmacology*, *16*: 545 (1977).
100. H. Rigter, *Science*, *200*: 83 (1978).
101. A. J. Kastin, E. L. Scollan, M. G. King, A. V. Schally, and D. H. Coy, *Pharmacol. Biochem. Behav.*, *5*: 691 (1976).
102. D. A. Gorelick, D. H. Catlin, R. George, and C. H. Li, *Pharmacol. Biochem. Behav.*, *9*: 385 (1978).
103. R. D. Olson, A. J. Kastin, G. F. Michell, D. H. Coy, and J. M. Montalbano, *Pharmacol. Biochem. Behav.*, *9*: 111 (1978).
104. H. Rigter, R. A.Jensen, J. L. Martinez, Jr. R. B. Messing, B. J. Vasquez, K. C. Liang, and J. L. McGaugh, *Proc. Natl. Acad. Sci. U.S.A.*, *77*: 3729 (1980).
105. D. DeWied, B. Bohus, J. M. van Ree, and I. Urban, *J. Pharmacol. Exp. Ther.*, *204*: 570 (1973).
106. D. DeWied, G. L. Kovacs, B. Bohus, J. M. van Ree, and H. M. Greven, *Eur. J. Pharmacol.*, *49*: 427 (1978).
107. M. LeMoal, G. F. Koob, and F. E. Bloom, *Life Sci.*, *24*: 1631 (1979).
108. P. Cushman, *N.Y. State J. Med.*, *71*: 1768 (1971).
109 B. J. Meyerson and L. Terenius, *Eur. J. Pharmacol.*, *42*: 191 (1977).
110. B. J. Meyerson and M. Berg, *Acta Pharmacol. Toxicol.*, *41*: 64 (1977)
111. B. P. Quarantotti, M. G. Corda, E. Paglietti, G. Biggio, and G. L. Gessa, *Life Sci.*, *23*: 673 (1978).
112. J. L. Veith, C. A. Sandman, J. M. Walker, D. H. Coy, and A. J. Kastin, *Physiol. Behav.*, *20*: 539 (1978).
113. A. Goldstein and R. W. Hansteen, *Arch. Gen. Psychiatry, 34:* 1179 (1977).
114. R. G. Browne and D. S. Segal, *Neuropharmacology*, *19*: 619 (1980).
115. H. N. Bhargava, *Pharmacol. Biochem. Behav.*, *9: 167 (1978).*
116. V. Frigeni, F. Bruno, A. Carenzi, R. Racagni, and V. Santini, *J. Pharm. Pharmacol.*, *30*: 310 (1978).
117. S. Amir, R. Blair, and Z. Amit, *Life Sci.*, *25*: 1407 (1979).
118. W. H. Gispen and V. M. Wiegant, *Neurosci. Lett.*, *2*: 159 (1976).
119. W. Gispen, V. Wiegant, A. Bradbury, E. Hulme, D. Smyth, and C. Snell, *Nature*, *264*: 794 (1976).
120. Y. F. Jacquet and N. Marks, *Science*, *194*: 632 (1976).
121. F. Bloom, D. Segal, N. Ling, and R. Guillemin, *Science*, *194*: 630 (1976).
122. K. Izumi, T. Motomatsu, M. Chretien, R. F. Butterworth, M. Lis, N. Seidah, and A. Barbeau, *Life Sci., 20:* 1149 (1978).

123. T. Motomatsu, M. Lis, N. Seidah, and M. Chretien, *Can. J. Neurol. Sci.*, *3*: 49 (1977).
124. N. P. Plotnikoff, A. J. Kastin, D. H. Coy, C. W. Christensen, A. V. Schally, and M. A. Spirtes, *Life Sci.*, *19*: 1283 (1976).
125. R. J. Katz and B. J. Carroll, *Prog. Neuropsychoparmacol.*, *3*: 395 (1979).
126. R. J. Katz, B. J. Carroll, and G. Baldrighi, *Pharmacol. Biochem. Behav.*, *8*: 493 (1978).
127. D. L. Margules, B. Moisset, M. J. Lewis, H. Shibuya, and C. B. Pert, *Science*, *202*: 988 (1978).
128. J. Rossier, J. Rogers, T. Shibasaki, R. Guillemin, and F. E. Bloom, *Proc. Natl. Acad. Sci. U.S.A.*, *76*: 2077 (1979).
129. S. R. Gambert, T. L. Garthwaite, C. H. Pontzer, and T. C. Hagen, *Science*, *210*: 1271 (1980).
130. L. Grandison and A. Guidotti, *Neuropharmacology*, *16*: 533 (1977).
131. T. L. Garthwaite, D. R. Martinson, L. F. Tseng, T. C. Hagen, and L. A. Menahan, *Endocrinology*, *107*: 671 (1980).
132. B. Brands, J. A. Thornhill, M. Hirst, and C. W. Gowdy, *Life Sci.*, *24*: 1773 (1979).
133. D. L. Margules, *Neurosci. Biobehav. Rev.*, *3*: 155 (1979).
134. G. DeCaro, L. G. Micossi, and F. Venturi, *Nature*, *277*: 51 (1979).
135. R. Arrigo-Reina and S. Ferri, *Eur. J. Pharmacol.*, *64*: 85 (1980).
136. P. Grevert and A. Goldstein, *Proc. Natl. Acad. Sci. U.S.A.*, *74*: 1291 (1977).
137. M. L. Billingsley and R. K. Kubena, *Life Sci.*, *22*: 897 (1978).
138. J. R. Vogel, B. Beer, and D. E. Clody, *Psychoparmacologia (Berl.)*, *21*: 1 (1971).
139. B. P. H. Poschel, *Psychopharmacologia (Berl.)*, *19*: 193 (1971).
140. P. Mitznegg, W. Domschke, W. Sprugel, S. Domschke, N. Subramanian, E. Wunsch, L. Moroder, and L. Demling, *Acta Hepato-Gastroenterol.*, *24*: 119 (1977).
141. S. J. Konturek, *Scand. J. Gastroenterol.*, *13*: 257 (1978).
142. H. Frenk, B. C. McCarty, and J. C. Liebeskind, *Science*, *200*: 335 (1978).
143. G. Urca, H. Frenk, J. C. Liebeskind, and A. N. Taylor, *Science*, *197*: 83 (1977).
144. J. G. Bajorek, W. Chesarek, M. Felmer, and P. Lomax, *Proc. West. Pharmacol. Soc.*, *21*: 365 (1978).
145. W. G. Clark, *Proc. Soc. Exp. Biol. Med.*, *154*: 540 (1977).
146. C. D. King, L. J. Hughey, J. M. Masserano, E. E. Codd, and W. L. Byrne, *Fed. Proc.*, *36*: 965 (1977).
147. H. Loh and C. H. Li, *Annu. N.Y. Acad. Sci.*, *297*: 115 (1977).
148. J. Florez and A. Mediavilla, *Brain Res.*, *183*: 585 (1977).
149. G. A. Olson, R. D. Olson, A. J. Kastin, F. X. Castellanos, M. T. Kneale, D. H. Coy, and R. H. Wolf, *Pharmacol. Biochem. Behav.*, *9*: 687 (1978).

chapter 8

Clinical Aspects

Lars Terenius

University of Uppsala
Uppsala, Sweden

I. INTRODUCTION

The endorphins were first discovered in 1974–1975, and since then research into their functional significance has been intensive. It was perhaps somewhat unexpected that such substances would be found in mammalian tissues since the administration of opioid antagonists such as naloxone or naltrexone had been shown to produce few effects in the morphine-naive human being (1–4). Research into the endorphins took a rather unusual course, since the technology for modulating the system was in fact developed before the endorphins were discovered. This state of affairs was a result of intensive research into the actions of opiate drugs. The early studies on the effects of the morphine antagonists were not primarily designed to detect or observe any functional significance of endorphins, and therefore more subtle effects of these substances may have been overlooked.

When the endorphins were detected and their structures identified (5), there was an interest in studies in humans for several reasons. One is of course the potential clinical usefulness of endorphins as strong analgesics with hopefully lower incidence of side effects and the other is the great difficulty of establishing adequate models for clinical pain in experimental animals. This is particularly true for chronic pain (6). Another matter of concern is that morphine is a psychopharmacological agent with both subtle and integrative effects on the central nervous system (CNS), again with severe difficulties of evaluation in an experimental animal. It might also be anticipated that in the human being there could be pathological conditions where deviations from normality could involve an endorphin system out of balance. Because of these considerations, and the previously existing broad knowledge of the action of opiates and to some extent their antagonists in the human being, the step to studies in humans was taken very rapidly. Probably there are very few historical parallels to the rapid development of clinical studies in the endorphin area. Thus studies *in vitro* in experimental animals and in humans were carried out almost simultaneously and not as usually occurs in succession. Thus results accumulated at a high pace. The clinical studies were also found to be not only of interest in their own right but also to contribute very considerably to the overall knowledge of endorphins and their actions.

II. OCCURRENCE AND DISTRIBUTION IN HUMANS

A. Chemistry

The information on the chemical structure of human endorphins is meager. Frederickson et al. (7) found a compound in human brain which behaved chromatographically and biologically like the porcine material, presumably enkephalin. No enkephalin has been isolated from humans. However, fractions reacting with specific antibodies in receptor assays or in vitro systems, and showing the expected relative activity in the different tests and the expected chromatographic behavior as the authentic enkephalins, have been observed in human brain and cerebrospinal fluid (8–9).

As in other species, the human pituitary contains β-endorphin which has been isolated and found to have the expected amino acid composition (10). Its structure has been verified by synthesis (11).

There are several reports on opiate receptor-active material which so far has not been fully characterized structurally. In the cerebrospinal fluid (CSF) several receptor-active components have been found (9, 12–14). The major components are not identical to the enkephalins or β-endorphin, but since they are at least partly degraded by proteolytic enzymes, they are probably peptides. They seem to be in the molecular weight range 800–1500. In human plasma Pert et al. (15) detected a low molecular weight substance, anodynin (molecular weight 600), with opiate receptor affinity which produced a long-lasting analgesia in experimental animals. The authors suggested that the compound was a peptide of pituitary origin. There have been confirmatory reports on the presence of opiate receptor-active material in blood and in urine as well from Schulz and coworkers (16, 17). However, it is uncertain whether the two groups have isolated the same material, since Schulz et al. found their active material to be resistant to enzymatic degradation. The activity of the material described by Pert et al. (15) and by Schulz and coworkers (16, 17) can be reversed by naloxone, and therefore it can be rightly considered to be an endorphin (15).

Another material, first isolated from rat brain and characterized by its affinity to morphine-directed antibodies (18), has also been found in human CSF (19). This material is resistant to enzymatic breakdown and its action it not reversed by naloxone. Its classification as an endorphin can therefore be discussed, although it was recently found that it affects morphine-sensitive adenylate cyclase (20).

B. Distribution

Very little is known about the fine distribution of enkephalins or β-endorphin in the human being. It is important that such studies are undertaken since it is by no means sure that experimental animal data can be extrapolated to the human situation. A recent example for the need of caution is the observation that in primates, in contrast to rodents, substance P neurons are abundant in the area postrema (21). Large concentrations of enkephalinlike immunoreactivity has been found in the antrum and the upper intestine (22). The distribution of the enkephalins and β-endorphin using radioimmunoassay in human brain and pituitary has also been published (23). (For a detailed discussion of the chemistry and distribution of endorphins, see Chap. 2 and 5, respectively).

III. PHYSIOLOGIC FUNCTION OF ENDORPHINS IN HUMANS

A. Experimental Approaches

As outlined earlier, essentially two approaches can be used in the evaluation of endorphin function in humans (24). The first is to use the classical pharmacological techniques, such as examining the actions of a receptor blocker. The second possibility is the chemical approach, that is, to measure the endorphin levels by chemical methods in a tissue or body fluid. Each of these possibilities have their inherent advantages and drawbacks, and both should be applied if a complete investigation of endorphins is to be conducted.

The pharmacological approach, using a receptor blocker and observing physiological changes, is applicable only if specific receptor blockers are available. The narcotic antagonists, naloxone and naltrexone, show very little agonistic (i.e., morphine-like) acitvity, but like any pharmacologic agent they may not be absolutely specific and may show effects unrelated to opiate receptor interaction. This possibility is more likely when doses are increased. As a further complication it is also known that the "opiate receptor" is really a mixed population of several receptors (25, 26), and one of these receptors requires approximately 10 times as much naloxone as another to antagonize the effects of morphine. The other principal disadvantage of using a receptor blocker is that it will only give rise to an effect if the system is already being stimulated at a high level. The tonic activity in endorphin systems seems to be rather low and it may be very difficult to observe "subnormal" activity.

The chemical approach is difficult because of the problems of access to the tissues, and samples can usually be obtained only at autopsy. Blood or urine present no problems of access and it might be possible to measure endorphins in these fluids, but the measure may be of little value since it is impossible to define whether they have originated from, for example, brain or intestinal tract tissues. Since endorphins can be measured in lumbar CSF (12, 14), this is the preferred biological fluid for the study of endorphin activity in the CNS. Evidence for the isolation of the CSF compartment from the periphery has been obtained by Jeffcoate and coworkers (27), who found similar β-endorphin levels in patients with normal or subnormal pituitary function. However, it may be difficult to determine whether a substance analyzed in lumbar fluid derives from sources in the brain, or whether it is of local spinal origin (28, 29).

B. The Pituitary System

The pituitary in humans, like that in other species, contains β-endorphin (9). The function of this system is entirely unknown. The targets for the pituitary endorphins are also unknown, although it seems possible that the pituitary itself may be a target. However, the capacity of FK 33-824, a synthetic analog of Met-enkephalin to raise plasma prolactin and growth hormone levels in humans (30, 31) is probably due to an effect on the hypothalamus (32). Since β-endorphin is a comparatively large molecule, it probably penetrates poorly into the brain if released into the general circulation. However, recent findings suggest that the pituitary secretes directly to the brain (33). β-Endorphin occurs in relatively high concentrations in rat plasma, whereas concentrations in human plasma are very low (34, 36). It is known that β-endorphin is formed from a protein of 31,000 daltons, called pro-opiocortin (37). This molecule can be split to form ACTH and β-lipotropin; the latter may then generate β-endorphin. It seems that in humans ACTH and β-lipotropin are the major release products and are released in roughly equimolar amounts. It is only in certain disease states such as Addison's disease, Cushing's disease, or chronic renal failure that levels of β-endorphin are significant (38). Also in pregnancy, high levels are observed in the third trimester, but it is possible that this increase is of placental origin (39 a and b). It is possible, however, that part of the changes depend on altered pituitary function, as is known to occur for other pituitary hormones.

One basic problem relates to the duality of pituitary and brain endorphin systems and their possible interrelationship. Probably, the two systems are independent, as suggested from work in several species, including humans. In humans, chemical hypophysectomy may produce almost immediate pain relief (40). The mechanism for this effect is not known and whether endorphins could be involved has recently been investigated. The results were negative, since naloxone did not reverse pain relief (41), nor were CSF endorphin levels altered (42). It has also been observed that hypopituitary function is not associated with lowered CSF β-endorphin levels (27).

C. The Central Nervous System

The classical morphine effect is analgesia, and therefore much attention has been focused on the role of endorphins in pain regulation. Endogenous pain control systems, inhibiting nociceptive information via centrifugal mechanisms, has been considered in the past. Reynolds (43) showed that descending inhibitory systems could be activated electrically. Whether such systems are operating normally may be difficult to assess experimentally since they may be part of the sensory habituation. To take an analogy, an adult human being in the civilized world is adapted to carrying a wristwatch on the left wrist, where it is not noticed. If the watch is moved to the right arm, it will immediately be recognized as foreign; it is not so easily handled as on the left wrist. Similarly, as part of the sensory adaptation to environment, pain and analgesia mechanisms reach a balance. The discrimination between pain and other sensory modalities, such as heat or touch, will depend on both the primary sensory-discriminative function and on a cognitive function, and in situations of threat or anxiety, also on an emotional component. It is possible that endorphins play a role in such sensory adaptation and processing. Several studies have attempted to investigate the role of endorphins in the

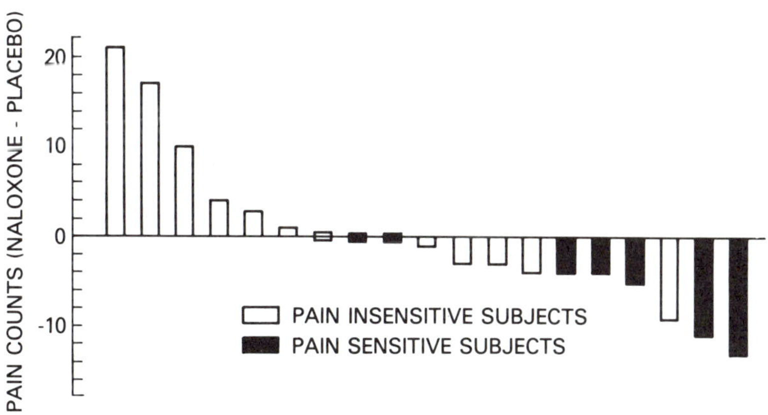

FIGURE 1 Naloxone differentially affects sensitivity to experimental pain in pain-insensitive or pain-sensitive but otherwise normal subjects. The effects are illustrated as the differences between naloxone and placebo. Thus, a positive difference represents individuals becoming more sensitive and a negative difference individuals becoming less sensitive with naloxone. The findings suggest that endorphins are involved in paid regulation in normal subjects. [From Buchsbaum et al. (47) with permission.]

adaptation to pain. In some early studies healthy volunteers were subjected to painful stimuli, and naloxone was given on a double-blind basis to inhibit endorphin activity. In the study of El-Sobky et al. (44), pain was elicited by electrical stimulation and pain thresholds were determined in a conventional way. Naloxone produced no significant effect. Negative results with naloxone were also reported by Grevert and Goldstein (45). Here pain was induced by ischemia. In these two studies the sensory threshold was measured by the method of ascending limits, but this variable has often been found to be an unreliable index of sensitivity to pain (46). In more elaborate studies, analyzing the response with the use of the signal detection theory, both the sensory-discriminatory function and the response factors are considered. With this experimental setup, naloxone has been shown to produce significant changes in sensitivity to radiant heat (47). Interindividual differences in pain sensitivity were observed; the pain-insensitive individuals reacted to naloxone with an increased pain sensitivity, as might have been expected. Paradoxically, pain-sensitive individuals reacted to naloxone with a decrease in pain sensitivity (Fig. 1). In fact, a bidirectional effect of naloxone on pain perception has been described earlier (48). More recent work has shown that naloxone produces hyperalgesia in the morning but not in the afternoon (49). This suggests that endorphins mediate the diurnal variation in the perception of pain (50) and may explain the clinical observation that patients with chronic pain report more intense pain during evening hours (51).

Another refinement in analysis of pain reactions (or sensory response in general) is to use the electroencephalogram (EEG) criterion, the average evoked potentials (EP) to electric shocks (47, 49) (for further details, see Ref. 52). Different individuals will show different stimulus-response relationships. The relatively pain-insensitive individual will show EP amplitudes that decrease or increase slowly with increasing stimulus intensity, whereas the pain-sensitive individual will show steeply increasing intensities. In the study mentioned earlier (47), the pain sensitivity was determined and the individuals were divided into pain-sensitive and pain-insensitive groups. The EP pattern differed between the groups as expected, and interestingly, naloxone markedly changed the response pattern of the sensitive group in the direction of sensitization while an opposite trend was seen in the sensitive group. Thus pain measures and EP responses varied in the same direction.

The studies discussed here show that provided that experimental conditions are adequate, naloxone will affect certain aspects of the response to experimentally induced pain, suggesting a physiological role for endorphins in pain regulation. None of the methods described will analyze the emotional aspects of pain (53), clearly an important component in clinical pain.

Any study on the effects of pharmacological treatment of pain is complicated by the placebo reaction, which by itself may be a powerful tool in pain control, particularly in the clinical situation (54). It is conceivable that part of the placebo response may be endorphin mediated and may therefore be sensitive to naloxone. This possibility should be amenable to experimental investigation. Several studies by Levine and collaborators (55, 56) have demonstrated that naloxone may increase pain ratings in placebo reactors, and concluded that endorphins mediate the placebo response. However, these studies have been criticized on logic and semantic grounds (57). Goldstein and Grevert (58) emphasize that the reason a nonreactor will not respond to naloxone might be the fact that his pains are already intense. A more recent observation by Levine and coworkers (59) is intriguing. Patients reporting more severe pain tended to respond better to placebo (intravenous saline injection). This could explain why placebo is more effective in the clinical situation (54) than against experimental pain, which can never replicate clinical pain. This observation, together with the observation that naloxone significantly enhances clinical pain in some patients (55), seems to argue rather strongly for endorphin participation in the placebo response, but factors such as suggestion may also play a role. It is likely that interindividual differences exist with regard to the extent and character of placebo reactivity. Endorphin activation is also possible under conditions of stress or strong arousal as in battlefield or sport situations, where subjects show paradoxical insensitivity to pain (60a). Particularly striking examples are reports that soldiers wounded in war may show remarkable tolerance to pain. No experiments in humans have as yet been conducted to determine whether this phenomenon involves endorphin activation.

Psychological approaches to pain management, such as behavior therapy or hypnotherapy, can produce adequate effects in some individuals. Hypnosis, in particular, can provide relief from pain, anxiety, and stress if motivation is high. Two studies (60b, 61) have failed to demonstrate an effect of naloxone administration on analgesia induced by hypnosis. In both studies, hypnosis induced a high degree of indifference to pain. Since no effect of naloxone could be discerned, the phenomenon would not be endorphin mediated. A pilot study by another investigator (62) demonstrated an effect by naloxone. Clearly, the results of this type of investigation will depend very much on the experimental design. For instance, all reported studies concern volunteer subjects. Experiments in patients ought to be done.

The effects of morphine on the CNS are very general and by no means confined to pain sensation. It might be anticipated therefore that endogenous opioids should have very general effects on the CNS, influencing mood and behavior. These aspects have not been adequately studied to date. The early literature on naloxone, naltrexone, and their effects in healthy individuals gave very little support for any major role of endorphins in maintaining the mental state (3, 4, 63). The most consistent finding has been those of slight changes in mood and attention (64).

Two investigations go into other aspects of CNS functions. Morphine and heroin are known to affect sleep variables, but naloxone fails to produce any effects (65). Another negative observation relates to sexual behavior, naloxone showing no effect on masturbation variables in the male (66). Both these studies are of a pilot character and can be criticized. Much work needs to be done to determine the role of endorphins on mood and behavior. These effects may be extensive, as suggested by the pronounced effects observed in pharmacological experiments.

The observations cited above merge in one point: naloxone (or naltrexone) shows only minor effects in the healthy individual under experimental conditions. That is not to say that the endorphin systems are unimportant, but that other parallel or counterdirected systems may exist so that pharmacologic intervention with the endorphin system produces very few overt effects. If the normal homeostasis is disturbed, which may be an unethical act in humans, endorphins may reach a level of activity corresponding to that given by analgesic doses of morphine.

D. The Periphery

Very little information is as yet available to evaluate the importance of enkephalin (enkephalinlike immunoreactivity) in the gastrointestinal tract (22). It may be of significance however, that early clinical trials with the enkephalin analogue FK 33-824 (see Sec. VII) reveal considerable effects on the gastrointestinal tract which were not blocked by nalorphine (30).

Other nonclassical effects were congestion of the nasal mucosa and facial flushings. In another study (67), it was observed that the FK-substance produced very intense flushing in patients with heredity for non-insulin-dependent diabetes, a syndrome associated with facial redness after alcohol in combination with chlorpropamide. Interestingly, in three subjects (two diabetics, one nondiabetic) the alcohol-induced flushings were reduced by naloxone, suggesting a role for endorphins in the pathophysiology of this disorder.

IV. ENDORPHINS AND STIMULATION-PRODUCED ANALGESIA

A. Intracerebral Stimulation

The work of Reynolds (43) indicated that surgical analgesia could be produced in rats by intracerebral electrical stimulation. Similar observations have been made in humans with intractable pain (68-71). The clinical success rate of the method is in the order of 75-80%, which merits its use in the treatment of severe cases resistent to other types of therapy. The reader is referred to references cited above for further details. Here we are only going to deal with the question of whether or not the pain relief is related to endorphin activation.

The most effective site for electric stimulation is in the areas close to the wall of the posterior third ventricle. Areas effective in rats, such as the periaqueductal gray, are not useful, since at this site in humans, noxious or unpleasant effects are produced (72). The reason for this discrepancy is not known but emphasizes the need for comparative neuroanatomical studies. In the rat, these paraventricular areas are very rich in enkephalin neurons (73).

There are two main observations which suggest a link between stimulation-produced analgesia and endorphins. One, and perhaps the strongest, is that naloxone is able to counteract stimulation-induced pain relief. In the study of Adams (74), the effect of naloxone was short, as expected from its rapid kinetics, and the induced pain relief returned. In fact, a session of 10–30 min stimulation in patients gives pain relief for 2–24 hr. Hosobuchi et al. (70) described six patients, five of which were clinical successes. These successful cases reported total naloxone reversal of pain relief, while a partial failure reported no effect of naloxone. Similarly, Richardson and Akil (69) reported inhibition of the pain relief by naloxone in five tested patients. However, observations by Meyerson et al. (75) indicated that the situation might be a little more complex. Here at least one subject reported good pain relief which was not affected by naloxone. However, in the majority of the cases, a clinically successful pain relief seems associated with a naloxone-reversible process.

Another observation that supports endorphin mediation of pain relief is the development of tolerance, a well-known phenomenon in morphine and also in endorphin pharmacology. Tolerance develops more rapidly if the stimulation is given frequently and for a long period (69, 70). The latter group reports on three patients, who responded very poorly to stimulation after 4–5 weeks of almost continuous use. Clearly indicating the similarity to opioid tolerance was the fact that larger quantities of narcotic analgesics were needed after than before the stimulation period. Furthermore, there are also reports that electric stimulation can substitute for narcotic analgesics in the chronic user (75). The development of tolerance can be largely abolished if stimulation sessions are shorter and stimulation is given at intervals.

In the clinical use of intracerebral electrical stimulation, the procedure causes pain relief, but hardly hypoalgesia or analgesia unless intensities are high (69, 75). Thus, even if analgesia is not obtained, tolerance is produced, indicating that tolerance mechanisms are able to operate also at a fairly low level of opioid receptor stimulation.

Quantitative analysis of endorphins in cerebrospinal fluid has been carried out in a few cases. Richardson and Akil (69) report six cases in which stimulation produced an elevation of the levels of enkephalinlike material. Similar observations have been done by Hughes and collegues in three patients (76). Meyerson et al. (75) found some cases to respond with elevated endorphin levels as measured in a radioreceptor-assay; treatment failures gave no similar response. More recent studies have shown increases of ventricular β-endorphin levels (77, 78). The case for endorphin involvement in intracerebral stimulation is therefore strong.

B. Peripheral Stimulation

The existence of ascending peripheral pain inhibitory mechanisms has been postulated in the past, largely based on empirical observations and not to put into a conceptual framework. However, in 1965 a theory was formulated by Melzack and Wall (79). In short, it was postulated that activation of large myelinated A-fibers would prevent noxious stimuli from reaching the spinal cord, by closing a "gate." Descending fibers from the brain could also activate such gates. This hypothesis has been of considerable heuristic value even if could not be verified in detail. Obviously, there are many old observations which could be interpreted in terms of activating endorphin systems, such as "counterirritation" massage or similar procedures. The ancient methods of acupuncture and moxa also fall into this category. In fact, Mayer et al. (80), recently showed that analgesia induced by acupuncture in humans could be reduced by naloxone. The study was done under strict double-blind conditions, and the results could hardly be explained by suggestion.

Acupuncture analgesia and the "gate control" theory led to the development of clinical maneuvres such as electroacupuncture or transcutaneous electrostimulation (TNS). The main difference between these techniques lies in the stimualtion parameters; electroacupuncture uses low-frequency, high-intensity stimulation, and TNS uses high-frequency, low-intensity stimulation. Already, etymology suggests an association between classic, Chinese, and electric acupuncture. In acupuncture, deep fibers are activated and a long period (10–30 min) of stimulation is required. Furthermore, pain relief induced by electroacupuncture can be reversed by naloxone and is accompanied by increasing CSF endorphin levels (81). Electroacupuncture may act both at spinal and at supraspinal levels. Support for the former site of action comes from temporal analysis of endorphin production.

The conventional TNS (82, 83) may be acting via other mechanisms and other more superficial fibers. This procedure, if applicable at all, offers advantages over electroacupuncture since the patient requires shorter sessions of stimulation and less discomfort during the stimulation period. Naloxone administration to a patient with maximum pain relief produces no antagonism (84, 85) or only a partial effect (86).

To summarize, one may influence the activity in the pain-conducting systems by stimulating peripheral sensory fibers. The stimulation parameters will determine which type of fibers are affected, and only under proper conditions will endorphin systems be activated. These observations also indicate that there may be several parallel pain inhibitory systems, and the role of endorphins in such a concerted action of several systems may be hard to define.

V. INVOLVEMENT OF ENDORPHINS IN DISEASE

A. Chronic Pain

When a pain syndrome becomes chronic, the patient will react with increasing anxiety and despair. The suffering seems endless and will change the person's emotional balance. Although problems with tolerance and dependence will limit their usefulness, narcotic analgesics can help considerably at this stage. In analogy, endorphin mechanisms may be involved in the adjustment or lack of adjustment to chronic pain. This problem is presently under investigation (87–91). A series of patients with chronic pain has been carefully investigated clinically with regard to neurologic and psychiatric symptoms. In all cases, CSF endorphin levels were measured with a receptorassay

(12). Most cases were also evaluated with regard to pain thresholds and average evoked potentials (EP) to visual stimuli.

The relationship between chronic pain syndromes and CSF endorphins is not simple. It appears that patients with organic, somatogenic pain tend to have lower than normal levels of endorphins, whereas in patients where the pain syndorme is better explained in psychologic terms, so-called psychogenic pain (92), levels are in the normal or slightly supernormal range (Table 1). Within a population of chronic pain patients these differences are highly significant and the lower than normal endorphin values are particularly characteristic of cases with pains of neurogenic origin (87). It is also known that naloxone has no effect on pain ratings in patients with chronic neurogenic pain (93). There is a significant positive correlation between endorphin levels and pain thresholds as well as a significant positive correlation between CSF endorphin levels and visual average EP (88, 89), indicating a functional relationship between the CSF endorphins and CNS endorphin activity. There is also a significant positive correlation between the levels of endorphin and the serotonin metabolite, 5-hydroxyindoleacetic acid (5-HIAA). 5-HIAA levels are very low in the neurogenic pain patients (90). It would therefore seem appropriate to attempt an explanation of these different groups of patients in functional terms. It is also significant that serotonin neurones have been attributed an important role in pain and analgesia (94).

The distinction between organic, somatogenic pain, and psychogenic pain syndromes is a hard task, since every pain syndrome will have a psychic component (95, 96). In practice, there is a tendency to " somatogenize" a pain syndrome, both by doctors and their patients (92). The psychogenic pain syndrome is probably related to depression and a generic relationship has been proposed (92, 97). In the series of patients described above, the cases with psychogenic pain had the higher depressive scores and CSF endorphin levels (87). On the other hand, there was no similar correlation to anxiety or motor retardation. More recent studies have indicated an even more extensive role for endorphins in mental states. Significant correlations exist be-

TABLE 1 Number of Patients with Mainly Somatogenic or Psychogenic Pain Syndromes at Various Endorphin Levels in Cerebrospinal Fluid

	Endorphin levels[a]		
Subjects	<0.6	0.6–1.2	>1.2
Somatogenic pain	28	5	0
Psychogenic pain	1	8	8
Healthy volunteers	3	12	4

[a]Expressed as picomoles/ml Met-enkephalin.
Source: From Refs. 12, 81, 87, and 107.

tween personality traits, (particularly sensation-seeking behavior) and endorphin levels (91).

In conclusion, patients with chronic pain seem to fall into at least two categories, differing diagnostically and with regard to endorphin involvement. In patients with organic, somatogenic pain, particularly when pain is elicited by deafferentation, CSF endorphin levels are very low and the patient has low pain thresholds. Although the causal relationships are not known, it may be that such pains are due to a loss in sensory input and an inadequate activation of the endogenous control mechanisms regulating pain sensitivity (98). In this regard, endorphins probably play an important role. In the patient with psychogenic pain there is a tendancy for rather higher than normal endorphin activity. This has also been observed in the primary diagnosis of endogenous depression (see Sec. V.D) and emphasizes the close relationship between depression and pain syndromes.

B. Migraine

It has been suggested that migraine and related types of essential headache are due to a central dysfunction of antinociceptive mechanisms (99). Sicuteri and coworkers (100) have already tested whether endorphin systems could be involved. Analysis of endorphins in the CSF with techniques previously described (12) was carried out in three patients with chronic headache, one patient with migraine (in the free period), and three neurological patients who did not suffer from essential headache. The levels were far lower in the cases with chronic headache than in the other cases. These observations, although preliminary, would support the hypotheses of attenuated endorphin activity in essential headache (101).

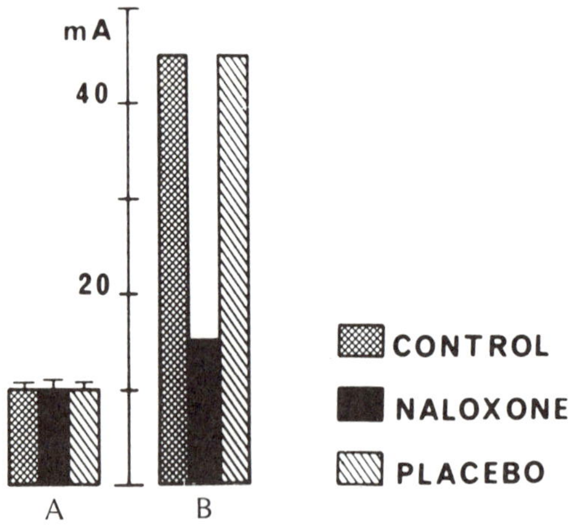

FIGURE 2 Effects of naloxone on pain thresholds in normal subject (A) and a patient with congenital insensitivity to pain (B). Note marked sensitivity to naloxone in patient which may be related to tonically hyperactive endorphin systems. [From Dehen et al. (103) with permission.]

C. Congenital Analgesia

This is a very unusual clinical syndrome with only about 100 cases known in the scientific literature. The peripheral neural system is usually intact and it has been postulated that the lesion is of central origin (102). It has recently been suggested that the syndrome may be related to an enhanced production and secretion of endorphins since naloxone produces considerably increased pain sensitivity (103, 104). A graphical representation of some results is found in Fig. 2.

D. Mental Disorders

The effect of morphine and its surrogates on mood and behavior are extensive. Jaffé (105) characterized the actions of morphine on the CNS as analgesia, drowsiness, changes in mood, and mental clouding. It is therefore conceivable that endorphins might produce essentially similar effects, particularly at high levels. On the other hand, subnormal endorphin activation may also lead to aberrant mood or behavior. An investigation into possible abnormalities in endorphin homeostasis in mental disorders may therefore be rewarding. To obtain objective data, the analysis of CSF endorphin was applied to various psychiatric patients (12, 106, 107). Marked deviations from the normal range were observed in unipolar depression, affective disorders, and schizophrenia (Fig. 3). In the schizophrenics there was some correlation between disease activity and endorphin levels. For instance, several cases showed very high levels in the untreated phase, but during the course of neuroleptic therapy a normalization of en-

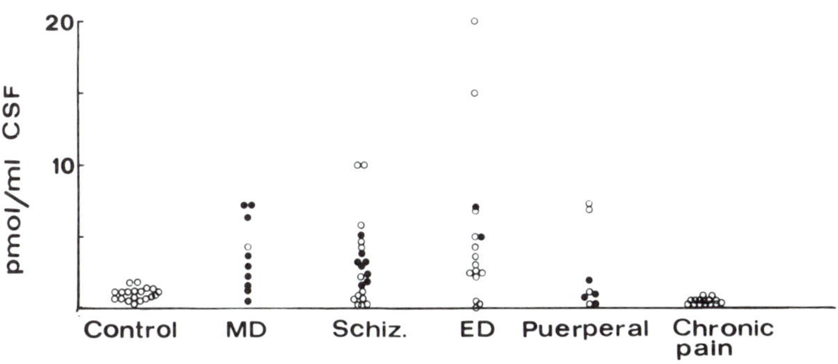

FIGURE 3 Endorphin fraction I levels in cerebrospinal fluid of healthy volunteers (control), manic-depressives (MD), schizophrenics (Schiz.), cases with endogenous depression (ED), puerperal psychosis and chronic pain. Closed circles represent patients under antipsychotic therapy, open circles patients without such treatment. [Data compiled for (12, 81, 107, 139).]

dorphin levels and a corresponding improvement in symptoms were observed (107). It was also noted that endorphin levels were statistically higher in acute cases than in chronic cases (108). Although the high endorphin values in some cases are spectacular, it should be noted that there are also cases where the levels tended to be normal or even subnormal. Certainly, there is no absolute correlation between CSF endorphin levels and disease activity. Also, in depression, cases with very high or very low levels were observed, although the former dominate. It may be recalled that pain insensitivity is quite common in psychiatric patients (109).

Although the results are intriguing as they stand, interpretation is not easy. The observed abnormal levels may be at the core of the illness but may also be a secondary phenomenon due to malfunctioning in other systems. However, it would seem possible that certain aspects of the pathologic changes in mood or thought content, which are characteristics of these diseases, may be mediated through changes in endorphin homeostasis. In principle, deviations can operate in two directions: against subnormal, inadequate function or against supernormal activity with development of tolerance and dependence (Fig. 4). Both the subnormally working and the tolerant system would be functionally inadequate according to this hypothesis and would explain why, for instance, patients with depression may have either very high or very low endorphin levels. Theoretically, one should be able to distinguish between these two groups of patients. In those with subnormal endorphin activity, supersensitivity to morphine (endorphins) might be expected and naloxone should produce no effects. In the other group, morphine (endorphins) should be relatively inactive and naloxone should provide a condition similar to narcotic withdrawal. In fact, a possible withdrawal effect has been observed in chronic schizophrenics on naloxone administration (110). More details on trials with naloxone or endorphins are described later.

A very provocative finding, which already has attracted much attention, is the observation of Wagemaker and Cade (111) that repeated treatment with hemodialysis

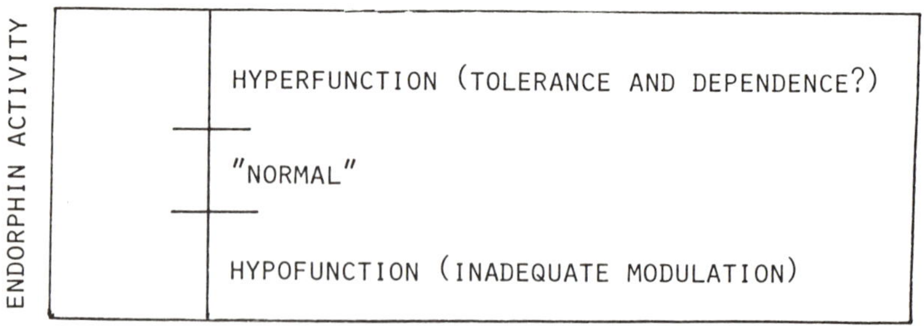

FIGURE 4 Schematic illustration of aberrant endorphin function and its possible consequences.

improves the symptoms in schizophrenics. The therapeutic effect depends on the dialysis procedure, since if it is temporarily stopped, recurrence is observed and the therapeutic effect can be reinstated by resumption of dialysis. The authors speculate that hemodialysis removes a substance from the bloodstream which is not removed by the kidneys. It has also been reported that an endorphinlike compound can be isolated in large quantities from the dialysate of patients treated by Wagemaker. The substance has been tentatively identified as Leu^5-β-endorphin (112, 113). In both the chromatographic properties and electrophysiological and behavioral effects, the isolated substance and the reference compound are similar. These observations were not confirmed in another study (114). If eventually confirmed they will lend additional strength to the endorphin hypothesis of mental disease. Since Leu^5-β-endorphin has not been isolated previously from natural sources, it might be an *abnormal* endorphin associated with the disease, a possibility suggested previously (115).

The potential use of dialysis in schizophrenia soon received public and professional acclaim. To find a reason for this may be a research topic in its own right. The placebo effect of such a procedure must be considerable. Moreover, the treatment procedure will give rise to a complex series of effects. The case clearly needs very careful investigation. There is a recent and timely publication of a protocol for blood purification/methods in chronic schizophrenics (116). Relevant in this connection may be the observation of elevated blood β-endorphin levels (37) and the wide array of somatic and psychic symptoms observed in patients with chronic renal failure.

E. Addiction

Addiction to various stimulants and drugs is peculiar to humans. Whether this is a result of a peculiar predisposition or to a result of a higher intellectual capacity (some would say foolishness) is not known. It may not be too far-fetched, however, to assume that endorphin mechanisms may be influenced by addictive drugs and that the process of addiction is related to endorphin systems. In the case of opiates the connection is obvious. An important question relates to the problem of whether in addition to exposure factors, there are also predisposition factors. The case for genetic factors in the development of alcoholism is rather strong (117). In other words, "addictive personality" might be defined in genetical and consequently biochemical terms. If we assume that endorphins act as "reward transmitters" (118), attenuated endorphin function may form an intrinsic part of these biochemical mechanisms. A more elaborate presentation of this hypothesis has been given elsewhere (119).

So far no data have appeared which could give support to this reasoning. It is of course quite difficult to carry out prospective studies, which attempt to identify factors that could make individuals vulnerable to developing addictive behavior. Once the individual has developed addictive behavior, it soon develops into a complex sociopsychological disorder with a number of secondary factors, such as changes in values and motivation, development of criminality, and poor nutrition. At this stage the picture is too complicated for a rational analysis in mechanistic terms. One of the intriguing factors of addiction in general, and opiate and alcohol addiction in particular, is its long duration and chronic character. Recurrence is always around the corner. This suggests that permanent mental changes may occur as the result of toxomania. No data are available to indicate what the nature of these changes might be, but it would seem possible that endorphins are involved. Further, there may be a link between certain aspects of toxomania and affective disorders.

VI. TRIALS OF NARCOTIC ANTAGONISTS IN DISEASE

If a disease process is thought to be associated with supranormal endorphin activity, a logical step would be a trial with narcotic antagonists (24, 120). The biochemical studies discussed earlier revealed high or very high levels of CSF endorphins in about half of the cases with schizophrenia or endogenous depression (Fig. 3). Consequently, trials were initiated in these diseases.

A. Schizophrenia

Besides the biochemical findings, another observation suggested naloxone trials in schizophrenia. Antagonist analgesics such as nalorphine (121), cyclazocine (122), and pentazocine (123, 124) were known to the pharmacologists to produce psychotomimetic effects, including hallucinations and dysreality phenomena. These phenomena never received much attention but were known to be relieved by naloxone in minutes (125). To test the "endorphin hypothesis," six chronic schizophrenics were selected and given 0.4 mg. of naloxone, i. v. versus physiological saline in a single-blind pilot study. All patients were well known to the experimenters. Since the hallucinations were thought to be a target symptom, the investigation was focused on that point. Four of the patients admitted hallucinating almost constantly, and the other two were thought to hallucinate. The result of this pilot study seemed to support the hypothesis, since in four patients, hallucinations were markedly reduced or abolished (115). Since these results were first made available to the scientific community at the CINP meeting in Quebec in July 1976 (24), a number of trials have been conducted with naloxone in schizophrenia. The design of the trials has been similar, focusing largely on hallucinations and other self-reported changes. Most studies have been done under double-blind conditions. A summary of the results is given in Table 2. Three groups were not at all able to replicate the results and report completely negative findings. One group (127) reports essentially negative results, although some patients reported unusual thoughts. Finally, five groups have reported positive results. In all, the summary covers 104 patients that have received one or more injections of naloxone, and in 36 cases there was a response supporting the endorphin hypothesis. It should be noted that in some patients, the total dosages of naloxone were considerable.

TABLE 2 Trials of Naloxone in Chronic Schizophrenia

Series	Dose (mg)	Number of responders/ Number of patients	Reference
1	0.4	4/6	115
2	0.4	0/7	126
3	0.4–10	0[a]/14	127
4	1.2	0/8	128
5	0.4–1.2	0/12	129
6	4.0	12/20	130
7	10	6/9	131
8	25	7/12	132
9	0.8	1/10	133
10	0.4	1/1	134
11	10	5/6	135[a]

[a]Several patients reported unusual thought content.

The case for endorphin involvement in the expression of certain symptons in schizophrenia will remain a matter of dispute for some time to come. The use of a short-acting parenteral compound such as naloxone, with a plasma half-life of less than one hour, gives severe methodological problems to the experimenter. Previous experience in clinical pharmacology of antipsychotic drugs has been from the use of long-acting compounds given chronically over weeks. With a short-acting drug, the selection of subjects becomes critical. The suggestible patient should be avoided; on the other hand, the patients should be communicable and capable of self-reporting. The importance of methodological studies has to be emphasized if further progress is to be achieved in the field (133). Another uncontrolled variable in most of the studies mentioned is background antipsychotic medication which might have obscured therapeutic effects. For instance, CSF endorphin levels are at a peak in the untreated phase and supranormal levels tend to decline under neuroleptic therapy (107, 108). Studies on naloxone as the sole therapeutical agent seem warranted. It is also possible that schizophrenia is a collective name for mechanistically different disease entities with similar clinical expression. One might therefore expect naloxone to be effective only in the appropriate subgroup.

Naltrexone is generally considered to be a very specific narcotic antagonist, although perhaps not as specific as naloxone. It has the important advantage of a longer plasma half-life and oral applicability (135[b]). A few pilot studies in schizophrenia have appeared so far, with essentially negative findings (133, 136, 137). This may be related to the essentially agonistic effects produced by this agent in clinically used doses (138).

B. Endogenous Depression

At first glance it may seem useless to try naloxone in depression. It is widely held that morphine is an euphoric agent, and presumably endorphins would also be euphoriants. Conversely, narcotic antagonists would produce dysphoria. An actual pilot trial (139) with multiple injections of naloxone in five patients with endogenous depression was also negative. In fact, two patients appeared worse after than prior to the treatment period. This is the predicted outcome if depression is associated with supranormal endorphins (Fig. 4). Clearly, this matter requires more extensive studies.

VII. EFFECTS OF ENDORPHIN ADMINISTRATION IN HUMANS

Since the endorphins are endogenously occuring substances, clinical evaluation is not delayed much by toxicological considerations. Unfortunately, the enkaphalins are metabolically so unstable in all mammalian species investigated that effects may be very difficult to observe. β-Endorphin, on the other hand, although much more metabolically stable, is costly to prepare and is not easily obtainable in large quantities from natural sources. To date, only a few studies have been carried out with synthetic β-endorphin, and due to shortness of supplies, the experiments have been largely of a pilot character.

In the study of Catlin and coworkers (140), two questions were asked; (1) whether β-endorphin is an analgesic in humans, and if so, whether it is indistinguishable from morphine in its actions. Three patients with advanced cancer were selected for analgesia testing. They all had a history of strong analgesic consumption; two received morphine injections at short intervals. A critical examination of the results reveals only one clear-cut β-endorphin responder. This patient reported less pain after β-endorphin (300 μg/kg). Of the other cases, one was a placebo reactor and the other responded to morphine (300 μg/kg) but not to β-endorphin (100 μg/kg). No adverse effects or euphoria was observed in any patient. Two addicts under withdrawal were given morphine, β-endorphin, or saline in that order on day 5, 7, 8 of abstinence, respectively. The subjects accurately identified morphine and found β-endorphin to be active in relieving abstinence but reported that it was qualitatively different from morphine. Saline was reported to be the least active. Kline and colleagues (141, 142) have administered β-endorphin to patients with various psychiatric disorders. Also included in these studies were the results of two injections of 9 mg of β-endorphin into one of the investigators. The investigator reported feelings of drowsiness, perplexity, and impaired concentration. The effects were distinct from those produced by morphine. In common with most of the patients, he also reported autonomic effects such as dry mouth. The patients, included four schizophrenics, two cases with unipolar depression, three with affective disorders, three with neurosis, one with mental deficiency, and one autistic patient. Injections of 1–10 mg of β-endorphin were given in an open study and several patients received more than one injection. Responses are generally described as being favorable, although this was not always clearly stated. The significance of several of these observed responses may be rather questionable, particularly since no placebo injections were made. Probably the most intriguing finding is that of "phase III effects," that is, effects that arise late and last long. These effects were most pronounced in two schizophrenics and in three patients with neurosis. If these findings can be confirmed, they indicate that some homeostatic mechanism can be reset on β-endorphin injection.

Pilot studies with the β-endorphin fragment des-Tyr^1-γ-endorphin have given very promising results in chronic schizophrenics (143). This compound is devoid of opioid receptor affinity (which requires N-terminal tyrosine). In animal tests, some of its actions resemble those of neuroleptics. However, the labeling of the compound as an endogenous neuroleptic seems premature. The clinical study involves two series of patients, six patients participating in an open trial and eight patients in a double blind, crossover study. In both series of patients, the ratings were less severe after treatment with drug. The effect had reached its maximum by the third day and in several cases seemed to outlast the treatment by several days or weeks.

The limited sources of β-endorphin or its fragments and the limitation inherent to the parenteral administration mode have led to the search for metabolically stable enkephalin analogs. However, since these analogs will no longer be the natural substances, they will have to undergo all the preclinical testing necessary for any new experimental drug. Also, when the first trials are done in humans it will have to be with rather low dosages and under very strict controls. A very active enkephalin analog, FK 33-824, has been tried in humans in dosages of 0.5–1.2 mg (30). This is in the same molar range as that used for β-endorphin. The substance was given to healthy volunteers, who showed and reported quite unexpected results. The symptoms included anaphylactoid effects on small vessels and gastrointestinal symptoms, atypical EEG, but not classical symptoms of the morphinelike analgesics, such as nausea or changes in emotional behavior. None of the effects observed was reversed by nalorphine, another indication that they are not morphinelike. The use of naloxone as an antagonist would give a more clearcut answer as to whether opiate ("morphine") receptors are involved in these effects at all. The absence of analgesia could be related to the doses used since the compound is a potent analgesic in animals, including monkeys, where it is morphinelike also in the sense that it produces tolerance, dependence, and substitutes for morphine in morphine dependence (144).

As indicated above, β-endorphin also produces autonomic side effects and it is possible that peripheral peptide receptors, which differ from those involved in analgesia mechanisms, are responsible. Endorphins are known to occur in certain ganglia (145, 146) and it may be that the non-morphine-like effects are elicited at the ganglion level via atypical receptors.

The FK compound stimulates pituitary secretion of prolactin and growth hormone in a dose-dependent manner (30). This effect is hightly significant and occurs at comparatively low doses. Similar effects have been reported for morphine (147). Measurements of plasma prolactin and growth hormone might be used to monitor therapy with endorphins or opioid antagonists, as has been suggested (148).

Two clinical studies in schizophrenia with FK 33-824 have been reported (149, 150). Both studies are open and nine patients entered into each study. In the first study, the substance was given in increasing doses for 3 days. Four patients showed a striking effect, which remained for 4-7 days after the final administration. In the second study, five patients responded. Three patients refused to have a second injection because of the side effects, which were of the character previously discussed. For this particular drug, double-blind studies will be difficult to carry out.

A common denominator for all the studies with endorphins or analogs in schizophrenia is the long-lasting character of the response. This speaks in favor of a modulatory or inductory role for the administered drug, as suggested for des-Tyr^1-γ-endorphin (143). It should be recalled that neuroleptics are slow in onset and produce effects long after withdrawal, indicating that they also act indirectly. In other words, there may be a link between neuroleptics and endorphins, a link that needs to be defined. The results support the endorphin hypothesis for schizophrenia. More work is needed, however, to define the mode of action of these drugs and which patient subgroups would be amenable to treatment.

VIII. CONCLUSIONS

A few years ago, reports that substances with morphinelike activity had been isolated from mammalian tissues were met with some scepticism. Now they are accepted, and news of the "body's own opiate" has received wide publicity. As research progresses it is apparent that there are a large number of endorphins, in the widest sense of the word, including several peptides and nonpeptides. The different systems in, for insstance, the pituitary, the intestine, and the brain may also differ mechanistically.

The physiologic effects of the endorphins may be very extensive, but research efforts have been concentrated largely on the role of endorphins in analgesia. It is not surprising that this line of research has been intensively followed since there was a wealth of background in the analgesic effects of the opiates, such as morphine.

There is now an increasing awareness, however, that the endorphins may also be involved in more general behavioral phenomena, and also in pathological conditions such as depression and schizophrenia. This aspect of endorphin function was enthusiastically pursued by many investigators (see also Refs. 151-153), and some of the early studies were limited in scope and size and may be criticized on methodological grounds. It is important that this area of research be investigated very carefully, since hurried or ill-designed experiments may fail to detect and charcterize important aspects of endorphin function. Further work must include improved methodology for functional tests and biochemical measurements of endorphin content in body fluids and, if accessible, in tissue. A prominent research strategy for the investigation of endorphin action has been the use of the morphine antagonists naloxone and naltrexone. However, it is important to note that these antagonists were synthesized to interfere with morphine action, and morphine may in fact reflect only the activity in some endorphin systems. Another limitation of the antagonist approach is that they may, in fact, under certain conditions have agonistic activity of their own in the absence of endogenous opioids.

To date, therapeutic attempts have been directed to pain and mental disorders. It is not yet known whether endorphin analogs would be superior to conventional drugs as analgesics. It may also be that some "nonclassical" actions such as the vascular effects may eventually be targets for the development of new drugs (154). The opiate antagonists may be of therapeutic or diagnostic potential as endorphin antagonists in some mental disorders or in pituitary dysfunction. One attractive feature of these drugs is their apparent safety.

To conclude, our picture of the physiological functions of endorphins and possible therapeutic applications is rather vague at the present moment. However, it seems clear that the endorphins can be activated and produce analgesia by various artificial procedures, such as electrical and physical stimulation. Endorphin action may also be an intrinsic part of certain pathologic conditions. Normally, the endorphins probably play a subtle but important modulatory role in a number of adaptive processes, which at least for the CNS may be difficult to observe with conventional experimental methodology. The endorphins may be just one example of numerous factors, peptides or nonpeptides, which serve to modulate various physiological functions.

ACKNOWLEDGMENT

Aided by the Swedish Medical Research Council (Research Grants 25x-3766 and 21x-5095).

REFERENCES

1. D. R. Jasinski, W. R. Martin, and C. A. Haertzen, *J. Pharmocol. Exp. Ther., 157:* 420 (1967).
2. W. R. Martin, D. R. Jasinski, and P. A. Mansky, *Arch. Gen. Psychiatry, 28:* 784 (1973).
3. A. Aroński, A. Kübler, A. Majda, and J. Jakubaszko, *Anaesthesiol. Resusc. Intens. Ther., 3:* 221 (1975).
4. E. R. Gritz, S. M. Shiffman, M. E. Jarvik, J. Schlesinger, and V. C. Charuvastra, *Clin. Pharmacol. Ther., 19:* 773 (1976).

5. A. Goldstein, *Science*, *193:* 1081 (1976).
6. D. Albe-Fessard, B. S. Nashold, Jr., and M. C. Lombard, *Pain Abstracts, 2nd World Congr. Pain*, Montreal, Canada, 1978, p. 268.
7. R. C. A. Frederickson, E. W. Schirmer, E. L. Grinnan, C. E. Harrell, and C. R. Hewes, *Life Sci.*, *19:* 1181 (1976).
8. J. Hughes, H. W. Kosterlitz, A. T. McKnight, R. P. Sosa, J. A. H. Lord, and A. A. Waterfield, in *Centrally Acting Peptides* (J. Hughes, ed.), Macmillian, London, 1978, 179.
9. A. Wahlström, L. Johansson, and L. Terenius, unpublished.
10. M. Chrétien, S. Benjannet, N. Dragon, N. G. Seidah, and M. Lis, *Biochem. Biophys. Res. Commun.*, *72:* 472 (1976).
11. C. H. Li, D. Yamashiro, L.-F. Tseng, and H. H. Loh, *J. Med. Chem.*, *20:* 325 (1977).
12. L. Terenius and A. Wahlström, *Life Sci.*, *16:* 1759 (1975).
13. A. Wahlström, L. Johansson, and L. Terenius in *Opiates and Endogenous Opioid Peptides* (H. W. Kosterlitz, ed.), Elsevier/North-Holland, Amsterdam, 1976, p.45.
14. Y. Sarne, R. Azov, and B. A. Weissman, *Brain Res.*, *151:* 399 (1978).
15. C. B. Pert, A. Pert, and J. F. Tallman, *Proc. Natl. Acad. Sci, U.S.A. 73:* 2226 (1976).
16. R. Schulz, M. Wüster, and A. Herz, *Life Sci.*, *21:* 105 (1977).
17. R. Schulz and M. Wüster, *Eur. J. Pharmacol.*, *43:* 383 (1977).
18. A. R. Gintzler, A. Levy, and S. Spector, *Proc. Natl. Acad. Sci., U.S.A.*, *73:* 2132 (1976).
19. S. Spector, J. R. Shorr, J. Finberg, and K. Foley, in *Endorphins in Mental Health Research* (E. Usdin, W. E. Bunney, Jr., and N. S. Kline, eds.) Oxford University Press, New York, 1979, p. 569.
20. A. J. Blume, J. Shorr, J. P. M. Finberg, and S. Spector, *Proc. Natl. Acad. Sci.*, U.S.A., *74:* 4927–4931 (1977).
21. T. Hökfelt, B. Pernow, G. Nilsson, L. Wetterberg, M. Goldstein, and S. L. Jeffcoate, *Proc. Natl. Acad. Sci. U.S.A.*, *75:* 1013 (1978).
22. J. M. Polak, S. N. Sullivan, S. R. Bloom, P. Facer, and A. G. Pearse, *Lancet, 1:* 972 (1977).
23. C. Gramsch, V. Höllt, P. Mehraein, A. Pasi, and A. Herz, *Brain Res.*, *171:* 261 (1979).
24. L. Terenius and A. Wahlström, Proc. Xth Colloq. Int. Neuropharmacol. Congr., Quebec, 1976 (P. Denicker, C. Radouco-Thomas, and A. Villeneuve, eds.), p. 453.
25. J. A. H. Lord, A. A. Waterfield, J. Hughes, and H. W. Kosterlitz, *Nature, 267:* 495 (1977).
26. L. Terenius, *Psychoneuroendocrinology, 2:* 53 (1977).
27. W. J. Jeffcoate, L. H. Rees, P. J. Lowry, L. McLoghlin, S. J. Ratter, J. Hope, and G. M. Besser, *Lancet, 2:* 119 (1978).
28. E. Garlis, S. N. Young, S. Lal, and T. L. Sourkes, *Brain Res.*, *79:* 9 (1974).
29. G. Curzon, B. D. Kantamaneni, J. R. Bartlett and P. K. Bridges, *J. Neurochem.*, *26:* 613 (1979).
30. B. von Graffenried, E. del Pozo, J. Roubicek, E. Krebs, W. Pöldinger, P. Burmeister, and L. Kerp, *Nature, 272:* 729 (1978).
31. M. S. Gold, D. E. Redmond, R. K. Donabedian, F. K. Goodwin, and I. Extein,

Am J. Psychiatry, 135: 11 (1978).
32. F. Labrie, L. Cusan, A. Dupont, L. Ferland, and A. Lemay, in *Characteristics and Function of Opioids* (J. M. van Ree and L. Terenius, eds.) Elsevier/North-Holland, Amsterdam, 1978, pp. 143–158.
33. R. B. Page, B. L. Munger, and R. M. Bergland, *Am. J. Anat., 146:* 273 (1976).
34. K. Nakao, Y. Nakai, S. Oki, K. Horii, and H. Imura, *Clin. Invest., 62:* 1395 (1978).
35. S. L. Wardlaw and A. G. Frantz, *J. Clin. Endocrinol. Metab., 48:* 176 (1979).
36. T. Suda, A. S. Liotta, and D. T. Krieger, *Science, 202:* 221 (1978).
37. R. E. Mains and B. A. Eipper, *J. Biol. Chem., 253:* 651 (1978).
38. D. T. Krieger, paper read at 13th Acta Endocrinol. Congr., Munich June 26–30, 1979.
39a. H. Akil, S. J. Watson, J. D. Barchas, and C. H. Li, *Life Sci., 24:* 1659 (1979).
39b. R. M. Bergland, S. L. Davis, and R. B. Page, Lancet, *2:* 276 (1979).
40. G. Moricca, *Adv. Neurol., 4:* 707 (1974).
41. D. S. Missfeldt and A. Goldstein, *N. Engl. J. Med., 297:* 1236 (1977).
42. J. Hughes, personal communication.
43. D. V. Reynolds, *Science, 164:* 444 (1969).
44. A. El-Sobky, J. O. Dostrovsky, and P. D. Wall, *Nature, 263:* 783 (1976).
45. P. Grevert and A. Goldstein, *Proc. Natl. Acad. Sci U.S.A., 74:* 1291 (1977).
46. C. R. Chapman, *Pain, 3:* 295 (1977).
47. M. S. Buchsbaum, G. C. Davis, and W. E. Bunney, *Nature, 270:* 620 (1977).
48. L. Lasagna, *Proc. R. Soc. Med., 58:* 978 (1965).
49. G. C. Davis, M. S. Buchsbaum, and W. E. Bunney, Jr., *Life Sci., 23:* 1449 (1978).
50. E. J. Rogers and B. Vilkin, *J. Clin. Psychiatry, 39:* 431 (1978).
51. C. J. Glynn and J. W. Lloyd, *Proc. R. Soc. Med., 69:* 369 (1976).
52. M. Buchsbaum, in *Biology of the Major Psychoses,* (D.X. Freedman, ed.), Res. Publ. Assoc. Res. Nerv. Ment. Dist., Vol. 54, Raven Press, New York, 1975.
53. C. R. Chapman and B. W. Feather, *Psychosom. Med., 35:* 330 (1975).
54. F. J. Evans, Adv. *Neurol., 4:* 289 (1974).
55. J. D. Levine, N. C. Gordon, and H. L. Fields, *Lancet, 2:* 654 (1978).
56. J. D. Levine, N. C. Gordon, and H. L. Fields, *Nature, 278:* 740 (1979).
57. P. Skrabanek, *Lancet, 2:* 791 (1978).
58. A. Goldstein and P. Grevert, *Lancet, 2:* 1385 (1978).
59. J. D. Levine, N. C. Gordon, J. C. Bornstein, and H. L. Fields, *Proc. Natl. Acad. Sci. U.S.A.,* in press (1979).
60a. R. Melzack, *The Puzzle of Pain,* Basic Books, New York, 1973.
60b. A. Goldstein and E. R. Hilgard, *Proc. Natl. Acad. Sci. U.S.A., 72:* 2041 (1975).
61. J. Barber and D. Mayer, *Pain, 4:* 1 (1977).
62. J. B. P. Stephenson, *Lancet, 2:* 991 (1978).
63. R. T. Jones and R. I. Herning, in *Endorphins in Mental Health Research* (E. Usdin, W. E. Bunney, Jr., and N. S. Kline, eds.), Oxford University Press, New York, 1979, p. 484.
64. S. Itwin, R. G. Kinohi, P. M. Cooler, and D. R. Bottomly, in Report on the

Thirty-sixth Annual Scientific Meeting Committee on Problems of Drug Dependence, Mexico City, 1974.
65. G. C. Davis, W. C. Duncan, J. C. Gillin, and W. E. Bunney, Jr., *Commun. Psychopharmacol. 1:* 489 (1977).
66. A. Goldstein and R. W. Hansteen, *Arch. Gen. Psychiatry, 34:* 1179 (1977).
67. R. D. G. Leslie, D. A. Pyke, and W. A. Stubbs, *Lancet, 1:* 341 (1979).
68. D. E. Richardson, in *IEEE Trans. Biomed. Eng., BME-23,* 304 (1976).
69. D. E. Richardson and H. Akil, *J. Neurosurg., 47:* 184 (1977).
70. Y. Hosobuchi, J. E. Adams, and R. Linchitz, *Science, 197:* 183 (1977).
71. B. A. Meyerson, J. Boëthius, L. Terenius, and A. Wahlström, 3rd Meet. Eurp. Soc. Stereotactic Functional Neurosurg., Freiburg, 1977.
72. D. E. Richardson and H. Akil, *J. Neurosurg., 47:* 178 (1977).
73. T. Hökfelt, R. Elde, O. Johansson, L. Terenius, and L. Stein, *Neuroscience Lett., 5:* 25 (1977).
74. J. E. Adams, *Pain, 2:* 161 (1976).
75. B. A. Meyerson, J. Boëthius, and A. M. Carlsson, personal communication.
76. J. Hughes, personal communication.
77. H. Akil, D. E. Richardsson, J. D. Barchas, and C. H. Li, *Proc. Natl. Acad. Sci. U.S.A., 75:* 5170 (1978).
78. Y. Hosobuchi, J. Rossier, F. Bloom, and R. Guillemin, *Soc. Neurosci. Abstr., 4:* 410 (1978).
79. R. Melzack and P. D. Wall, *Science, 150:* 971 (1965).
80. D. J. Mayer, D. D. Price, and A. Rafii, *Brain Res., 121:* 368 (1977).
81. B. Sjölund, L. Terenius, and M. Eriksson, *Acta Physiol. Scand., 100:* 382 (1977).
82. C. N. Shealy and D. Maurer, *Surg. Neurol., 2:* 45 (1974).
83. R. Melzack, *Pain, 1:* 357 (1975).
84. B. Sjölund and M. Eriksson, Brain Res., *173:* 295 (1979).
85. B. G. L. Almay and F. Johansson, personal communication.
86. C. R. Chapman and C. Benedetti, *Life Sci., 21:* 1645 (1977).
87. B. G. L. Almay, F. Johansson, L. von Knorring, L. Terenius, and A. Wahlström, *Pain, 5:* 153 (1978).
88. L. von Knorring, B. G. L. Almay, F. Johansson, and L. Terenius, *Pain, 5:* 359 (1978).
89. L. von Knorring, B. G. L. Almay, and L. Terenius, *Neuropsychobiology, 5:* 322 (1979).
90. B. G. L. Almay, F. Johansson, L. v. Knorring, G. Sedvall, and L. Terenius, *Psychopharmacology, 67:* 139 (1980).
91. F. Johansson, B. G. L. Almay, L. v. Knorring, L. Terenius, and M. Åström, *Psychiatry Res., 1:* 231 (1979).
92. R. A. Sternbach, in *Pain Patients,* Academic Press, New York, 1974.
93. U. Lindblom and R. Tegńer, *Pain,* in press.
94. R. B. Messing and L. D. Lytle, *Pain, 4:* 1 (1977).
95. H. Merskey and F. G. Spear, *Pain,* Ballière, Tindall , London, 1967.
96. T. S. Szasz, *Pain and pleasure: A Study of Bodily Feelings,* Tavistock, London, 1957.

97. L. von Knorring, *"The experience of pain in patients with depressive disorders: a clinical and experimental study,"* Umeå University Medical Dissertations, New series, No. 2, Umeå, Sweden, 1975.
98. R. Melzack and J. D. Loeser, *Pain, 4:* 195 (1978).
99. F. Sicuteri, *Headache, 16:* 145 (1976).
100. F. Sicuteri, B. Anselmi, C. Curradi, S. Michelacci, and A. Sassi, *Adv. Biochem. Psychopharmacol., 18:* (1978).
101. F. Sicuteri, *Headache, 17:* 253 (1978).
102. D. C. Thrush, *Brain, 96:* 591 (1973).
103. H. Dehen, J. C. Willer, S. Prier, F. Boureau, and J. Cambier, *Pain, 5:* 351 (1978).
104. H. Yanagida, *Lancet, 2:* 520 (1978).
105. J. H. Jaffé, in *The Pharmacological Basis of Therapeutics* (L. S. Goodman and A. Gilman, eds.) Macmillan, New York, 1975, p. 284.
106. L. Terenius, A. Wahlström, L. Lindström, and E. Widerlöv, *Neurosci. Lett. 3:* 157 (1976).
107. L. H. Lindström, E. Widerlöv, L. -M. Gunne, A. Wahlström, and L. Terenius, *Acta Psychiatr. Scand., 57:* 153 (1978).
108. R. Rimon and L. Terenius, in preparation.
109. N. Geschwind, *N. Engl. J. Med., 296:* 1480 (1975).
110. M. Gitlin and M. Rosenblatt, *Am. J. Psychiatry, 135:* 377 (1978).
111. H. Wagemaker and R. Cade, *Am. J. Psychiatry, 134:* 684 (1977).
112. R. M. Palmour, F. R. Ervin, H. Wagemaker, and R. Cade, in *Endorphins in Mental Health Research* (E. Usdin, W. E. Bunney, Jr., and N. S. Kline, eds.), Oxford University Press, New York, 1979, p. 581.
113. B. M. Cox, M. Ross, A. Goldstein, and R. M. Palmour, *Brain Res., 165:* 311 (1979).
114. R. V. Lewis, L. D. Gerber, S. Stein, R. L. Stephen, B. I. Grosser, S. F. Velick, and S. Udenfriend, *Arch. Gen. Psychiatry, 36:* 237 (1979).
115. L. -M. Gunne, L. Lindström, and L. Terenius, *J. Neural Transm., 40:* 13 (1977).
116. H. Hippius, N. Matussek, N. Nedopil, A. Strauss, G. D. v. Zerssen, H. Emrich, W. J. Kolff, and H. J. Gurland, Artif. Organs, *3:* 104 (1979).
117. D. W. Goodwin, F. Schulsinger, N. Møller, L. Hermansen, G. Winokur, and S. B. Guze, *Arch. Gen. Psychiatry, 31:* 164 (1974).
118. J. D. Belluzzi and L. Stein, *Nature, 266:* 556 (1977).
119. L. Terenius, in *The Basis of Addiction* (J. Fishman, ed.), Dahlem Konferenzen Berlin, 1978, pp. 513–526.
120. L. Terenius and A. Wahlström, in *Centrally Acting Peptides* (J. Hughes, ed.), Macmillan, London, 1978, p. 161.
121. L. Lasagna and H. K. Beecher, *J. Pharmacol. Exp. Ther., 112:* 356 (1954).
122. L. Lasagna, T. J. de Kornfield, and J. W. Pearson, *J. Pharmacol. Exp. Ther., 144:* 12 (1964).
123. W. H. Forrest, Jr., E. G. Beer, J. W. Bellville, B. J. Ciliberti, E. V. Miller, and R. Paddock, *Clin. Pharmacol. Ther., 10:* 468 (1969).
124. D. R. Jasinski, W. R. Martin, and R. D. Hoeldtke, *Clin. Pharmacol. Ther., 11:* 385 (1970).

125. D. R. Jasinski, W. R. Martin, and J. D. Sapira, *Clin. Pharmacol. Ther., 9:* 215 (1968).
126. J. Volavka, A. Mallya, S. Baig, and J. Perez-Cruet, *Science, 196:* 1227 (1977).
127. G. C. Davis, W. E. Bunney, Jr., and E. G. de Fraites, *Science, 197:* 74 (1977).
128. D. S. Janowsky, D. S. Segal, A. Abrams, F. Bloom, and R. Guillemin, *Psychopharmacology, 53:* 295 (1977).
129. A. A. Kurland, L. McCabe, T. E. Hanlon, and D. Sullivan, *Am. J. Psychiatry, 134:* 1408 (1977).
130. H. M. Emrich, C. Cording, S. Pirée, A. Kölling, D. v. Zerssen, and A. Herz, *Pharmakopsychiatr. Neuro-psychoparmakol., 10:* 265 (1977).
131. P. A. Berger, S. J. Watson, H. Akil, and J. D. Barchas, in *Endorphins in Mental Health Research* (E. Usdin, W. E. Bunney, Jr., and N. S. Kline, eds.), Oxford University Press, New York, 1979, p. 423.
132. H. M. Emrich, C. Cording, S. Pirée, A. Kölling, H. –J. Möller, D. v. Zerssen, and A. Herz in *Endorphins in Mental Health Research* (E. Usdin, W. E. Bunney, Jr., and N. S. Kline, eds.) Oxford University Press, New York, 1979, p. 452.
133. L. –M. Gunne, L. Lindström, and E. Widerlöv, in *Endorphins in Mental Health Research* (E. Usdin, W. E. Bunney, Jr., and N. S. Kline, eds.) Oxford University Press, New York, 1979, p. 547.
134. M. Orr and C. Oppenheimer, *Br. Med. J., 1:* 481 (1978).
135a. H. Lehmann, N. P. V. Nair, and N. S. Kline, *Am. J. Psychiatry, 136:* 762 (1979).
135b. M. J. Kogan, K. Verebey, and S. J. Mulé, *Res. Commun. Chem. Pathol. Pharmacol., 18:* 29 (1977).
136. D. H. Mielke and D. M. Gallant, *Am. J. Psychiatry, 134:* 1430 (1977).
137. G. M. Simpson, M. H. Branchey, and J. H. Lee, *Curr. Ther. Res., 22:* 909 (1977).
138. J. Volavka, A. Mallay, J. Bauman, J. Pernik, D. Cho, D. Reker, B. James, and R. Dornbush, *Adv. Ext. Med., 116:* 291 (1979).
139. L. Terenius, A. Wahlström, and H. Ågren, *Psychopharmacology, 54:* 31 (1977).
140. D. H. Catlin, K. K. Hui, H. H. Loh, C. H. Li, *Commun. Psychopharmacology, 1:* 5 (1977).
141. N. S. Kline and H. E. Lehmann, A. Lajtha, E. Laski, and T. Cooper, *Arch. Gen. Psychiatry, 34:* 1111 (1977).
142. N. S. Kline and H. E. Lehmann, in *Endorphins in Mental Health Research* (E. Usdin, W. E. Bunney, Jr., and N. S. Kline, eds.), Oxford University Press, New York, 1979, p. 500.
143. W. M. A. Vernoeven, H. M. van Praag, J. M. van Ree, and D. DeWied, *Arch. Gen. Psychiatry, 36:* 294 (1979).
144. D. Romer, H. H. Buscher, R. C. Hill, J. Pless, W. Bauer, F. Cardinaux, A. M. Closse, D. Hauser, and R. Huguenin, *Nature, 268:* 547 (1977).
145. J. Hughes, H. W. Kosterlitz, and T. W. Smith, *Br. J. Pharmacol. 61:* 639 (1977).
146. M. Schulzberg, J. Lundberg, T. Hökfelt, L. Terenius, R. P. Elde, and M. Goldstein, *Neuroscience, 3:* 1169 (1979).
147. G. Tolis, J. Hickey, and H. Guyda, *J. Clin. Endocrinol. Metab., 41:* 797 (1975).

148. M. S. Gold, D. E. Redmond, and R. K. Donabedian, *Lancet, 1:* 323 (1978).
149. A. Jørgensen, R. Fog, and B. Veilis, *Lancet, 1:* 935 (1979).
150. N. Nedopil and E. Rüther, *Pharmakopsychiat. Neuro-psychopharmacol., 12:* 277 (1979).
151. H. M. Emrich, *Arzneim.-Forsch./Drug Res., 28:* 1270 (1978).
152. K. Verebey, J. Volavka, and D. Clouet, *Arch. Gen. Psychiatry, 35:* 877 (1978).
153. S. J. Watson, H. Akil, P. A. Berger, and J. D. Barchas, *Arch. Gen. Psychiatry, 36:* 35 (1979).
154. J. Moreley, *Annu. Rev. Pharmacol., 20:* 81 (1980).

Author Index

Numbers in parentheses are reference numbers and indicate that an author's work is referred to although his name is not cited in the text. Italic numbers give the page on which the complete reference is listed.

Subject Index